Problem Solving in Apheresis Medicine

Ilknur Kozanoglu
Editor

Problem Solving in Apheresis Medicine

Springer

Editor

Ilknur Kozanoglu
Adana Adult BMT Center
Baskent University
Adana, Türkiye

Acibadem Labmed Medical Laboratories
Hematology Laboratories
Istanbul, Türkiye

ISBN 978-3-031-74080-0 ISBN 978-3-031-74081-7 (eBook)
https://doi.org/10.1007/978-3-031-74081-7

This Springer imprint is published by the registered company Springer Nature Switzerland AG
The registered company address is: Gewerbestrasse 11, 6330 Cham, Switzerland

Contents

Part I

Principles of Apheresis

History of Apheresis

1

Omur Kayikci and Emre Tekgunduz

1.1 Introduction

The term apheresis is a Greek word, which means to separate or remove. The idea of changing the blood composition and removing a presumed pathological substance from the blood to treat various diseases mainly through bloodletting goes back to 1000 years BC [1]. Apheresis is a process or treatment modality by which blood is being removed from a patient/subject, desired component is collected, and the rest is returned to the donor [2]. Modern apheresis is a complex, technology-dependent field involved in the treatment of a broad spectrum of diseases belonging to various disciplines including but not restricted to hematology, oncology, rheumatology, hematopoietic stem cell transplantation (HSCT), infectious diseases, intensive care, cardiology, nephrology, neurology, and solid organ transplantation. This fact is reflected by steady increase of indications where apheresis can be used as either a standalone or adjuvant treatment option.

Apheresis may be used for the separation of blood products like whole blood for transfusion of components or for the treatment of patients (therapeutic apheresis). The former use of apheresis is closely associated with transfusion medicine, whereas the latter has a wide range of clinical applications. History of apheresis reflects the development of instrumentation. It is not the scope of this review to discuss all the achievements regarding apheresis, but rather its milestones and current state will be summarized.

1.2 Early Efforts Regarding Cell Separation

In 1914 Abel, Rowntree, and Turner used manual apheresis in an animal model (performed in phlebotomized dogs) where they separated plasma from whole blood through centrifugation [3]. The return of red blood cells to the animal prevented undesirable effects of bleeding and was later found to be cost-effective in harvesting horse-derived antiserum [4]. Manual plasmapheresis was successfully used for the treatment of a patient presenting with Waldenström macroglobulinemia-associated hyperviscosity in 1952 [5]. Harvesting platelet concentrates by using repeated manual plasmapheresis from

O. Kayikci
Memorial Bahçelievler Hospital Adult Hematology and BMT Clinic, Istanbul, Turkey
e-mail: omur.kayikci@memorial.com.tr

E. Tekgunduz (✉)
Memorial Bahçelievler Hospital Adult Hematology and BMT Clinic, Istanbul, Turkey

Division of Hematology, Department of Internal Medicine, Maltepe University Medical School, Istanbul, Turkey
e-mail: emre.tekgunduz@memorial.com.tr

I. Kozanoglu (ed.), *Problem Solving in Apheresis Medicine*,
https://doi.org/10.1007/978-3-031-74081-7_1

blood donors was first described in 1961 [6]. Colman was the first to report on therapeutic thrombocytapheresis decreasing the platelet count in a patient with myeloproliferative neoplasm [7].

1.3 Blood Cell Separators

The basic principle behind the technology of modern blood cell separator devices relied on the principle of Dr. Carl Gustaf Patrik De Laval, who invented a cream separator through continuous flow centrifugation [8]. In the early 1950s, Dr. Edwin Cohn developed a method for the purification of plasma albumin from pooled human plasma that is used for the resuscitation of wounded soldiers. Dr. Cohn envisioned a device to separate online donor plasma during whole blood donation, which was actually more useful in deglycerolizing frozen red blood cells rather than the intended purpose [9]. By improving the design of the Cohn's centrifugal element, Alan Latham developed Haemonetics model 30 as the first apheresis device designed for intermittent-flow platelet donation and therapeutic apheresis (TA) [10].

An important step for the development of therapeutic apheresis technology came from the National Cancer Institute. George Hudson, an IBM engineer, whose son was being treated for chronic myeloid leukemia (CML), worked with Dr. Emil Freireich who envisioned a device designed for collecting excess leucocytes from CML patient and the later use of these cells for supporting neutropenic patients. The result of this collaborative effort was the development of Cobe Spectra instrument, which is widely used for therapeutic apheresis worldwide since the late 1980s [9]. Herbert Cullis and Yoichiro Ito devised an independently sealless centrifuge mechanism designed for third-generation continuous flow cell centrifugal separators [2].

1.4 Red Blood Cell Procedures

Red blood cell (RBC) exchange, erythrocytapheresis, and RBC depletion are different apheresis modalities used to decrease the RBC mass in the donor/apheresis product or replace patient RBSc with donor erythrocytes [11]. Manual RBC exchange involves serial phlebotomies, followed by colloid/crystalloid infusions. Meanwhile, automated RBC exchange is performed using apheresis instruments where donor RBCs are selectively removed and replaced with healthy donor RBC or colloid/crystalloid solutions. RBC exchange is frequently used to treat acute/chronic complications of sickle cell disease [12], to decrease the pathogen load in malaria [13] and babesiosis [14], and to decrease acute and long-term consequences in ABO-mismatched allogeneic hematopoietic stem cell transplantation [15].

1.5 Therapeutic Plasma Exchange

Therapeutic plasma exchange (TPE) is the most frequently used modality in therapeutic apheresis. Acquired thrombotic thrombocytopenic purpura (aTTP) is the prototype disease indicating the life-saving role of TPE, which is characterized by autoantibody-associated inhibition of von Willebrand cleaving protease (ADAMTS13). The efficacy mechanism of TPE in aTTP depends on the removal of autoantibody and restoration of normal enzyme activity. Rubinstein was the first who successfully treated a child with aTTP with exchange transfusion in 1959 [16]. Similar observations were made by Bukowski, who hypothesized that the success of plasma exchange was related to the removal of a soluble toxic substance in the plasma of aTTP patients [17]. Bukowski has successfully treated two aTTP patients with TPE alone, which supported this hypothesis [18].

In their landmark study, Rock et al. showed the superiority of TPE over plasma infusion in the treatment of aTTP, which made TPE a standard of care [19].

1.6 Peripheral Blood Stem Cell Collection

HSCT is an established treatment modality with a curative potential frequently used in patients presenting with hematological malignancies, inborn errors of metabolism, solid tumors, immunodeficiency states, and collagen vascular disorders. There is a noted steady and global increase in the use of HSCT for more than three decades. [20, 21] The use of peripheral blood as a source of hematopoietic stem cells revolutionized the application of HSCT. Lansky was able to collect sufficient number of pluripotent hematopoietic cells from normal donors by apheresis in 1982 [22]. Kessinger showed the ability of peripheral blood-derived hematopoietic progenitor cells to restore normal hematopoiesis after chemotherapy-associated aplasia in breast cancer patients [23]. Barlogie et al. used autologous bone marrow-derived HSCT in refractory multiple myeloma [24]. Due to faster engraftment kinetics, similar efficacy, and not necessitating general anesthesia, peripheral blood is found to be the preferred source for almost 80% of HPCT procedures, especially in adults presenting with malignancies [20, 21].

1.7 Evidence-Based Application of Apheresis

As therapeutic apheresis is not free of complications, rational use of the procedure is of utmost importance to provide clinical benefit without placing the patient at unnecessary risks. Before evaluating a patient for therapeutic apheresis, every step of McLeod's criteria should be considered: (1) Pathogenesis of the disease (there must be a clear rationale justifying the use of therapeutic apheresis). (2) Correction (the pathology/abnormality may be corrected with the procedure). (3) Clinal benefit (therapeutic apheresis should confer clinical benefit to the patient) [25, 26]. Beginning with the fourth edition of American Society for Apheresis (ASFA) guideline in 2007, ASFA regularly publish guidelines by using evidence-based approach in grading and categorization of indications regarding therapeutic apheresis. The most recent ASFA guideline was published in 2019 [27]. The development of ASFA guidelines is an important step and valuable effort for the global standardization of apheresis procedures regarding evidence-based medicine.

Conflict of Interest Statement All authors declare that they do not have any potential conflict of interest that could inappropriately influence the present study.

References

1. van Tellingen C. Bleeding—edge technology in cardiology—or the mixed blessings of phlebotomy throughout the ages. Neth Heart J. 2010;18:2128–2.
2. Corbin F, Cullis HM, Freireich EJ, et al. Development of apheresis instrumentation. In: McLeod BC, Szczepiorkowski ZM, Weinstein R, Winters JL, editors. Apheresis: principles and practice. 3rd ed. Bethesda: AABB Press; 2010.
3. Abell J, Rowntree L, Turner B. Plasma removal with return of corpuscles (plasma-pheresis). J Pharmacol Exp Ther. 1914;5:625–41.
4. Taft EG. Application history. In: McLeod BC, Szczepiorkowski ZM, Weinstein R, Winters JL, editors. Apheresis: principles and practice. 3rd ed. Bethesda: AABB Press; 2010.
5. Adams WS, Blahd WH, Bassett SH. A method of human plasmapheresis. Proc Soc Exp Biol Med. 1952;80:377–9.
6. Kliman A, Gaydos LA, Schroeder LR, et al. Repeated plasmapheresis of blood donors as a source of platelets. Blood. 1961;18:303–9.
7. Colman RW, Sievers CA, Pugh RP. Thrombocytapheresis: a rapid and effective approach symptomatic thrombocytosis. J Lab Clin Med. 1966;68:389–99.
8. De Laval CGP. Inventor. US Patent 247,804. 1881.
9. McLeod BC. Therapeutic apheresis: history, clinical application, and lingering uncertainties. Transfusion. 2010;50:1413–26.

10. Tullis JL, Tinch RJ, Baudanza P, et al. Plateletpheresis in a disposable system. Transfusion. 1971;11:368–77.
11. Stussi G, Buser A, Holbro A. Red blood cells: exchange, transfuse and deplete. Transfus Med Hemother. 2019;46:407–16.
12. Kernoff LM, Botha MC, Jacobs P. Exchange transfusion in sickle cell disease using a continuous-flow blood cell separator. Transfusion. 1977;17:269–71.
13. Yarrish RL, Janas JS, Nosanchuk JS, et al. Transfusion malaria. Treatment with exchange transfusion after delayed diagnosis. Arch Intern Med. 1982;142:187–8.
14. Cahill KM, Benach JL, Reich LM, et al. Red cell exchange: treatment of babesiosis in a splenectomized patient. Transfusion. 1981;21:193–8.
15. Rowley SD, Donato ML, Bhattacharyya P. Red blood cell-incompatible allogeneic hematopoietic progenitor cell transplantation. Bone Marrow Transplant. 2011;46:1167–85.
16. Rubinstein MA, Kagan BM, MacGillivray MH, et al. Unusual remission in a case of thrombotic thrombocytopenic purpura syndrome following fresh blood exchange transfusions. Ann Intern Med. 1959;51:1409–19.
17. Bukowski RM, Hewlett JS, Harris JW, et al. Exchange transfusions in the treatment of thrombotic thrombocytopenic purpura. Semin Hematol. 1976;13(3):219–32.
18. Bukowski RM, King JW, Hewlett JS. Plasmapheresis in the treatment of thrombotic thrombocytopenic purpura. Blood. 1977;50(3):413–7.
19. Rock GA, Shumak KH, Buskard NA, et al. Comparison of plasma exchange with plasma infusion in the treatment of thrombotic thrombocytopenic purpura. N Engl J Med. 1991;325(6):393–7.
20. Passweg JR, Baldomero H, Chabannon C, et al. Hematopoietic cell transplantation and cellular therapy survey of the EMBT: monitoring of activities and trends over 30 years. Bone Marrow Transplant. 2021;56:1651–64.
21. Auletta JJ, Kou J, Chen M, et al. Current use and outcome of hematopoietic stem cell transplantation: CIBMTR summary slides; 2021. http://www.cibmtr.org.
22. Lasky LC, Ash RC, Kersey JH, et al. Collection of pluripotential hematopoietic stem cells by cytapheresis. Blood. 1982;59:822–7.
23. Kessinger A, Armitage JO, Landmark JD, et al. Reconstitution of human hematopoietic function with autologous cryopreserved circulating stem cells. Exp Hematol. 1986;14:192–6.
24. Barlogie B, Alexanian R, Dicke KA, et al. High-dose chemoradiotherapy and autologous bone marrow transplantation for resistant multiple myeloma. Blood. 1987;70:869–72.
25. McLeod BC. An approach to evidence-based therapeutic apheresis. J Clin Apher. 2002;17:124–32.
26. Schwartz J, Winters JL, Padmanabhan A, et al. Guidelines on the use of therapeutic apheresis in clinical practice-evidence-based approach from the Writing Committee of the American Society for Apheresis: the sixth special issue. J Clin Apher. 2013;28:145–284.
27. Padmanabhan A, Connelly-Smith L, Aqui N, et al. Guidelines on the use of therapeutic apheresis in clinical practice-evidence-based approach from the Writing Committee of the American Society for Apheresis: the eighth special issue. J Clin Apher. 2019;34:171–354.

2 The Basics of Apheresis

Kaatje le Poole, Marleen M. Neyrinck, and Hans Vrielink

2.1 Introduction

Blood components from donors and patients can be collected via whole blood and apheresis donation. The word apheresis is derived from the Greek language, which means "to take away." However, apheresis does not only mean to take away. Apheresis is also described as a medical technology in which the blood of a donor or patient is separated into its component parts, the desired component is removed, and the remaining components are returned to the donor or patient [1]. For this separation, specific blood separating machines are available. Usually, the apheresis procedure is named after the blood component that is collected, e.g., plasmapheresis when plasma is collected and HPC apheresis when human progenitor cells (HPCs) are the aim of the collection.

K. le Poole · H. Vrielink (✉)
Department of Transfusion Medicine, Sanquin Blood Supply, Amsterdam, The Netherlands
e-mail: k.lepoole@sanquin.nl; h.vrielink@sanquin.nl

M. M. Neyrinck
Department of Hematology, AZ Delta, Roeselare, Belgium
e-mail: marleen.neyrinck@azdelta.be

2.2 History of Apheresis

As early as 400 years BC, Hippocrates suggested that a proper balance of the four bodily fluids maintained the health of the human being. It was postulated that disease is an expression of misbalance. Based on this hypothesis, he was convinced that bloodletting could correct the balance and therefore cure the disease. For many centuries, this principle was followed. In the end of the nineteenth century, the Swedish scientist Karl Gustaf Patrik de Laval developed the earliest continuous flow centrifugation device and patented this as centrifugal milk-cream separator.

"Selective bloodletting" with the removal of plasma and return of blood cells to the person (= plasmapheresis) was described and practiced in the USA in 1914 [2]. A unit of whole blood was drawn and mixed with citrate. With centrifugal technique, cells were separated from the plasma and returned to the donor. This can be interpreted as a manual apheresis procedure during which the unit of whole blood is collected in a bag. The bag is disconnected from the needle after donation. The whole blood is separated into components, and the not desired components are returned to the donor. At present, in the western world, this process is obsolete because of the risk of mixing up collected units of cells of different donors.

To collect sufficient volumes of plasma for wounded soldiers on the battle fields, selective

I. Kozanoglu (ed.), *Problem Solving in Apheresis Medicine*,
https://doi.org/10.1007/978-3-031-74081-7_2

bloodletting was used by Edwin Joseph Cohn and colleagues during and after World War II. They started with the collection of whole blood glass bottles containing a citrate solution. After centrifugation of the bottles, the cells were returned to the donor, and the albumin fraction was isolated from the plasma, or the plasma was stored until use. Cohn also planned a device that would separate donor plasma—the desired component—immediately and "online" during the whole blood donation process. Allen Latham (inventor of the Latham centrifuge bowl and founder of Haemonetics Corporation) thereafter turned this idea into a working apheresis machine. A second group of clinicians and scientists interested in blood cells and the reduction of cells in leukemia patients developed a second line of apheresis equipment in the 1960s. The latter equipment is the basis for the present apheresis machines of Fresenius Kabi (Amicus Cell Separation Platform™) and Terumo BCT (Cobe Spectra® and Spectra Optia®) [3].

Because of their work, de Laval and Cohn are considered as the founding fathers of the modern-day practice of apheresis science and medicine and therefore honored by the World Apheresis Association with an award. This award is given to recognize individuals who have made major contributions to the discipline of apheresis [4].

2.3 Background and Principle of Apheresis

Apheresis procedures are performed in donors and in patients as well (see Table 2.1).

Based on the blood component requested, apheresis procedures for donors can be separated into as follows:

1. Plasmapheresis
2. Cytapheresis
   (a) Platelets (plateletpheresis)
   (b) Erythrocytes (erythrocytapheresis)
   (c) Cells for cellular therapies (leukocytes) (it must be noted that when a patient is donating for him/herself, the patient is usually named (autologous) donor, e.g., autologous stem cell donor.)
   - Therapeutic cells
     - Lymphocytes (lymphocytapheresis)
     - Monocytes (monocytapheresis)
     - Granulocytes (granulocytapheresis)
   - Hematopoietic progenitor cells (HPC apheresis)
3. Multicomponent apheresis (apheresis procedure in which more than one blood component is collected, e.g., platelets and red blood cells (RBCs)).

Table 2.1 An overview of apheresis procedures

Donor apheresis	Patient apheresis[a]
Collection of components – Plasma – Platelets – Lymphocytes – Human progenitor cells (HPCs) – Monocytes – Granulocytes – Erythrocytes	*Therapeutic apheresis procedures* – Reduction of cells – Platelets – Leukocytes – Erythrocytes – Exchange of blood components – Plasma – Erythrocytes

[a] When a patient is donating for him/herself, the patient is usually named (autologous) donor, e.g., autologous stem cell donor

In one apheresis procedure, one or more volumes of the total blood volume of a donor can be processed to achieve the requested cell amount or plasma volume. Because of this, the apheresis procedure can take several hours, depending on the type of machine and the procedure to be performed. The most performed apheresis procedures in blood donors (plasmapheresis and plateletpheresis) take approximately 30–90 min.

Besides donor procedures, apheresis procedures can also be of applied in patients as therapeutic procedure. In case a patient is donating cells for further cellular therapy, e.g., CD34+ cells, this is not a therapeutic apheresis procedure, but a donor apheresis procedure. The aims of these therapeutic apheresis procedures are to reduce the pathogenic substances in plasma (e.g., autoantibody removal and plasma exchange), remove A/B-antibodies in ABO-incompatible organ transplants, and reduce myeloblasts in an acute myeloid leukemia (AML) patient suffering from leukostasis. In other situations, therapeutic apheresis is applied to "make space" for sufficient volume infusion of donor blood components, e.g., functional ADAMTS13 containing plasma for patients with thrombotic thrombocytopenic purpura (TTP) or exchange of red blood cells (RBCs) in sickle cell crisis. In a special issue of the *Journal of Clinical Apheresis*, on a regular basis, indications for therapeutic apheresis are reviewed [5].

2.4 Apheresis Procedures

As said above, in principle, manual and automated apheresis procedures can be performed.

2.4.1 Manual Apheresis

A standard whole blood donation is the starting point of a manual apheresis procedure. The collection bag with citrated whole blood is disconnected after the donation, but the needle remains in situ. Clotting of the needle will be prevented by maintaining a saline drip (0.9% NaCl). The collection bag with whole blood is centrifuged; the desired blood component is pressed into a component collection bag, and the remainder of the blood is returned intravenously to the donor. By repeating this process a few times, like mechanical/automated apheresis procedures, up to 750–850 mL of plasma can be collected in one donation. If by accident the wrong blood components are returned to the donor, it can lead to fatal consequences. Therefore, in the developed world, this technique has been abandoned. Currently, almost all apheresis procedures are performed with automated/mechanical apheresis equipment.

2.4.2 Mechanical Apheresis

Mechanical apheresis techniques are performed with specially developed machines. Plasmapheresis is the simplest apheresis procedure. Since plasmapheresis in donors is globally the most frequently performed procedure, specific plasmapheresis machines are produced by most manufacturers to reduce costs.

Most producers of apheresis machines have patented single-use apheresis disposable collection sets that fit only one type of machine. For most procedures, special disposal models are available. The sterile disposable, incorporating collection bags, bacterial and/or separation filters and/or centrifuge chambers, etc., is placed in the machine. To prevent clotting in the system and collection bag, the patients/donors' whole blood is mixed with an anticoagulant solution (usually trisodium citrate) in a specific whole blood-to-anticoagulant ratio. To add these anticoagulation solutions close to the needle, a port is available on the inlet line. Since part of the anticoagulated blood is returned to the donor/patient, trisodium citrate will also be administered to the person on the apheresis machine.

For the collection or removal of the desired blood component, the whole blood needs to be separated in different components. Various separation techniques have been developed.

2.4.2.1 Filtration Techniques

In 1943, Willem Johan Kolff presented the first hemodialysis machine (artificial kidney) using an animal-derived membrane to filter plasma. The plasma of kidney patients contains a lethal amount of waste products and pathogenic substances due to kidney failure, which can be swept via the filtering membrane and thus be removed from the body of the kidney patient. Similar to that principle, semipermeable filtration membranes are used for apheresis procedures. The pore size of the membrane is used to separate blood components based on their size. Water and small solutes can pass, but for larger blood proteins and blood cells, the membrane acts as a sieve. Filtration technique can be used solely for plasmapheresis. A substantial part of the plasma is pushed through the pores in the membrane and guided to the waste collection bag. The remainder of the plasma and the blood cells are returned to the patient together with a volume of plasma-replacing fluids in an isovolumic way.

2.4.2.2 Centrifugal Techniques

Anticoagulated whole blood flows into the centrifuge chamber of the apheresis machine. Here,

Table 2.2 Specific weight and size of various blood components

	Specific weight (kg/m^3)	Size (μm)
Plasma	1.026	
Platelets	1.040	1–4
Lymphocytes	1.050–1.061	6–10
Monocytes	1.077	10–30
Basophils	1.080	10–15
Eosinophils	1.082	9–15
Neutrophils	1.088	12–15
Erythrocytes	1.100	6–8

based on the specific weight of the various blood cells and not the size of the cells, the blood is separated into various blood components (see Table 2.2). Important in this are the time in the centrifuge chamber, the radius of the centrifuge, and the number of rotations per minute (G-forces in the centrifuge chamber). During the centrifugation process, various blood cells in the blood will be positioned in layers enriched with various blood components. The sequence in centrifugal techniques of apheresis is always plasma—platelets—lymphocytes—HPCs (if present)—monocytes—granulocytes and finally the erythrocytes. The apheresis machine is equipped with a software that allows the operator to decide which components need to be collected and returned to the donor.

2.4.2.3 Combination of Filtration and Centrifugation Techniques

Besides the separation of blood components by centrifugation, a membrane separation is also employed. Usually, the membrane is located in the centrifuge chamber. Examples of this principle are the separation technology in the Autopheresis C™ and Aurora™ plasmapheresis system from Fresenius Kabi for the collection of donor plasma.

2.4.2.4 Elutriation Techniques

In elutriation techniques, we make use of two opposite forces, the centrifugal force and the flow of plasma. The centrifugal forces achieve a first separation of the cells based on the specific weight of the cells. In the product collection line, a specific elutriation chamber is placed in which the heavier cells are pushed to the centrifuge wall; meanwhile, with an opposite force caused by a fluid flow, a second separation of the blood cells based on the size of these cells is forced.

The platelets are the smallest cells and will leave the elutriation chamber prior to all other cells. The sequence of the various blood components with elutriation techniques is plasma—platelets—erythrocytes—lymphocytes—HPCs (if present)—granulocytes—monocytes. Elutriation in apheresis techniques is applied not only to achieve leukoreduction of the collection of specific mononuclear cells (lymphocytes and monocytes) but also to reduce the donor's platelet loss due to the apheresis procedure.

2.4.2.5 Adsorption Techniques

The adsorption technique can be used to remove substances out of the plasma (e.g., specific (auto) antibodies) by binding them to the surface of a solid-phase column (adsorber). During an apheresis procedure, plasma is separated by filtration or centrifugal techniques and led via an adsorber before it is returned to the donor or patient with the blood cells. With antigen-specific immunoadsorption, selected cells, lipids, or immunoglobulins can be removed by binding to absorber fibers in columns.

2.5 Apheresis Disposables

As described earlier, product- and machine-specific apheresis disposables are used. Based on the composition of the disposable, it can be categorized as an open or a closed system.

2.5.1 Closed Versus Open Apheresis Disposables

A closed apheresis disposable is one which is completely assembled by the manufacturer and ready for use. Within the disposable, no connections need to be made. Connections between the machine and disposable (e.g., pressure lines) are fitted with bacterial filters. Also, the anticoagulant solution is spiked using an inline bacterial filter. In a closed system only, the venipuncture is performed without a bacterial filter.

All other disposables are open systems. Disposable systems may be delivered completely assembled by the manufacturer but are classed as open systems when, for instance, there is no bacterial filter in the anticoagulant line incorporated. More often, open apheresis disposables are not completely assembled by the manufacturer. Prior to use, the apheresis operator needs to connect one (e.g., the needle) or more parts, e.g., needle, lines, centrifuge chamber, and collection bag(s).

According to international guidelines, products that are collected in open systems should be used or processed within 24 h after donation. Usually, blood components that are applied for direct patient care (e.g., fresh frozen plasma (FFP), platelets, RBCs, etc.) should be collected in closed systems, with one exception. Plasma used to produce plasma-derived blood products (e.g., intravenous immunoglobulin G (IVIG), clotting factor VIII (FVIII), albumin, etc.) can be collected in sterile open systems.

When a closed system is opened, (e.g., change of needle, second venipuncture with the same disposable), by definition, the system becomes an open system, and the collected blood component should be transfused within 24 h after donation.

2.6 The Apheresis Procedure

The apheresis procedure is started by performing the venipuncture. Next to the needle, the donor's blood is anticoagulated by adding an anticoagulant solution. In donor apheresis, usually, trisodium citrate is used as an anticoagulant, either as a simple solution trisodium citrate solution or in mixtures such as acid citrate dextrose (ACD-A) solution or citrate phosphate dextrose (CPD) solution. Using the lines of the disposable set, the anticoagulated whole blood is guided to the separation part. After separation, the requested blood component is stored in a collection bag, and the remaining components are returned to the donor including a specific volume of the anticoagulant used. During an automated apheresis procedure, the volume of anticoagulation is controlled by the apheresis machine and balanced to the drawn blood volume from the donor.

2.6.1 Continuous and Discontinuous Flow Techniques

An apheresis procedure can be performed using a continuous flow technique or a discontinuous flow technique. With continuous flow techniques, the blood is drawn, processed, and returned at the same time. In consequence, an inlet and a return line to the patient or donor are needed. Venous access can be obtained by placing two peripheral venous catheters or a double-lumen central venous line. In donor procedures, the venipuncture is usually performed in the antecubital fossa of both arms; hence, the donor is stalled for the duration of the apheresis procedure. Therefore, in some cases, for the return access, one of the veins in the forearm can also be used. In patients, double-lumen central venous catheters placed in femoral, jugular, or subclavian veins are often used.

In discontinuous flow techniques, only one venipuncture is needed. During the draw period, whole blood is drawn from the donor and enters the separation part of the disposable set. Here, the requested blood component is separated from the other blood components and stored in a collection bag. The remaining blood components are temporarily stored in a reservoir of the disposable. When the reservoir is full, the return phase of the procedure is then initiated, and the contents of the reservoir are returned to the donor/patient via the same needle. After this, the cycle of draw, separation, and return is repeated until the desired volume is reached.

In discontinuous techniques, two variants are seen: (1) return of the complete volume of all components collected in the reservoir of the disposable, followed by an iteration of the entire procedure until the target volume of requested blood components is achieved, or (2) after fully filling the collection and separation system, draw and return of small volumes of blood is performed intermittently; thus, the separation of the blood components is performed almost continuously. Usually, in the first variant, the centrifuge is completely stopped (including loss of the separation); meanwhile, in the second variant, the centrifuge remains working at normal levels, or the number of rotations per minute is slightly decreased. The benefit of this technique is that the separation of blood cells in the system remains intact, thus reducing the procedure time to achieve a new full separation. One of the advantages of continuous apheresis techniques versus the discontinuous technique is a smaller extracorporeal volume.

2.7 Anticoagulant

There are at least four requirements for anticoagulation solutions used in apheresis practice:

1. Blood should not clot during a procedure.
2. The effect of the anticoagulant should also be sufficient to prevent clotting during storage and transfusion of the blood component.
3. The effect of the anticoagulant should have no or as little as possible activation of the platelets or clotting factors.
4. The anticoagulant should be as safe as possible for the donor and patient.

Three important types of anticoagulation can be distinguished:

2.7.1 Local Anticoagulation with a Citrate Solution

Citric acid (Fig. 2.1) occurs naturally in citrus fruits. In biochemistry, it is an intermediate in the citric acid cycle, which occurs in the metabolism of all aerobic organisms and is present in all body cells. The anticoagulation effect of citrate is based on the chelation of calcium, which is necessary for the coagulation cascade (Fig. 2.2). With the binding of ionized calcium in the system and the collection bag, there is no free calcium for the calcium-dependent reactions in the clotting cascade resulting in clotting prevention.

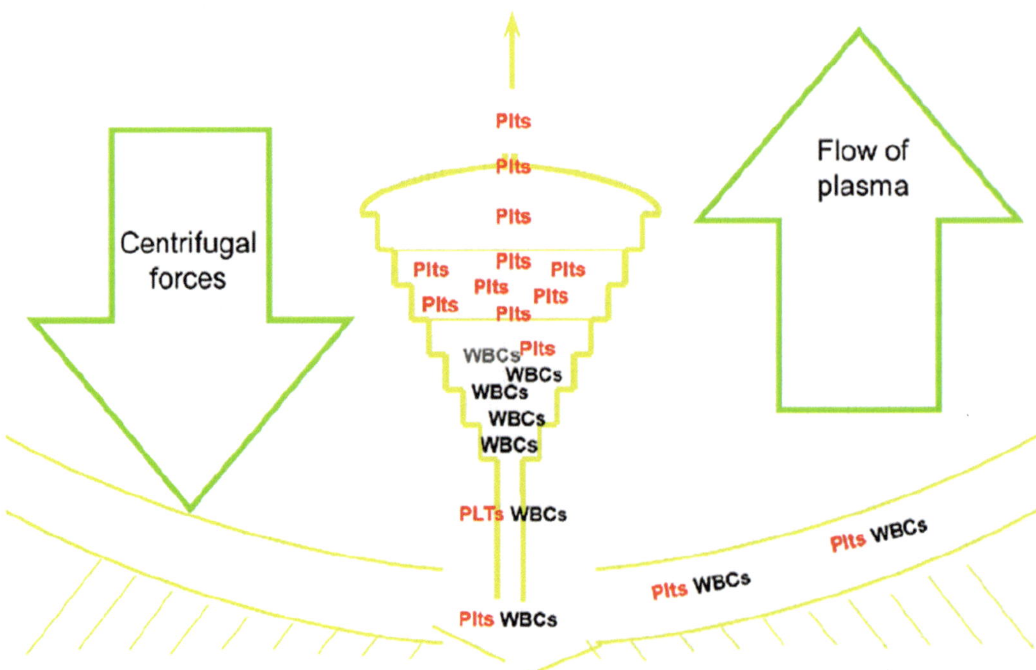

Fig. 2.1 Elutriation in the leukoreduction process during platelet apheresis with Trima Accel® Automated Blood Collection System (Terumo BCT)

Citrate can therefore be applied as an anticoagulation limited to the extracorporeal apheresis circuit. When citrate anticoagulation is utilized during an apheresis procedure, only the blood in the machine and the collected product are anticoagulated. The volume of citrate that is returned to the donors' or patients' bloodstream is rapidly metabolized and excreted. In patients and donors with normal kidney and liver function and calcium and pH levels within normal range, no effects on clotting status are to be expected.

In the human body, 99% of the calcium is bound to hydroxyapatite, giving the structural function of the bones. A small quantity of calcium in the bones can be mobilized rapidly in case of hypocalcemia. Approximately 1000 mg of extracellular calcium is available in the plasma (2.2 mmol/L = 9 mg/dL). The amount of calcium in the cells is negligible. Of plasma calcium, 40% is protein bound (to albumin), and 13% forms complexes with ions such as citrate, phosphate, and lactate. The remaining 47% is unbound and is named ionized (iCa) or free calcium. A normal iCa level in the blood is essential for the functioning of cells. A decrease in free calcium in the blood will release calcium from the skeleton and increased (re)absorption in kidney and intestine. This is controlled by parathyroid hormone (PTH) and vitamin D. Parathyroid hormone (parathormone) is secreted by the chief cells of the parathyroid glands, and PTH levels rise 5–10 min after the start of an apheresis procedure due to lowering of the ionized calcium levels.

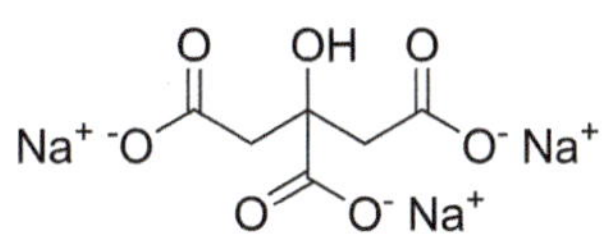

Fig. 2.2 Trisodium citrate

In donor apheresis procedures, citrate is the preferred anticoagulant. In cytapheresis, additional substrates are needed to improve blood cell survival. In ACD-A, for example, citric acid and dextrose are added to the citrate to improve the quality of the platelets, while phosphates and dextrose are added to a citrate solution to improve storage of erythrocytes (CPD = citrate, phosphate, dextrose) (Fig. 2.3).

Increase of citrate use during an apheresis procedure may lead to adverse reactions in the donor or patient due to hypocalcemia caused by the citrate. Acute hypocalcemia can result in severe symptoms, such as paresthesia, muscle spasms, cramps, tetany, circumoral numbness, and seizures [6]. Citrate levels in the donors/patients'

Fig. 2.3 Systematic scheme of the steps within clotting system showing the points of influence of calcium

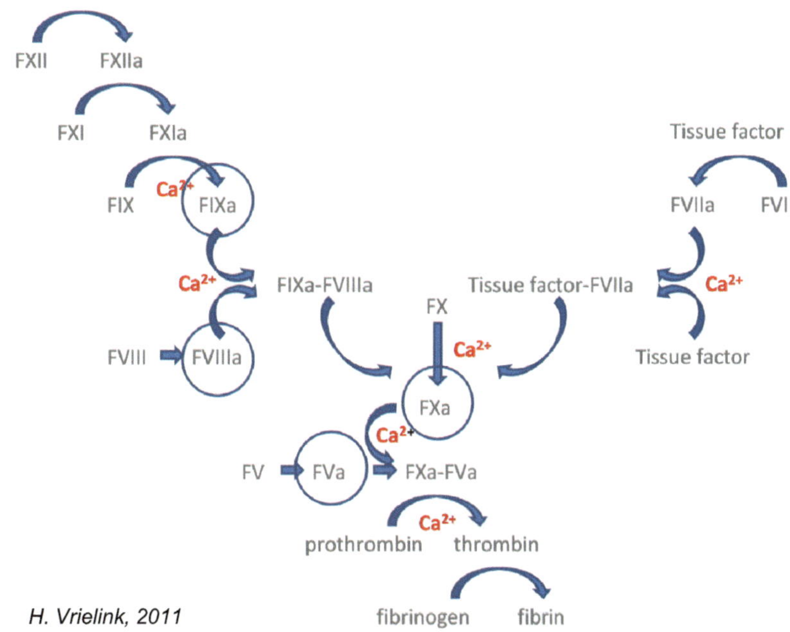

Table 2.3 Various citrate solutions used in apheresis

• Sodium citrate 4%	Bags of 250 mL with 40 g/L trisodium citrate solution	Used in plasmapheresis procedures
• ACD-A 2.2%	Bags of 500 or 750 mL with 22 g/L trisodium citrate solution. The solution also contains citric acid (8 grams per liter) and dextrose	Used for platelet apheresis, leukocytapheresis, and combinations of these, e.g., with the collection of RBCs
• CPD-50	Bags with a 39.5 g/L trisodium citrate solution. The solution also contains phosphates and dextrose	Used for erythrocytapheresis

serum and urine usually normalize within 4 h after completion of the apheresis procedure.

Examples of citrate solutions and their use are shown in Table 2.3.

During the apheresis procedure, the citrate solution is added to the donors/patient's whole blood just next to the needle. Since the concentration of citrate in a citrate solution can vary, the manufacturer of the apheresis equipment recommends different blood-to-anticoagulant ratios per procedure type, depending on the citrate concentration of the anticoagulant. This anticoagulant-to-whole-blood ratio varies between the different techniques from 1:8 (1 mL of anticoagulant per 8 mL of whole blood) to 1:25. Modern apheresis machines accurately titrate the addition of citrate solution to the whole blood within safe limits. The volume of anticoagulant during an apheresis procedure added to the donors' or patients' blood is closely monitored and, in many machines, limited to a specific citrate volume per minute and per kilogram of bodyweight of the person on the system.

Citrate does not bind to blood cells but will be completely dissolved in the plasma. The occurrence of hypocalcemia due to citrate in donor or patient depends, among other things, on the procedure performed. If more plasma is returned during an apheresis procedure, the donor receives more citrate, and this, in turn, increases the chance of a hypocalcemia.

2.7.2 Anticoagulation with Heparin

Heparin can also be used as an anticoagulant in apheresis procedures. However, heparin is not the anticoagulant of first choice. Heparin binds to the inhibitor antithrombin III and is causing its activation. The activated antithrombin then inactivates thrombin and other proteases involved in blood clotting, most notably factor Xa. Heparin works instantly, and this characteristic makes it suitable for apheresis procedures. But because of its longer half-time survival in the human body, it causes systemic anticoagulation in the donor/patient and increases the risk for bleeding. The increased bleeding risk is seen as a disadvantage, thus making the use of heparin less preferred for blood donor apheresis procedures. However, in patient apheresis, a mixture of citrate with a limited international units of heparin is used to reduce the citrate load of the patient..

Another disadvantage of heparin is that its anticoagulation effect is neutralized by normal plasma. In case of donor apheresis, the consequence is that the product must be processed or transfused rapidly after collection. Also, the use of heparin is associated with an infrequent but serious side effect: the formation of autoantibodies directed to platelets. This can cause thrombocytopenia and is called heparin-induced thrombocytopenia (HIT).

In patient apheresis, a combination of ACD-A plus heparin can also be applied. This is especially performed for apheresis procedures in small children to reduce the citrate load for the pediatric patient. The reduced citrate-depleting capacities of the pediatric liver are associated with an increased risk of citrate toxicity in children. Furthermore, children may not be able to express the symptoms of citrate intoxication. When ACD-A and heparin are used in combination, less citrate is needed. The heparin is added to the ACD-A, and a whole-blood-to-anticoagulant ratio of 1:20–25 is used.

2.7.3 Anticoagulation with Vitamin K Antagonists

Coumarins act through inhibition of the enzyme vitamin K epoxide reductase, which catalyzes the γ-carboxylation of the so-called vitamin K-dependent coagulation factors (II, VII, IX, and X). The anticoagulant effect can take 3–4 days to sort effect due to the long half-lives of the preexisting coagulation factors. Therefore, coumarin derivatives are not of any use in apheresis.

2.8 Leukoreduction of Blood Components Collected by Apheresis

In many countries, there is a policy of exclusively leukocyte-reduced blood supply of cellular blood products, a policy which is generally referred to as universal leukodepletion. The leukocytes must be reduced prior to storage. According to the European guidelines, the remaining leukocytes should not exceed 5×10^6 per unit.

In apheresis, the method of leukocyte reduction varies between manufacturers and types of apheresis equipment. For instance, in platelet apheresis with the Trima Accel (Terumo BCT), a special leukocyte reduction system (named LRS chamber; Fig. 2.1) is incorporated into the disposable. Other systems employ an inline leukocyte reduction filter which is incorporated in the disposable. Also, leukocyte reduction can be achieved by separation through the centrifugal forces in the centrifuge chamber, sometimes in combination with a membrane in the centrifuge chamber.

2.9 Safety of Apheresis Equipment

Modern apheresis machines are computer-controlled devices with multiple safety features for both the donor and collected product.

2.9.1 Pressure Monitoring

To protect the veins of the donor, pressure monitors are installed on the draw and return lines. With these detectors, it should be avoided that a too high or too low pressure in the needle will harm the vein. If the pressure exceeds the predetermined values set by the manufacturer, the process stops and sounds an alarm. To avoid bacterial contamination of the blood inside of the disposable, the disposable is connected to the machine with an inline bacterial filter. Pressure monitors can also be available to protect the complete system for too high pressures avoiding leakages of the disposable. The pressure monitors are also used to check correct installation of the disposable and for leakages by opening and closing various valves during an installation check.

2.9.2 Air Detectors

Of course, when the disposable is installed, the disposable is filled with sterilized air. With the filling up of the disposable with blood or other fluids, the air is lead to a specific bag included into the disposable. When returning the remaining blood in the disposable set to the donor/patient during or at the end of the apheresis procedure, the disposable is filled with air again. To prevent an air embolism due to infusion of air to the donor or patient, one or more air detectors are included in the apheresis equipment. Air detectors are acoustic detectors. Through hearing, they can detect air bubbles. In case air is detected, a warning alarm is given, and a light extinguishes on the detector where the air is detected. The procedure is stopped automatically.

2.9.3 Extracorporeal Volume

In most apheresis equipment, prior to the apheresis procedure, the gender, height, and body weight of the donor or patient must be entered into the software of the apheresis machine. Based on this information, the machine calculates the total blood volume of the person on the machine. By monitoring the volume of donor/patient blood processed and collected by the machine, the donor/patient is protected by the apheresis machine from removing more than 15% of the donor's total blood volume. The machine stops, and a warning alarm is given on the display.

2.9.4 Maximal Volume Collected in Donor Apheresis Procedures

The software of the apheresis machine is parameterized so that a predetermined maximum allowable volume of blood component can be drawn.

2.9.5 Fluid Detectors in Centrifuge Chamber

Fluid leakage in a centrifuge chamber is detected by sensors. If leakage in the centrifuge chamber occurs, the process stops and an alarm sounds.

2.10 Technical Problems

During an apheresis procedure, various technical challenges can occur. The problems may be caused by disposables, equipment, the apheresis operator, or the donor.

1. Disposables
   (a) Leaks or faults in the disposable system.
   (b) If a leak or defect in the disposable is not noted prior to the start of the apheresis procedure, blood can leak outside the disposable. This can lead to an infection risk and can be stressful for donors and patients. As the procedure must be aborted, the contents of the disposable cannot be returned to the donor or patient. This will result in donors' unintentional blood cell donation with a longer delay/interval until the next donation. Proper checking of the disposable prior to its installation can prevent most cases. Also, a valuable product can be lost for use, e.g., an HPC component needed for progenitor cell transplant.
   (c) Coagulation or clotting in the disposable system, despite the addition of a sufficient volume of anticoagulant. The cause is not always clear.
2. Equipment

   Whatever equipment is used, several problems can be seen:
   (a) Software problems in the device
   (b) Technical problems with the device
   (c) Loss of electricity supply
3. Apheresis operator

   Despite good training, education, and maintaining knowledge and skills to operate the equipment, several problems can arise which are determined by the staff's performance. Some examples are wrong operation of the equipment, improper installation of the disposable or failure to adequately check the disposable prior to the procedure, and difficulties to achieve adequate venous access.
4. Donor
   (a) Poor venous access or development of a hematoma.
   (b) Medical problems directly or indirectly related to the apheresis procedure, such as hypovolemia (especially in low-weight persons), fainting, and hyperventilation.
   (c) Hypocalcemia is also named as citrate reactions or citrate intoxication.
   (d) Low total blood volume for the apheresis equipment leading to too large ECV. According to the guidelines, a maximum of 15% is allowed.

References

1. Hematopoietic cellular therapy accreditation manual, 8th ed. 2021.
2. Anstee DJ, Klein HG. Mollison's blood transfusion in clinical medicine, 12th ed. 2014.
3. McLeod BC. Therapeutic apheresis: history, clinical application, and lingering uncertainties. Transfusion. 2010;50:1413–26.
4. https://worldapheresis.org.

5. Padmanabhan A, Connelly-Smith L, Aqui N, Balogun RA, Klingel R, Meyer E, Pham HP, Schneiderman J, Witt V, Wu Y, Zantek ND, Dunbar NM. Guidelines on the use of therapeutic apheresis in clinical practice—Evidence-based approach from the writing Committee of the American Society for Apheresis: the eighth special issue. J Clin Apher. 2019;34:171–354.
6. Fong J, Khan A. Hypocalcemia: updates in diagnosis and management for primary care. Can Fam Physician. 2012;58:158–62.

Apheresis Mathematics

3

Marleen M. Neyrinck and Hans Vrielink

3.1 Introduction

Working at an apheresis unit, logistics can be challenging. Not all procedures can be scheduled, and in case of a medical emergency, you must perform procedures immediately. Think of a total plasma exchange (TPE) in a newly diagnosed TTP (thrombotic thrombocytopenic purpura) patient. Prior to the start of the procedure, it is important that you can make an estimation of the volume of the replacement fluid you will require, since sufficient units of plasma need to be thawed, or bottles of albumin available. To calculate this, you need to know the TBV, the TPV, and the hematocrit (Hct) of your patient.

Mathematics can be of help for the logistics in an apheresis collection center. Think of scheduling apheresis staff and equipment, but also in specific apheresis procedures. In a stem cell transplant procedure, for instance, the hematologist requests the collection of a minimally required number of CD34-positive cells per kilogram of the patients' bodyweight. The estimated number of cells that can be collected when processing a specific volume of the patients' blood can be calculated. With this outcome, you can estimate whether it is needed to organize a one-, two-, or three-day collection. This is also important since your patient needs to be mobilized for a CD34-positive cell collection. With other formulas, the volume to process for achieving a specific number of cells can be estimated. You can decide to process not "the usual" 3× the TBV, but, for instance, 2× the TBV or less. Therefore, with a good estimate, you can avoid the donor/patient unnecessarily connected to the apheresis device and excessive numbers of cells need to be stored.

Various calculations in apheresis are needed to perform the procedures correctly without harming the donor or patient. In this chapter, we will discuss how to calculate the TBV, the TPV, the ECV, and the ECRV. We also pay attention during the calculation of the CE, which is an important quality parameter for your collection unit. In relation to that, we discuss how many TBVs should be processed to collect a specific number of cells and what is the estimated product yield when you process a specific blood volume during your procedure. Finally, we describe how many RBCs to remove in case of an RBC reduction to achieve a target Hct and how to calculate the Hct level, when you only know the Hb level.

M. M. Neyrinck (✉)
Department of Hematology, AZ Delta,
Roeselare, Belgium
e-mail: marleen.neyrinck@azdelta.be

H. Vrielink
Sanquin Blood Supply, Amsterdam, The Netherlands
e-mail: h.vrielink@sanquin.nl

I. Kozanoglu (ed.), *Problem Solving in Apheresis Medicine*,
https://doi.org/10.1007/978-3-031-74081-7_3

3.2 Calculation Methods

3.2.1 Total Blood Volume

1. Nadler's formula to calculate the TBV of a human being based on gender, height, and weight [1].

   For males: TBV = (0.3669*Ht3 in M) + (0.03219*Wt in kgs) + 0.6041

   For females: TBV = (0.3561*Ht3 in M) + (0.03308*Wt in kgs) + 0.1833

   * Ht in M = Height in meters, * Wt in kgs = Bodyweight in kilograms
2. Gilcher's rule of fives (Table 3.1)
3. TBV in relation to age (Table 3.2)
4. TBV in relation to the BMI (Table 3.3)
5. Nomogram for estimation of pediatric patients [2]

Asking in general how much blood human beings have, many people answer that the TBV of an adult person is approximately 5 L. However, this is not similar in everybody. All persons are different. Looking around, we see a lot of differences in persons in terms of weight and height. Because of the differences between various human beings, for a more precise estimation of the total blood volume, various formulas are published. Well known are Nadler's formula and Gilcher's rule of fives, but there are also other formulas to calculate the approximate TBV.

Nadler's formula is a complex formula [1], considering the height, bodyweight, and gender of a person. Most apheresis equipment uses this formula to calculate the TBV. That is the reason that we must fill in the gender, height, and bodyweight of the donor/patient prior to

Table 3.1 Calculate the figure in the table with the bodyweight of your patient for an estimation of the TBV

Gilcher's rule of fives				
	Blood volume (mL/kg of body weight)			
Patient	Obese	Thin	Normal	Muscular
Male	60	65	70	75
Female	55	60	65	70
Infant/Child	–	–	80/70	–

Table 3.2 Calculate the figure in the table with the bodyweight of your patient for an estimation of the TBV

Age-group	Approximate blood volume (mL/kg)
Premature infant, at birth	90–105
Term newborn infant	80–90
Children >3 months	70–75
Adolescents and adults	
Male	70
Female	65

Table 3.3 Calculate the figure in the table with the bodyweight of your patient for an estimation of the TBV

	BMI <18.5	BMI 18.5–24.9	BMI 25–29.9	BMI >30
Blood volume	80 mL/kg	70 mL/kg	65 mL/kg	55 mL/kg

BMI = Wt/H^2, H = Height in meters, Wt = Bodyweight in kilograms the procedure into the parameter settings of the machine. It is important to know that this formula cannot be used for children <25 kg. For children, Linderkamp et al. [2] published, in 1977, a model to predict the blood volume depending on the age and gender of the child. He constructed his nomogram based on determining the TBV of 160 infants and children between 1 h and 14 years of age. This estimation of the TBV of pediatrics is based on the age and gender of the child and is easy to use. By drawing a line from the bodyweight to the height in the nomogram, you can read the TBV of the child on the line based on the gender and age of the child.

In Gilcher's rule of fives, a difference is made between a male, female, and pediatric person, and they take the physics of the person into account. Is the person obese, thin, normal, or muscular? Depending on the group the patient belongs to, you calculate the TBV by multiplying the bodyweight with a number given in the table. The difference in physics of the person is based on the difference in vascularization between fat and muscle tissue.

In the calculation methods based on the age of the person, you calculate the TBV by multiplying the bodyweight with a figure given in the table. In the group of adolescents and adults, a difference is made between men and women.

In the last calculation method, the body mass index (BMI) is considered. Based on the BMI of the person, the bodyweight is multiplied by a number given in the table to achieve the TBV. To calculate the BMI, you divide the bodyweight in kilograms by the square height in meters.

Looking at all the different calculation methods used to calculate the TBV, you can see similarities. In most of the methods, the TBV of an adult man is calculated by multiplying the bodyweight with 70 and 65 for a woman. In Gilcher's rule of fives and the method considering the BMI, they also look at the physics of the body. These two calculation methods correspond the most with Nadler's formula. In case you need a quick calculation of the TBV of someone, as a rule of thumb, the easiest calculation method is multiplying the bodyweight with 70 in men and with 65 in women. Having a more obese person, the TBV can be calculated by multiplying the bodyweight with 60 in men and 55 in women.

3.3 Total Plasma Volume (TPV)

1. $\text{TPV} = \text{TBV} \times (1 - \text{Hct})$
   Hct is given as decimal
2. $\text{TPV} = \text{TBV} \times (1 - \text{Hct} / 100)$
   Hct is given as percentage

Also, the TPV is not the same for everyone. To calculate the TPV, you need to know the TBV and the hematocrit (Hct). The Hct is, per definition, the volume percentage of RBCs in the TBV. Normally in females, we find a hematocrit between 36 and 46% (0.36–0.46 L/L); meanwhile, in men, it is between 41 and 53% (0.41–0.53 L/L). Based on the clinical situation of the patient, the Hct can be different from the normalized values. In chronic anemia, the red cell volume is decreased, while the TBV is normal or even somewhat higher, so the Hct is decreased. For our therapeutic plasma exchange (TPE) patients, we mainly find a decreased red cell volume. As said, to calculate the TPV, we need to know the TBV and the Hct. Having a patient with a TBV of 5000 mL and Hct of 50%, the TPV will be 2500 mL (5000 mL × 0.5 = 2500 mL). If the same patient has an Hct of 30%, the TPV will be 3500 mL (5000 mL × 0.7 = 3500 mL). So even when having two patients with the same TBV, the TPV can be different based on the Hct. With a lower Hct, the plasma volume is higher compared with a higher Hct. In patients for TPE with a lower Hct, there is a higher plasma volume, and a larger volume needs to be exchanged. In our example, there is a difference of 1000 mL. If you must do a plasma exchange of twice the TPV in this patient, with an Hct of 50%, you must exchange 5000 mL of plasma; meanwhile, with an Hct of 30%, you must exchange 7000 mL of plasma, thus influencing procedure time and exchange volume. Prior to the start of a TPE, it is important to make a calculation of the TBV and the TPV of the patient, so you can order the correct volume of exchange fluids.

Also, in plasma collections in blood donors, the Hct is an influencing factor in the procedure. In donor plasmapheresis, discontinuous apheresis systems are usually used, and a fixed volume of plasma is collected. During the procedure, the plasma will be separated from the blood cells. The plasma is led to the plasma collection bag, while the concentrated blood cells prior to the return are temporarily stored in a reservoir in the disposable set. The component in the reservoir has an Hct of 60–80% depending on the plasmapheresis equipment. In donors with a higher Hct, the reservoir will be filled much more rapidly compared with donors with a lower Hct. Let us assume we have a reservoir of 200 mL and in case the machine concentrates to an Hct of 80% in the reservoir, we will have around 160 mL of RBC and 40 mL of plasma. In case the donor's Hct is 50%, you will need to process approximately 320 mL of anticoagulated whole blood to collect approximately 120 mL of plasma in the collection bag per cycle before the reservoir is completely filled (50% of the 320 mL processed volume is 160 mL of cells). With a donor Hct of 35%, you need to process 460 mL to collect the 160 ml of RBCs in the reservoir, but you will then collect 260 mL of plasma per cycle. In conclusion, when the donors' Hct is higher, you need to process more donor blood to achieve the same collection volume compared to donors with a lower Hct, resulting in a longer procedure time.

3.4 Extracorporeal Volume

The extracorporeal volume (ECV) is the volume of blood which is outside of the body. Besides the anticoagulated blood in the disposable, you have also the volume of the collected blood component and the volume of tubes collected before or after the procedure. For the safety of the donor or patient, it is advisable that the ECV is maximally 15% of the TBV. So, to be aware of the ECV avoiding hypovolemia, you must not only know the TBV of your patient/donor but also the volume of the disposable and the volume of the collected tubes. Working with Spectra Optia® (Terumo BCT), the volume of the disposable is different depending on the procedure you performed. Working with Optia's MNC procedure to collect mononuclear cells, the volume of the disposable is 151 mL; using the continuous MNC (cMNC) procedure, the volume is 285 mL. The volume content of a disposable set, together with the thought to work safe with ECVs at maximum 15%, is important when performing procedures in children and smaller persons with a low TBV. Let us assume that you would use the cMNC procedure with the volume of the disposable at 285 mL and you collect 300 mL without volume compensation; the ECV will be 285 + 300 mL = 585 mL. This 585 mL is 15% of 3900 mL, which could be a problem in persons with a TBV <3900 mL. Many of the apheresis machines will warn you in case of suspected ECVs of <15% of the TBV.

3.5 Extracorporeal Red Cell Volume

Especially in pediatric apheresis, the extracorporeal red cell volume (ECRV) is of importance. Also, here is a maximum of 15% of the TBV advised to avoid too low Hcts during apheresis procedures. The RBCs of the patients are present in the disposable during a procedure and in the test tubes taken. To calculate the RBC volume, you need to know the patients' TBV and Hct. Calculation of the RBC volume can be of importance to decide whether priming of the disposable with donor RBCs is needed.

To give an example how to calculate: You have a female patient with a TBV of 2900 mL and an

Hct of 20%. The RBC volume is 580 mL (2900 × 0.2). The maximal ECRV is then 87 mL (580 × 0.15).

Let us assume that you would like to do a CD34+ cell collection in a 6-year-old child with a calculated TBV of 1800 mL. This child has an Hct of 20%, so the RBC volume is 360 mL (1800 × 0.2). Using the Optia's MNC protocol with a disposable volume of 151 mL and a blood warmer of 45 mL, you increase the child's TBV from 1800 to 1996 mL (1800 + 151 + 45). Starting the procedure with a saline or albumin prime, the child's RBCs are being divided in 1996 mL of "blood volume" instead of 1800 mL, so you decrease the Hct from 20 to 18% and will have a ERCV of 35 mL, which is 19.4% of the RBC volume. For this child, a blood prime should be suggested.

3.6 Hemoglobin (Hgb) g/dL ↔ mmol/L

1. $1\,g/dL = 0.62\,mmol/L$
2. $1\,mmol/L = 1.61\,g/dL$

Inside the RBC, we have the iron-containing oxygen-transporting protein named hemoglobin. Depending on the center or country, there can be a variation in the unit for the Hgb level. Some labs work with gram per deciliter (g/dL), while others with millimoles per liter (mmol/L). To convert from g/dL to mmol/L, you should be aware that 1 g/dL is 0.62 mmol/L and 1 mmol/L is 1.61 g/dL.

3.7 Calculating Hemoglobin into Hematocrit

1. $g/dL \rightarrow Hct(\%) = 3 \times Hgb$
2. $mmol/L \rightarrow Hct(\%) = ((Hgb \times 10)/2) - 2$

As mentioned before, the Hct is the volume percentage of RBCs in the TBV, or the volume percentage of the blood being taken by RBCs.

Sometimes, you only know the Hgb level; however, our apheresis machines ask for the Hct, and we need to be able to calculate the plasma volume of a patient. An estimation of the Hct can be made by taking 3× the Hgb level in case of g/dL or multiplying the Hgb level with 10, dividing it by 2, and extracting 2 from the outcome in case of mmol/L.

As an example, you have a person with a Hgb level of 16.1 g/dL = 10 mmol/L. To estimate the Hct level, you multiply 16.1 with 3, and you will have an Hct result of 48%. If you make the calculation with 10 mmol/L, you multiply 10 with 10, divide it by 2, and extract 2 from the outcome. Also here, you have an outcome for the Hct of 48%.

3.8 Volume ↔ Weight

1. Gram to mL: Mass (gram)/Density (Specific gravity)
2. mL to gram: Volume (mL) × Density (Specific gravity)

There is a noted correlation between the volume and the weight of fluids/blood. If we only know the weight of the collected product, we can calculate the collected volume by taking the net weight of the bag (tarra weight = weight component without the weight of the empty bag) divided by the specific weight of the collected component. Knowing the volume, we can calculate the weight by multiplying the volume of the collected product with the specific weight of the collected component.

As an example, we have a bag of plasma weighing 500 g. To calculate the volume, we divide the 500 g by the specific weight of the plasma that is 1.026. With this calculation, we know that the volume of this bag of plasma weighing 500 g is 487.3 mL (500/1.026 = 487.3).

When the volume of the bag plasma is 500 mL, we can calculate the weight by multiplying the 500 with 1.026, and so we know that the weight of the bag plasma is 513 g (500 × 1.026 = 513).

3.9 Collection Efficiency (CE)

1. $CE_1 = \text{Cells product} / \left(\left(\text{Pre PB count} + \text{Post PB count} \right) / 2 \right) \times \left(\text{TBV processed} - \text{AC volume} \right) * \right) \times 100$

2. $CE_2 = \text{Cells product} / \left(\text{Pre PB count} \times \left(\text{TBV processed} - \text{AC volume} \right) * \right) \times 100$

   **the TBV processed – AC volume in liters*

In summary, the CE of a machine is the number of cells collected as a percentage from the number of cells in the patient prior to the procedure. For instance, when the donor had 100 × 10e6 CD34+ cells per liter in his peripheral blood and the apheresis machine collects 50 × 10e6 CD34+ cells from every processed liter of uncoagulated blood, the CE is 50%. The CE can be used as a critical performance indicator in the collection center. Several apheresis machines, and also operators, can be compared to each other. Moreover, the performance of an apheresis machine in time can be observed. Besides this, with the knowledge of the mean CE in specific diseases, the number of particular cells that can be expected in your collection bag in a determined processed volume can be estimated, leading to a more personalized donor collection procedure (not standard 3× TBV) and logistics on the apheresis center.

It is important to understand that you should calculate what is processed with the uncoagulated whole blood volume (= processed anticoagulated volume − anticoagulant (AC) volume used) since the cells are only found in the donors' whole blood and not in the AC used. Furthermore, you should know that the concentration of specified cells in the donors peripheral blood is not constant during a procedure (you usually know only the concentration prior to the procedure). How the concentration exactly is during a procedure (increasing or decreasing, and if so how much) is unknown. This can influence the CE enormously.

Here, two formulas to calculate the CE are given. In the first formula, you need to know the peripheral blood (PB) cell count in your donor before and after the procedure. Furthermore, you need to know the processed volume without the AC volume and the cell count in your collection bag. The problem is that you do not always know the post-cell count in the donor. In these cases, you need to use the second formula. However, since the cell count during a procedure is changing, the CE with the second formula is less accurate than with the first one.

This formula can be used for all variations of cell collections, for instance, platelet, RBC, or CD34+ collections.

Example 3.1 CE of a Platelet Collection In our plateletpheresis, we collected a product with a platelet concentration of 350 × 10^9 cells/unit. The donors' pre-count was 280,000/μL (280 × 10^9/L), and the post-count was 200,000. We processed a blood volume of 2000 mL without AC. Since we know the pre and post platelet count, we can use the CE_1 formula. The CE_1 is 350,000/((280,000 + 200,000)/2) × 2)) × 100 = 72.9%. So for this plateletpheresis, the CE_1 is 72.9%.

Example 3.2 CE for a CD34 Collection A CD34 collection in a donor with a CD34+ count of 30 × 10^6/L is performed. In total, 15 L of the TBV (without AC) is processed. In this procedure, 4 × 10^6/kg of the patients' bodyweight (70 kg) was collected. In this case, to calculate the CE, we need to use the CE_2 formula, since the post PB CD34+ count is unknown. It is important to take the absolute number of CD34+ cells in the collection bag. So if we know that we collected 4 × 10^6/kg, the absolute number of CD34+ cells in the collection bag is 4 × 70 kg or 280 × 10^6. The CE for this CD34 collection is 280/(30 × 15) × 100 = 62.2%.

By calculating the CE for all the different cell collections of your center, you can calculate a mean CE for every specific cell collection.

It should be noted that the mean CE is usually based solely on the pre-procedure cell count in the donor (CE_2). However, it is wrongly assumed that the cell concentration in the donors' peripheral blood is constant throughout the procedure (see Fig. 3.1). Therefore, it is better to calculate the CE on the pre- and post-procedure cell count (CE_1), assuming there's a linear reduction of cells during the procedure. The CE_1 gives a somewhat better estimation of the CE, but still this gives an unrealistic outcome. However, using a pessimistic CE, most of the times, we will not fail to collect sufficient cells [3].

As shown with the donors' pre- and post-cell counts, the cell concentration will drop but not via a linear line, but via a curved one. How steep this curve is, is not exactly known. Therefore, it would be more realistic to use a linear regression model to calculate CEs based on the normalized yield per liter of whole blood processed by the apheresis machine [4]. This will give a more accurate estimation on how to proceed with a collection procedure avoiding an over- or under-concentrated cell outcome in your collected component. To calculate the formula for your center or even for your various machines, divide per procedure the cell yield per liter of processed whole blood (you can use the data from previous collections (years)). Plot subsequently the cell pre-procedure count of

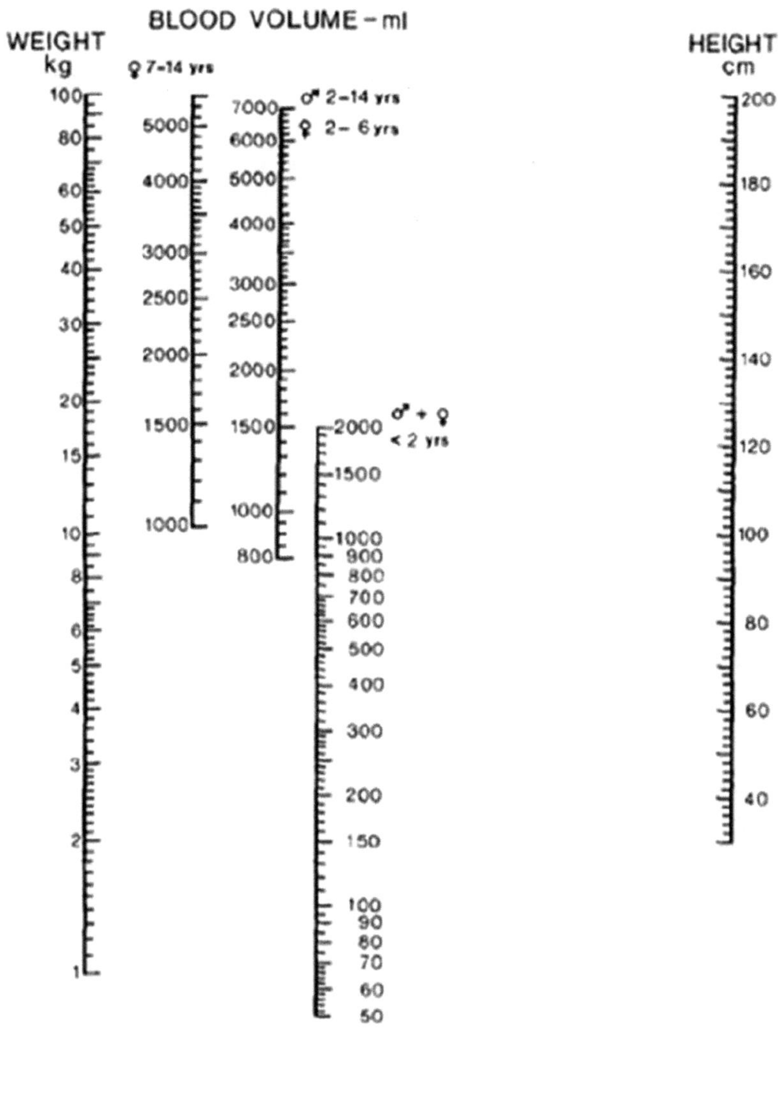

Fig. 3.1 Nomogram Linderkamp et al. [2]

the donor against the outcome of the yield per liter in a statistical program. The program will then give a linear regression formula with the regression index (R^2) (see Fig. 3.3). The linear regression formula will be *Cells collected/Liter WB = 0.4706 × Cell pre-count + 6.3936*; in other words, for this example, you get the formula for a CD34+ collection:

$$\text{Liters WB to process} = \text{Target CD34+}/\text{kg} \times \text{kg recipient}/\left(\left(0.4706 \times \text{CD34+ pre}\right) + 6.3936\right)$$

By using this formula in the given example of hospital A, you will have with 87.2% reliability (R^2) the number of requested cells when the calculated liters of whole blood will be processed.

To give an example:

- The CD34+ pre-count is 30×10^6/L
- By processing 15 L of uncoagulated blood, you collected 270×10^6 CD34+ cells
- Yield per liter = $270 \times 10^6/15 = 18 \times 10^6$
- In a statistical program (also the graphic part of Excel® can be used), you plot the yield per liter (=18) versus the pre-count in the donor (=15) of, for instance, 50 different procedures, and you will get a graph as shown in Figs. 3.2 and 3.3.

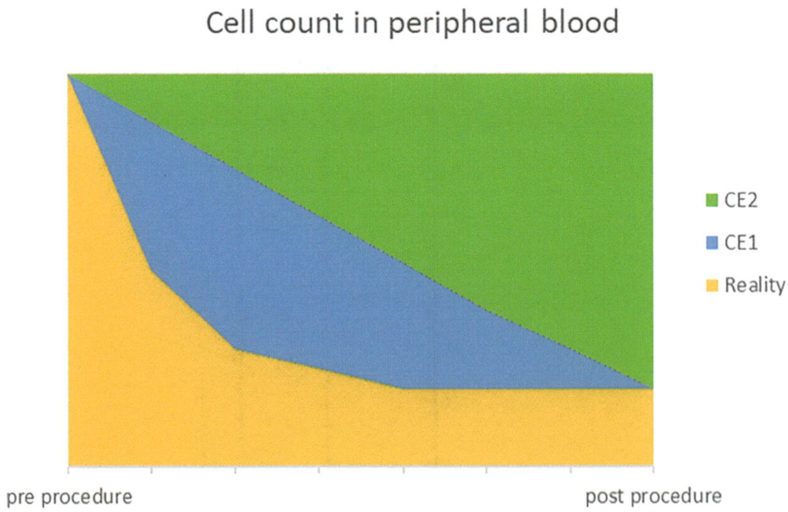

Fig. 3.2 Cell count in the peripheral blood during an apheresis procedure (Adapted from Joseph Roig (2016) [4] (with permission))

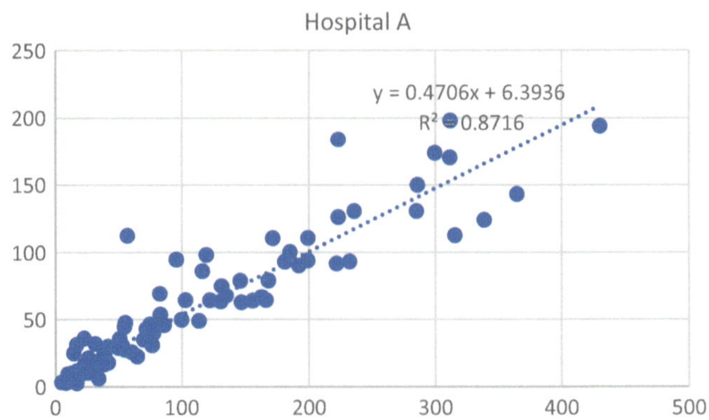

Fig. 3.3 CD34+ collection concentration per liter of the processed whole blood versus CD34+ pre-procedure count in the donors' peripheral blood. X-axis: CD34+ concentration per liter of the whole blood processed. Y-axis: CD34+ concentration pre-procedure in the donors' peripheral blood

3.10 TBV to Process During a Collection Procedure

1. TBV to process = Absolute number of cells needed/Cells of interest in PB × mean CE

   By knowing the mean CE of your apheresis collections for the specific cell, you can calculate what volume of blood should be processed to collect a specific number of cells. It is totally not needed to process always 3× the TBV or always the standard 15 L. By using this formula, you can sometimes see that one procedure will not be sufficient and that a second procedure is needed to collect the requested number of cells. This can be important for the logistics and practical organization of the apheresis collection facility. For this calculation method, it is important that you know the pre-cell count in your donor and the requested number of cells needed to be collected. Let us assume that we must perform a CD34+ collection in an allogeneic donor. The patient's attending physician is requesting a product with 3×10^6 CD34+ cells/kg of the patient's bodyweight, which is 65 kg. The CD34+ pre-count of the donor is 35×10^6/L. From previous collections, we know that the mean CE of our center is 45%. In making the calculation, you will see that you need to process 12.5 L of uncoagulated blood to achieve the request number of cells ((3 × 65)/(35 × 0.45) = 12.5 L).

   As said earlier, this calculation can be helpful in the logistics of your apheresis center. Probably, you can avoid a procedure the next day by processing 2 L, but you will also have information on the volume to process when a second day is needed.

3.11 Expected Product Yield

1. Expected product yield = (Cell count donor × processed TBV × mean CE)/1000

   Prior to the start of a cell collection procedure, you can calculate the expected product yield, when the cell count in the donor, the TBV to process, and the mean CE are known. Let us give an example. You want to perform a CD34+ collection and decide to process 3× the TBV of the donor with a TBV of 5600 mL. The CD34+ pre-count is 35×10^6/L. From previous procedures, you know that the mean CE of your center is 45%. By placing this data in the formula, you can make an estimation of what the absolute number of CD34+ cells in your collection product:

$$\frac{35 \times 5600 \times 3(\text{you will process 3x TBV}) \times 0.45(\text{mean CE})}{1000} = 265 \times 10^6 \text{ CD34+ cells in your product}$$

When the recipient has a bodyweight of 65 kg, you need to divide the outcome of 265 by 65, and you will achieve a product of 4×10^6/kg. When the hematologist requests an outcome of $>3 \times 10^6$/kg, you can assume that one procedure of 3× TBV in this donor probably is sufficient.

3.12 Red Cell Exchange: Volume RBCs to Remove

1. Volume to remove (VR) = (Hct start − Hct target)/79 × TBV

   In case of RBC reductions in, for instance, polycythemia or hemochromatosis patients, you can calculate the volume to be removed to achieve the target Hct. For this calculation, you abstract the target Hct of the start Hct and divide the outcome by 79 (which is the Hct of the removed product). The outcome will then be multiplied with the TBV of the patient.

   To give an example: You would like to reduce the ferritin level of a hemochromatosis patient by taking a volume of RBCs. The patient has an Hct of 49% and a TBV of 5000 mL. You aim at a post-procedure Hct of

40%. For calculating the volume of RBC to remove, you calculate ((49 – 40)/79) × 5000 resulting in a removal of 570 mL of concentrated RBCs to achieve the target Hct of 40%.

3.13 Summary

In this chapter, we discussed a few calculation methods which are helpful in various apheresis procedures, as well in cell collection in therapeutic procedures. By making these calculations, it gives our work as apheresis nurses at an apheresis facility more value, makes the apheresis procedure safer for donors and patients, and improves the logistics of an apheresis center. We discussed the TBV of a human being and the understanding that this varies per person. Also, the TPV is varied since it is based on the TBV and the Hct. For the safety of the donor/patient, it is important to take the ECV into consideration. Especially in pediatric patients, the red cell volume is also important to consider. It is possible to make an estimation of the Hct level when solely the Hb is known. If we only have the weight of a collection bag, we can calculate the volume and vice versa; when you have the volume of a collection bag, it is possible to calculate the weight. The CE is a very valuable quality parameter for your procedures and collection center. By calculating the mean CE, it is possible to make an estimation of the TBV to process for the collection of a specific number of cells or to make an estimation of the expected product yield when you processed a specified TBV of the donor or patient. Finally, we discussed the volume of red cells that need to be removed to achieve a target Hct during RBC reductions.

References

1. Nadler SB, Hidalgo JH, Bloch T. Prediction of blood volume in normal human adults. Surgery. 1962;51:224–32.
2. Linderkamp O, Versmold HT, Riegel KP, Betke K. Estimation and prediction of blood volume in infants and children. Eur J Pediatr. 1977;125:227–34.
3. Rosenbaum ER, O'Connell B, Cottler-Fox M. Validation of a formula for predicting daily CD34+ cell collection by leukapheresis. Cytotherapy. 2012;4:461–6.
4. Roig JM. Prediction algorithms for cell therapy collections, J. Roig WAA 2016.pptx. LinkedIn.

4 Apheresis Team and Job Descriptions

Nina Worel and Annika Malmborg Kisch

4.1 Background

Apheresis is a highly specialized area in the healthcare system [1–3]. According to the aim of the apheresis procedure, either blood components are collected (i.e., preparative apheresis) or, in case of therapeutic apheresis (TA), pathological components are discarded (i.e., depletion) or exchanged. The vast majority of preparative apheresis is performed to collect plasma or platelets from volunteer donors at a blood center, which may take up to 100–120 min. TA, in contrast, is an extracorporeal therapy often performed in critically ill patients requiring a close cooperation of involved medical specialties [4]. TA is done almost exclusively in hospital-based facilities, and treatment times exceed the duration of preparative apheresis procedures. Peripheral blood stem cell (PBSC) collection is a distinct form of preparative apheresis performed not only in patients mainly with hemato-oncologic diseases but also in volunteer donors who may be related or unrelated. Besides adults, pediatric patients and, under some circumstances, pediatric donors also undergo PBSC collection. These procedures are characterized by a long duration time of up to 5–6 h during which three to five times the total blood volume may be processed, which might be up to 30 L of blood in adults.

This implies that the staff responsible for TA and PBSC collection not only needs a comprehensive knowledge of the underlying disease or condition but also has general skills on how to perform an apheresis procedure to avoid the exposure of the patient or donor to a risk or harm and a technical understanding of the equipment used [4–6].

4.2 General Considerations

4.2.1 Organization of Centers

Depending on the scope of the apheresis facility—only therapeutic apheresis or also preparative procedures—governmental regulations have to be followed. In European Union (EU) member states, both hematopoietic progenitor cells (HPCs) and T-cells fall under the European Directive 2004/23/EC on "quality and safety for the donation, procurement, testing, processing, preservation, storage and distribution of tissues and cells" and the implementing directives 2006/17/EC and 2006/86/EC. National or state

N. Worel (✉)
Department of Transfusion Medicine and Cell Therapy, Medical University of Vienna, Vienna, Austria
e-mail: nina.worel@meduniwien.ac.at

A. M. Kisch
Lund University Cancer Centre, Lund, Sweden
e-mail: annika.kisch@med.lu.se

I. Kozanoglu (ed.), *Problem Solving in Apheresis Medicine*,
https://doi.org/10.1007/978-3-031-74081-7_4

laws and regulations may require registration and/or certification by competent authorities or may need accreditation from professional organizations for the activities performed within the facility. In the EU, the competent authorities in the member states ensure that all tissue establishments including cell collection facilities have been accredited, designated, authorized, or licensed and that these establishments have implemented the EU directive and/or other national regulations. Additionally, apheresis centers can seek accreditation from other bodies to express their accordance to specific quality standards at least for collection activities. One example is an accreditation according to the FACT-JACIE (Foundation for the Accreditation of Cellular Therapy—Joint Accreditation Committee of the International Society of Cellular Therapy (ISCT) and European Society of Blood and Marrow Transplantation (EBMT)) International Standards for Hematopoietic Cellular Therapy Product Collection, Processing, and Administration [7]. Therapeutic apheresis procedures are normally not regulated by competent authorities.

Apheresis units, irrespective of performing only preparative or also therapeutic procedures, should provide adequate conditions as described in the national guidelines or recommendations of scientific organizations (e.g., European Society for Hemapheresis (ESFH), American Society for Apheresis (ASFA), and German Society for Transfusion Medicine and Immunohematology (DGTI)). This implies, among others, adequate size of the apheresis area to allow for safe practice and, in case of emergencies, allow for adequate room for resuscitation. The space used for collection procedures and TA should be well-defined and leave enough space for the preparation of the apheresis device and storage of reagents and equipment. For emergency situations, it is essential that apheresis facilities have access to an intensive care unit (ICU) or emergency services to protect patient's and donor's safety in rare emergency situations.

4.2.2 Apheresis Staff

The medical director of an apheresis facility is normally board-certified in an appropriate medical discipline (e.g., transfusion medicine, internal medicine/hematology, pediatrics, etc.). Physicians and operators, which can be nurses or technicians, need to be experienced in extracorporeal procedures and educated in emergency medicine. Therefore, all staff members must be trained and retrained in regular intervals at least in basic life support (BLS).

Overall, there is little published in the field of apheresis nursing education so far. This makes it difficult for institutions worldwide to design and create a structured educational program that encompasses the needs of the apheresis newcomers and existing/senior staff. A literature review in 2015 found that the European Union and United States Joint Task Force had developed a 3-day modular apheresis educational program and certification [8]. The program and certification courses were designed for nurses and operators. Also, a small group of nurses and physicians in Asian countries participated in this modular program designed by the Joint Task Force [8].

4.2.3 Specific Skills for Apheresis Operators

For an optimal performance of a preparative or therapeutic apheresis procedure, a thorough knowledge about each procedure with all onsite available technical devices is necessary, irrespective of working in a donor center or in a hospital-based apheresis facility covering donors and patients or in apheresis centers with patients only. The operators must be qualified and competent to perform all procedures, that is, having hands-on experience with an adequate number of apheresis treatments per apheresis device, and continuously update their education. Most often, initial training is given by the medical device company with special focus on the technical equipment.

However, this training often does not focus on the specific needs of patients or characteristics of diseases and does not consider possible comorbidities of patients. In some countries, a train-the-trainer approach can be followed where the medical device company and national regulations allow specific trained staff members to disseminate their knowledge on a specific procedure among their colleagues.

The definition of an adequate number of procedures is not easy as it depends on the respective indication for TA. Symptomatic hyperleukocytosis in leukemic diseases, for example, is rare; therefore, the annual number of leukocyte depletion procedures maybe less than 1–5. The same is true for the treatment of sickle cell crisis in regions where this disease is not endemic. The DGTI section on preparative and therapeutic apheresis recommends that physicians performing TA should possess hands-on experience of at least 10 apheresis treatments per apheresis system and continuously update their training to perform each procedure safely [6]. Other organizations (e.g., FACT-JACIE) request the minimum numbers of preparative apheresis procedures to be performed for an accreditation which are given for a whole center and not for individual apheresis staff members itself; this requires five cellular therapy product apheresis collection procedures to be observed within 12 months for the apheresis medical director [7].

An operator should not perform more than two TA procedures in parallel, depending on the clinical situation of the patient. In critically ill patients, it even may not be possible to take care of an additional contemporary procedure. All technical equipment including apheresis devices and secondary separation systems (selective/specific removal procedures) should be approved for their respective application, CE-certified (or similar, depending on the region), and handled according to national legislation [6].

Apheresis centers, especially those performing preparative procedures, need an established quality management system (QMS). However, facilities with only therapeutic procedures would only profit off of a QMS. An integral part of a QMS are standard operating procedures (SOPs) describing, in detail, all procedures to ensure the safety of the procedure itself and the quality not only of the TA performed (i.e., does the procedure as it is performed lead to the expected outcome?) but also the quality of the collected blood components (i.e., adequate cell numbers, low number of contaminating cells, etc.). Every staff member working in the apheresis facility must be trained on the QMS and shall work according to the respective SOPs. The apheresis staff must be aware of the content in the SOPs and be familiar with the QMS [8].

More or less frequently, serious adverse events (SAE) can occur during each apheresis procedure. In majority of cases, these SAEs are mild or moderate and mainly related to the anticoagulation fluid (citrate toxicity). In exchange (e.g., plasma exchange) and depletion procedures (e.g., in hyperleukocytosis), the substitution fluid or loss of specific components can lead to SAEs. More detailed information regarding SAEs in apheresis and how to interact is given in Chap. 15.

4.2.4 Specific Apheresis Societies

In 1984, the European Society for Hemapheresis (ESFH) was founded with the aim of gathering European physicians, scientists, and allied health personnel working in the field of hemapheresis with a vision to improve donor and patient care. The mission of ESFH is to advance knowledge in apheresis techniques through education, to consolidate and spread proven methods, and to open new paths in the collection of blood cells and treatment of diseases by apheresis (www.esfh.eu).

Two years later, in 1986, the World Apheresis Association (WAA), an umbrella organization of national and international professional societies, was funded, and it has been devoted to the scientific, medical, administrative, and educational aspects of apheresis (https://worldapheresis.org). The seven founding societies of the WAA were the American Society for Apheresis (ASFA), Canadian Apheresis Group (CAG), ESFH, Group Latino America Hemapheresis (GLHEMA), International Society for Artificial Organs (ISAO), Japan Society of Therapeutic Plasmapheresis (JSTP), and Societe Francais d'Enchanges Plasmatiques (SFEP). A major activity of the WAA is an international data registry with the goal to collect data on the routinely used therapeutic apheresis procedures performed worldwide, to gain more information about their effects and side effects, and to have a basis for knowledge, transfer, technique, and a common registry to perform retrospective and prospective studies. The WAA-registry is available to all member societies and includes over 80,000 apheresis procedures in more than 20,000 patients.

Importantly, the ASFA publishes, on a regular basis, internationally recommended guidelines on the use of therapeutic apheresis in clinical practice based on evidence-based medicine. The most recent guidelines have been released in 2023 [9].

4.2.5 Patient and Donor Perspective on Hematopoietic Stem Cell Donation

HPCs can be either donated by patients (i.e., a person with a serious disease) themselves or donors, i.e., persons donating HPCs to a patient in need of an allogeneic hematopoietic stem cell transplantation (HSCT). When taking care of a patient before, during, and after apheresis, it is important to see the person and meet the individual needs. Patients usually have gone through several treatments and might have symptoms and side effects to be considered and cared for during and in connection to apheresis. Donors can be related; most often siblings but also parents or children to the recipient since haplo-identical HSCTs are increasing or unrelated (i.e., registry donors) [10, 11]. Standards, guidelines, and recommendations concerning suitability, donor safety, and obtaining informed consent of donors are stated in several documents from international organizations and experts; moreover, emotional and ethical aspects are also pointed out [7, 12–15].

There is a big difference between being an unrelated or a related donor: when an unrelated donor has voluntarily signed up to be a donor for an unknown recipient somewhere in the world, while a related donor is being asked to become a donor and, at the same time, has a relation with the recipient. We know very little or nothing about on the quality of the relationship. Experiences of potential donors and donors have been elucidated in qualitative research, showing a significant variety of feelings and thoughts, from related as well as unrelated stem cell donors before, during, and after donation [16–26]. Both positive and negative experiences have been reported, and that they often feel abandoned after donation with a wish for more support [16, 17, 20–22]. Related and unrelated donors have reported great worry about themselves of being a donor and for the recipient and the outcome of the HSCT [27, 28].

In HSCT, there are ethical and psychological/psychosocial challenges to be aware of. Apheresis staff has two individuals, the recipient, and the donor, to focus on, thereby highlighting the importance of securing confidentiality and autonomous choices of each individual [7, 12, 14]. Healthy donors are exposed to drugs without personal therapeutic benefit, and the donation is often associated with side effects and the risk of severe complications; additionally there is no guarantee about the outcome for the recipient [29–32]. It is important to point out that HpC donation is not a risk-free procedure; the transplant community has the responsibility to minimize the risks and provide donors with exhaustive information, and health and well-being of the donors must be a priority [31–33].

The situation with a pediatric donor needs certain specific considerations about minimizing toxicity, ethical issues, and informed consent procedure, including interactions with the family. Children are donors to seriously ill siblings but are also increasingly considered as haploidentical donors to their parents, and they can be minor as well as adolescents. In the case of a pediatric donor, the whole family is involved in the HSCT, and the parents are usually caregivers as well as legal guardians of the minor donor, making it more complex especially in information and informed consent procedures. Even though there is a strong recommendation for donor advocates for minor donors, many transplantation centers still do not have a donor advocate regularly available [34–36]. Research on pediatric stem cell donation including children's experiences is scarce. However, existing literature has showed that it is a great challenge to obtain true informed consent from a minor donor [37]; girls older than 13 years have the highest risk for short-term side effects and pain, including pain at 1-year after donation [38]; also, significant decreases in health-related quality-of-life (HRQoL) after donation, especially among donors aged 5–7 years, have been highlighted [39–43].

The abovementioned aspects illustrate the importance of awareness of the patient and donor perspective among apheresis operators, thereby highlighting the importance of education and training in how to deal with and take care of patients and donors optimally, including pediatric patients, donors, and their parents and how to interact with families.

As suggested, education for apheresis operators should be continuous and repeated, including emotional and ethical aspects in stem cell donation. Education should involve social training in how to meet patients and donors respectfully with the goal of a good experience from the donation process and no decrease in HRQoL following the donation. The training should include specific considerations before, during, and after apheresis following the updated recommendations and guidelines [7, 12–15].

4.3 Summary

Apheresis procedures should only be carried out by well-trained and experienced teams after careful evaluation of the indication and balance of the risks and benefits for patients but also for donors. Especially in pediatric patients, this can be crucial and should be an absolute requirement. In preparative procedures, legal requirements should be followed; meanwhile, in therapeutic procedures, scientific guidelines or recommendations should be followed. Continuous education and training of all individuals involved in an apheresis procedure is a prerequisite to ensure safety.

References

1. Karr EG. Advantages of joining a professional apheresis organization. Transfus Apher Sci. 2016;55:371–3.
2. Kala S, Isaramalai S, Pohthong A. Electronic learning and constructivism: a model for nursing education. Nurse Educ Today. 2010;30:61–6.
3. Nemec R. Apheresis education: one center curriculum design experience. Transfus Apher Sci. 2017;56:263–7.
4. Gerogianni SK, Panagiotou MC, Grapsa EI. The role of nurses in therapeutic plasma exchange procedure. Int J Caring Sci. 2015;8:194–200.
5. Neyrinck MM, Vrielink H. Performance of an apheresis procedure: the apheresis nurse-operator and nursing aspects. Transfus Apher Sci. 2019;58:296–9.
6. Worel N, Mansouri Taleghani B, Strasser E. Recommendations for therapeutic apheresis by the section 'preparative and therapeutic hemapheresis' of the German Society for Transfusion Medicine and Immunohematology. Transfus Med Hemother. 2019;46:394–406.
7. FACT-JACIE International Standards for Hematopoietic Cellular Therapy. 2021. http://www.factwebsite.org/HCT8thEdStandards/. Accessed 10 Apr 2022.
8. Neyrinck M, Vrielink H. Apheresis training for nurses and physicians around the world. J Clin Apher. 2015;30:32–7.
9. Connelly-Smith L, Alquist CR, Aqui NA, et al. Guidelines on the use of therapeutic apheresis in clinical practice—Evidence-based approach from the Writing Committee of the American Society for Apheresis: the ninth special issue. J Clin Apher. 2023;38:77–278.
10. Niederwieser D, Baldomero H, Bazuaye N, et al. One and a half million hematopoietic stem cell trans-

plants: continuous and differential improvement in worldwide access with the use of non-identical family donors. Haematologica. 2022;107:1045. https://doi.org/10.3324/haematol.2021.279189.
11. Passweg JR, Baldomero H, Chabannon C, et al. Hematopoietic cell transplantation and cellular therapy survey of the EBMT: monitoring of activities and trends over 30 years. Bone Marrow Transplant. 2021;56:1651–64.
12. Worel N, Aljurf M, Anthias C, et al. Suitability of haematopoietic cell donors: updated consensus recommendations from the WBMT standing committee on donor issues. Lancet Haematol. 2022;9:e605–14.
13. WHO guiding principles on human cell, tissue and organ transplantation. Transplantation. 2010;90:229–233.
14. National Marrow Donor Program/Be The Match® 24th edition standards and glossary notice and disclaimer NMDP/Be The Match standards. 2018. https://bethematch.org/workarea/downloadasset.aspx?id=10093. Accessed 10 Apr 2022.
15. World Marrow Donor Association WMDA International Standards Unrelated Hematopoietic Stem Cell Donor Registries. 2021. https://wmda.info/wp-content/uploads/2021/01/Amendment-1-to-2020-Std_AM1_Jan2021.pdf. Accessed 10 Apr 2022.
16. Christopher KA. The experience of donating bone marrow to a relative. Oncol Nurs Forum. 2000;27:693–700.
17. Kisch A, Bolmsjö I, Lenhoff S, Bengtsson M. Being a haematopoietic stem cell donor for a sick sibling: adult donors' experiences prior to donation. Eur J Oncol Nurs. 2015;19:529–35.
18. Kisch AM, Forsberg A. Sibling stem cell donors' perceptions of experiences of donation. Clin Nurs Stud. 2017;5:23.
19. Kisch AM, Forsberg A. The core of sibling stem cell donation—A grounded theory study. Open Nurs J. 2017;11:73–83.
20. Munzenberger N, Fortanier C, Macquart-Moulin G, et al. Psychosocial aspects of haematopoietic stem cell donation for allogeneic transplantation: how family donors cope with this experience. Psychooncology. 1999;8:55–63.
21. Pillay B, Lee SJ, Katona L, et al. The psychosocial impact of haematopoietic SCT on sibling donors. Bone Marrow Transplant. 2012;47:1361–5.
22. Williams S, Green R, Morrison A, Watson D, Buchanan SS. The psychosocial aspects of donating blood stem cells: the sibling donor perspective. J Clin Apher. 2003;18:1–9.
23. Zomerdijk N, Turner J, Hill GR, Gottlieb D. Experiences and unmet needs of family members requested to donate haematopoietic stem cells to an ill relative: findings from a prospective multi-centre study. Support Care Cancer. 2021;29:635–44.
24. Billen A, Madrigal JA, Scior K, Shaw BE, Strydom A. Donation of peripheral blood stem cells to unrelated strangers: a thematic analysis. PLoS One. 2017;12:e0186438.
25. Holroyd E, Molassiotis A. Hong Kong Chinese perceptions of the experience of unrelated bone marrow donation. Soc Sci Med. 2000;51:29–40.
26. Wanner M, Bochert S, Schreyer IM, Rall G, Rutt C, Schmidt AH. Losing the genetic twin: donor grief after unsuccessful unrelated stem cell transplantation. BMC Health Serv Res. 2009;9:2.
27. Switzer GE, Bruce JG, Kiefer DM, et al. Health-related quality-of-life comparison of adult related and unrelated HSC donors: an RDSafe study. Biol Blood Marrow Transplant. 2020;26:2365–71.
28. Winterling J, Pahnke S, Lagnebjörk J, et al. Worries and psychological Well-being in potential hematopoietic stem cell donors before donation—A Swedish National Study. Transplant Proc. 2023;55:242–8.
29. Halter J, Kodera Y, Ispizua AU, et al. Severe events in donors after allogeneic hematopoietic stem cell donation. Haematologica. 2009;94:94–101.
30. McCullough J, Kahn J, Adamson J, et al. Hematopoietic growth factors-use in normal blood and stem cell donors: clinical and ethical issues. Transfusion (Paris). 2008;48:2008–25.
31. Liumbruno GM, Petrini C. Ethical issues and concerns about the use of biosimilar granulocyte colony-stimulating factors for the mobilisation of stem cells in normal donors. Blood Transfus. 2012;10:550–2.
32. Moalic-Allain V. Medical and ethical considerations on hematopoietic stem cells mobilization for healthy donors. Transfus Clin Biol. 2018;25:136–43.
33. O'Donnell PV, Pedersen TL, Confer DL, et al. Practice patterns for evaluation, consent, and care of related donors and recipients at hematopoietic cell transplantation centers in the United States. Blood. 2010;115:5097–101.
34. Recommendation CM/Rec(2020)6 1 of the Committee of Ministers to member States on establishing harmonised measures for the protection of haematopoietic progenitor cell donors. www.coe.int/cm.
35. American Academy of Pediatrics Committee on Bioethics. Children as hematopoietic stem cell donors. Pediatrics. 2010;125:392–404.
36. Pentz RD, Chan KW, Neumann JL, Champlin RE, Korbling M. Designing an ethical policy for bone marrow donation by minors and others lacking capacity. Camb Q Healthc Ethics. 2004;13:149. https://doi.org/10.1017/S0963180104132064.
37. Fleck LM. Children and organ donation: some cautionary remarks. Camb Q Healthc Ethics. 2004;13:161. https://doi.org/10.1017/S0963180104132088.
38. Pulsipher MA, Logan BR, Kiefer DM, et al. Higher risks of toxicity and incomplete recovery in 13- to 17-year-old females after marrow donation: RDSafe Peds results. Biol Blood Marrow Transplant. 2019;25:955–64.
39. Zając-Spychała O, Pieczonka A, Barańska M, Wachowiak J. Long-term recipient health-related quality of life and donor-recipient relationship following sibling pediatric hematopoietic stem cell transplantation. Biol Blood Marrow Transplant. 2020;26:401–6.

40. Hutt D, Nehari M, Munitz-Shenkar D, Alkalay Y, Toren A, Bielorai B. Hematopoietic stem cell donation: psychological perspectives of pediatric sibling donors and their parents. Bone Marrow Transplant. 2015;50:1337–42.
41. Hoag J, Igler E, Karst J, Bingen K, Kupst MJ. Decision-making, knowledge, and psychosocial outcomes in pediatric siblings identified to donate hematopoietic stem cells. J Psychosoc Oncol. 2019;37:367–82.
42. D'Auria JP, Fitzgerald TM, Presler CM, Kasow KA. Through the eyes of young sibling donors: the hematopoietic stem cell donation experience. J Pediatr Nurs. 2015;30:447–53.
43. Switzer GE, Bruce J, Kiefer DM, et al. Health-related quality of life among pediatric hematopoietic stem cell donors. J Pediatr. 2016;178:164–170.e1.

Part II

ASFA Guide 2019

5 How to Read ASFA Guideline

Bilgen Hulya

5.1 Introduction

The American Society for Apheresis (ASFA) was formed in 1982, with a mission to advance apheresis sciences and set a stage for physicians and allied healthcare workers to share their knowledge [1]. The decision to treat a patient with therapeutic apheresis (TA) depends on multiple factors. These include the following: what does the patient most likely have (diagnosis), is the diagnosis amenable to treatment with TA, what is the harm-versus-benefit ratio of TA in this patient, and what are the internal and external issues associated with receiving this treatment? The "Guidelines on the Use of Therapeutic Apheresis in Clinical Practice—Evidence-based Approach from the Writing Committee of the American Society for Apheresis" addresses these issues and helps aid in clinical decision-making [2]. The ASFA Journal of Clinical Apheresis Special Issue Writing Committee has periodically published guidelines for the use of therapeutic apheresis since 1986. The most recent update is the ninth special issue published in 2023 and is available for clinical use [3].

B. Hulya (✉)
İstanbul Medipol University, Vocational School of Health Services, İstanbul, Turkey

Medipol Mega University Hospital, Therapeutic Apheresis Center, İstanbul, Turkey
e-mail: hulya.bilgen@saglik.gov.tr

TA is usually performed via several FDA- or CE-cleared continuous or semi-continuous automated cell separators (apheresis machines). In addition to common procedures such as therapeutic plasma exchange (TPE) and RBC exchange, several specialized apheresis machines are also available to remove blood elements including low-density lipoprotein (LDL) cholesterol (LDL apheresis) or immunoglobulins (immunoadsorption; or remove, treat, and return blood elements (extracorporeal photopheresis (ECP)).

McLeod's criteria are used to determine the success of TA in a disease's treatment. It consists of three components: (1) Understanding of the disease pathogenesis enables a clear rationale for TA. (2) The abnormality should be able to be corrected by TA. (3) There should be evidence that TA is clinically beneficial [3]. Since 1986, to help clinicians apply McLeod's criteria in evaluating apheresis requests, ASFA has published evidence-based guidelines. While preparing these guidelines, the committee reviews the literature and the recommendations of Choosing Wisely committee. The ASFA Choosing Wisely recommendations encourage apheresis practitioners, patients, and donors to discuss and prioritize best clinical practices that avoid harm and waste while optimizing clinical benefit [4].

The Journal of Clinical Apheresis (JCA) Special Issue Writing Committee presented the ninth edition of the JCA Special Issue in

I. Kozanoglu (ed.), *Problem Solving in Apheresis Medicine*,
https://doi.org/10.1007/978-3-031-74081-7_5

2023. This edition was delayed for a year from the scheduled 2022 release due to the tremendous impact of the COVID-19 pandemic on the apheresis community, the provision of healthcare, and the population of the entire world.

This latest edition of evidence-based guidelines for therapeutic apheresis is based on a careful review of up-to-date literature, analysis of the quality of evidence, and the strength of recommendation derived from this evidence [3].

ASFA guidelines help provide comprehensive, yet condensed, information with extensive references to share with patients and clinical services involved in the care of the patients undergoing apheresis. However, the guidelines do not describe all the diseases for which TA had been applied or all the potential conditions that TA might be used. It only describes the diseases that have sufficient published evidence to support (or not support) the use of TA. ASFA guidelines organize diseases and their therapies into category and grading systems.

Category describes the efficacy and priority of apheresis in the treatment of a disease, while grading describes the quality of evidence to support apheresis treatment of a disease [1].

In every 3 years, new fact sheets are added. To meet the criteria for a new fact sheet, the committee required a minimum of ten cases published in the last decade in peer-reviewed journals, ideally by more than one group.

Our role as apheresis practitioners and clinicians is to read these guidelines for the best interest of the patients. The fact sheet is a very useful tool. The design of the fact sheet and the explanation of the information in it are included in Fig. 5.1.

Fact sheet format. (A) This section requires the name of the disease/condition. (B) This section lists the incidence or prevalence of the disease. For certain diseases with insufficient data on incidence or prevalence, other terms such as rare or unknown are used. The reader is cautioned to use this information only as a general indicator of disease incidence or prevalence. For some diseases, this may vary by geographical area. (C) This indication section refers to the use of apheresis in specific situations encountered in the disease/condition (e.g., antibody-mediated rejection [indication] in the setting of "Transplantation, heart" [disease]). (D) The type of therapeutic apheresis procedure is listed here. For certain diseases, there are several apheresis-based modalities available. In such instances, more than one type of procedure is listed (e.g., "Transplantation, lung" includes both TPE and ECP). (E) This section notes the category recommendation. (F) Grade recommendation is assigned to each categorized entity based on the Grading of Recommendations Assessment Development and Evaluation (GRADE) system. (G) This section lists the number of patients reported in the literature who were treated with TA. The committee used the following three categories: fewer than 100, between 100 and 300, and more than 300. This entry will help readers in judging how often this entity was reported to be treated with TA. However, the number of patients treated is often less important than the quality of the scientific reports. (H) This section lists the randomized controlled trials (RCT) (Patient counts should not be regarded as exact figures of all existing literature, but reflecting the magnitude of published evidence for a particular indication and representing the major source of evidence used to assign category and grade recommendation.). This part indicates the number of RCTs and the total number of patients studied. For example, 4 (250) indicates that there were 4 RCTs with 250 enrolled patients. The patient count includes all patients irrespective of randomization to either treatment group (with TA) or the control arm. The minimum requirement for these studies was randomization to a control arm and a test arm. The quality of this study is not reflected here. Example: Two randomized studies with 50 patients in each of the 2 arms and 1 randomized study with 75 patients in each of the 2 arms are denoted as 3 (350). (I) This section lists the controlled trials (CT) (Patient counts should not be regarded as exact figures of all existing literature, but reflecting the magnitude of published evidence for a particular indication and representing

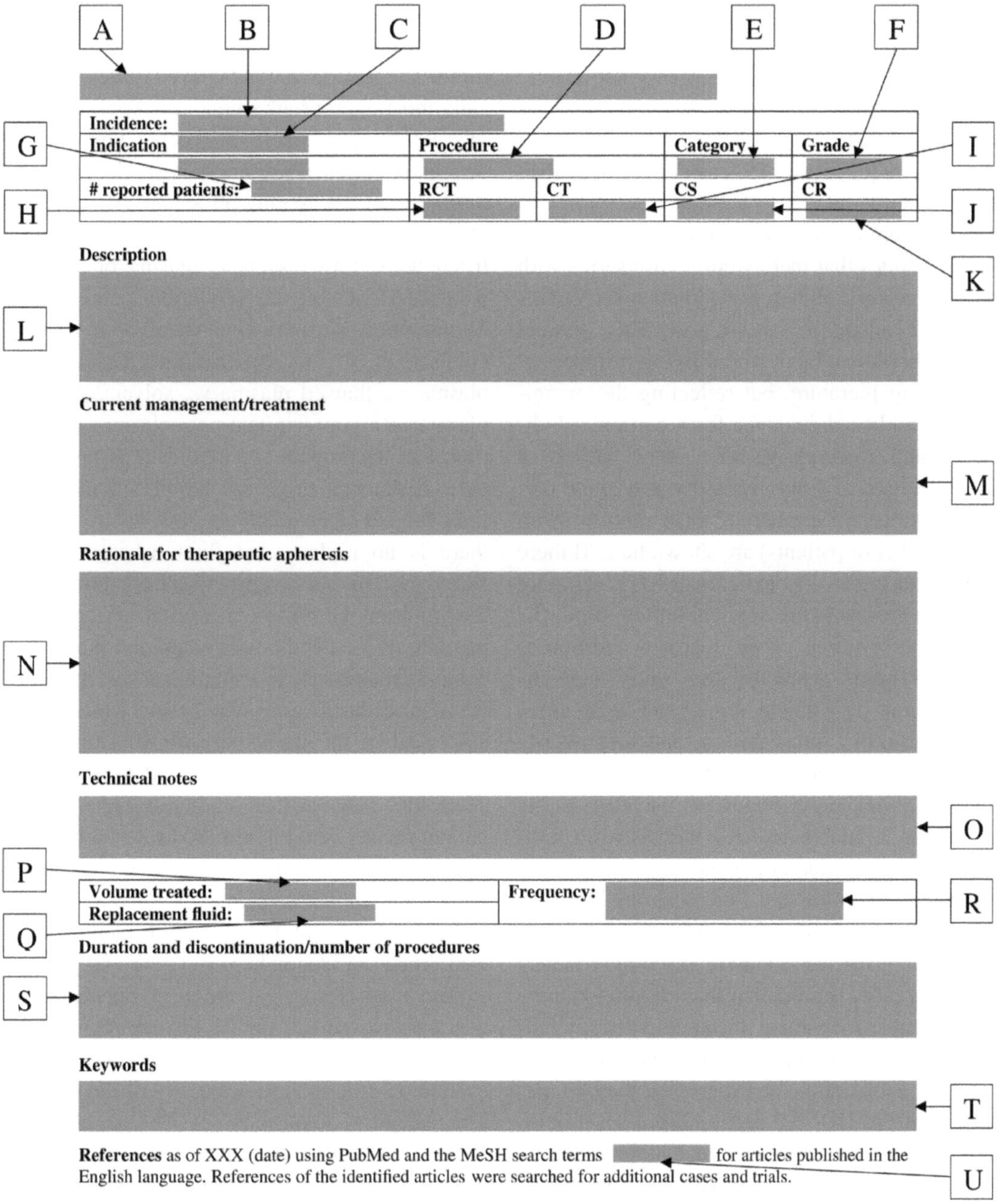

Fig. 5.1 The format of the fact sheet. *This figure is adapted from reference [3]

the major source of evidence used to assign category and grade recommendation.). The notation is similar to that of RCTs. Studies listed here were not randomized. The control group could be historical or concurrent to the treatment group. (J) This section indicates the case series (CS) (Patient counts should not be regarded as exact figures of all existing literature, but reflecting the magnitude of published evidence for a particular indication and representing the major source of evidence used to assign category and grade recommendation.). The number of case series are reported here (with total number of patients reported). If there were greater than 300 patients in RCT and/or CT studies, NA (not applicable) was used. If there were more than 10 case series with more than 200 patients, >10 (>200) was used. We required that the case series described at least three patients. Case series with two patients were included in case reports. Example: 4 (56) implies that there were 4 case series with the total number of 56 reported patients. (K) This section requires the case report (CR) (Patient counts should not be regarded as exact figures of all existing literature, but reflecting the magnitude of published evidence for a particular indication and representing the major source of evidence used to assign category and grade recommendation.). Number of case reports (with total number of patients) are shown here. If there were greater than 100 patients in RCT, CT, and/or CS studies, NA (not applicable) was used. (L) A brief description of the disease/condition is provided here. Typically, this entry contains information on clinical signs and symptoms, pathophysiology, presentation, and the severity of the disease/condition. (M) This section provides a brief description of the therapeutic modalities available to treat the disease/condition. The committee attempted to cover all reasonable modalities (e.g., medications, surgical procedures, etc.); however, this section is not intended to provide extensive discussion of any specific treatment modality. In addition, for some entities, the management of standard therapy failure is discussed (e.g., steroids), especially when the failure of established therapies may trigger the use of TA. (N) This section discusses a rationale for TA use in the disease and summarizes the evidence in this area. (O) This section briefly describes technical details relevant to the treated disease, which the committee believed were important to improve the quality of care or increase the chances of a positive clinical outcome. Not all diseases may have specific technical notes. (P) This section specifies commonly used volumes of plasma or blood treated. (Q) The proposed frequency of treatment is listed here. The frequency reported was typically based on data from published reports. However, in some settings, due to significant variability in treatment schedules reported by different groups, the committee suggested what is believed to be the clinically most appropriate frequency. Application of this information may vary depending on the patient and clinical presentation and is left to the discretion of the treating physician. (R) The type of replacement fluid most frequently used is listed here. Terms such as plasma or albumin were used to denote the type of replacement fluid. No attempt was made to include all possible variations (e.g., 4% vs. 5% albumin; fresh frozen plasma vs. thawed plasma vs. solvent/detergent plasma vs. cryoprecipitate-poor plasma). In addition, blood component modifications are listed here, if relevant (e.g., red blood cell modifications for red cell exchange). "NA" is used when there is no replacement fluid necessary (e.g., ECP). (S) This section provides basic criteria for the duration and discontinuation of apheresis procedures (i.e., end points/outcomes, both clinical and laboratory). In some instances, the number of procedures/series which may be reasonably employed in the particular clinical situation is suggested based on currently available data. The committee believes that a thoughtful approach to patient management is required to establish reasonable and scientifically sound criteria for discontinuation of treatment. (T) Keywords are listed here. (U) The terms used to identify relevant articles are listed here.

The ninth edition of the JCA Special Issue contains fact sheets for 91 diseases/conditions. To decide to perform TA for a patient, the main evaluation criteria is the category of the disease. The category definitions for TA are listed in Table 5.1. (Reference [3] describes the classic category definitions, and we are obliged to understand these categories in order to read the ASFA guidelines.)

Each disease/condition, indication, and procedure is assigned a grade (Table 5.2) as well as a category recommendation. The grade can be used in support or against the use of the therapeutic intervention. This recommendation grade reflected the committee's clinical judgment as well as the quality of the available literature on TA for that specific indication.

Table 5.1 Category definitions for therapeutic apheresis [3]

Category	description
I	Disorders for which apheresis is accepted as first-line therapy, either as a primary standalone treatment or in conjunction with other modes of treatment
II	Disorders for which apheresis is accepted as second-line therapy, either as a standalone treatment or in conjunction with other modes of treatment
III	Optimum role of apheresis therapy is not established. Decision-making should be individualized
IV	Disorders in which published evidence demonstrates or suggests apheresis to be ineffective or harmful. IRB/Ethics Committee approval is desirable if apheresis treatment is undertaken in these circumstances

Table 5.2 Grading recommendations, strength, and quality of evidence [3] (In order to read ASFA category and grading)

Recommendation	description	Methodological quality of supporting evidence	Implications
Grade 1A	Strong recommendation, high-quality evidence	RCTs without important limitations or overwhelming evidence from observational studies	Strong recommendation can apply to most patients in most circumstances without reservation
Grade 1B	Strong recommendation, moderate quality evidence	RCTs with important limitations (inconsistent results, methodological flaws, indirect, or imprecise) or exceptionally strong evidence from observational studies	Strong recommendation can apply to most patients in most circumstances without reservation
Grade 1C	Strong recommendation, low-quality or very low-quality evidence	Observational studies or case series	Strong recommendation but may change when higher-quality evidence becomes available
Grade 2A	Weak recommendation, high-quality evidence	RCTs without important limitations or overwhelming evidence from observational studies	Weak recommendation, best action may differ depending on circumstances or patients' societal values
Grade 2B	Weak recommendation, moderate-quality evidence	RCTs with important limitations (inconsistent results, methodological flaws, indirect, or imprecise) or exceptionally strong evidence from observational studies	Weak recommendation, best action may differ depending on circumstances or patients' societal values
Grade 2C	Weak recommendation, low-quality or very low-quality evidence	Observational studies or case series	Very weak recommendations; other alternatives may be equally reasonable

RCT randomized controlled trial

5.2 Diagnosis

The guidelines assume the user understands the diseases presented and has made a correct diagnosis. There is information in the "description of the disease" section to help the user, which highlights key diagnostic as well as treatment and outcome information [2].

5.3 TA Treatment

With each special issue edition, the authors have continued to drill down on specific disease states to better apply the guidelines to particular patient presentations. The fact sheet helps to assess where in the disease course TA should be applied (e.g., early, after treatment failure, if the disease is severe, if the disease is mild). There are diseases that require emergency TA although the guidelines do not specify any details. In this medical decision-making, evaluating the patient and their clinical status is needed to make this determination. For some diseases, it is better to perform TA and then wait to confirm the diagnosis, such as thrombotic thrombocytopenic purpura (TTP). The fact sheet also helps in understanding which TA procedures should be used or TA alternatives, such as intravenous immunoglobulin (IVIG), and how they compare to TA [2].

In the technical notes section, particular risks are highlighted, for example, in patients with liver failure, there is a need for plasma replacement and to decrease the amount of citrate anticoagulant infused. These should be considered when assessing a patient's risk versus benefit from the procedure and how to make the procedure safer. Thus, the entire fact sheet should be used, not just the ASFA category and recommendation grade.

While using the fact sheets to approach apheresis consultations, there are several issues to consider and answer prior to the initiation of any TA procedure:

1. Prior to the agreement to perform procedure:
   (a) Rationale for using TA: Is the presumed diagnosis the most likely diagnosis? Is there a clear rationale for the use of TA? Does the use of TA correct the abnormality, and is there clinical evidence that TA benefits the patients? Have the usual or standard treatments failed or are contraindicated in the patient? Are there other alternatives that achieve equal efficacy as apheresis but are less expensive and/or invasive than apheresis?
   (b) Impact: What effect does TA have on the patient's comorbidities and medications? Does apheresis harm the patient?
2. After the decision of starting apheresis:
   (a) Technical issues: What anticoagulant, replacement fluid, vascular access, and volume of blood processed should be used? When, where, and how many total procedures and at what frequency should TA be performed?
   (b) Clinical and/or laboratory endpoints: What clinical and/or laboratory endpoints should be used to determine the efficacy of TA? What is/are the criteria for discontinuation? [1].

The ASFA guidelines can be helpful in answering many of the above questions and are essential for a best application.

5.4 Conclusions

The ASFA guidelines are published every 3 years with the goal to provide the most up-to-date, practical, and evidence-based guidance for the use of TA procedures. The medical literature is ever expanding with new reports coming out constantly. Therefore, it is important to review the medical literature and all the information in the relevant fact sheet (not just the ASFA category and the recommendation grade) prior to initiating any TA procedure. The ASFA guidelines help clinicians and patients minimize overuse in their own practice and treatment [5]. Choosing wisely should be our goal. The delivery systems and clinical practices should begin to develop beyond the recommendations [4, 6]. Practitioners of therapeutic apheresis should strive to establish a firm evidential basis for what they do.

References

1. Pham HP, Schwartz J. How to approach an apheresis consultation using the American Society for Apheresis guidelines for therapeutic apheresis procedures. 2015 International Society of Blood Transfusion, ISBT Science Series. 2015;10(Suppl. 1):79–88.
2. Shaz BH, Schwartz J, Winters JL. How we developed and use the American Society for Apheresis guidelines for therapeutic apheresis procedures. Transfusion. 2014;54:17–25.
3. Connelly-Smith L, Alquist CR, Aqui NA, et al. Guidelines on the use of therapeutic apheresis in clinical practice–evidence-based approach from the Writing Committee of the American Society for Apheresis: the ninth special issue. J Clin Apher. 2023;38(2):77–278.

4. Connelly-Smith L, Tanhehco YC, Chhibber V, et al. Choosing wisely for apheresis. J Clin Apher. 2018;33:576–9.
5. McLeod BC. An approach to evidence-based therapeutic apheresis. J Clin Apher. 2002;17:124–32.
6. Cassel CK, Guest JA. Choosing wisely: helping physicians and patients make smart decisions about their care. JAMA. 2012;307(17):1801–2.

6 American Society for Apheresis Indication Categories and Indications

Jeffrey L. Winters

6.1 Introduction

The American Society for Apheresis (ASFA) publishes clinical guidelines on the use of therapeutic apheresis in the treatment of human diseases. These guidelines are published approximately every 3 years, with the first guidelines published in 1986 [1], with the guidelines available at the time this chapter was written being published in 2019 [2]. The next ASFA guidelines are scheduled to be published in mid-2023.

The driving factor behind the initial creation and regular revision of the ASFA guidelines is the fact that most diseases treated by apheresis are considered "orphan" diseases, which are defined by the Food and Drug Administration (FDA) as a disease affecting 200,000 or fewer individuals in the United States. This means that for most of these diseases, it is difficult to perform a randomized, controlled, clinical trial. As a result, the majority of the literature published concerning the use of apheresis consists of case series or case reports with few controlled and randomized controlled trials [3]. Even when randomized controlled clinical trials have been performed, many of these trials fall short due to the small number of patients enrolled [3]. While the number of manuscripts concerning apheresis has increased with time, unfortunately, the number of randomized controlled trials has remain limited and represents the minority of these publications [3].

To address the shortcomings in the medical literature, ASFA created evidence-based guidelines written by a committee of experts selected through a competitive application process. These experts were assigned specific diseases/disorders and tasked with performing a comprehensive review of the available medical literature for each, to create a single-page fact sheet that provides the essential information, derived from the literature, necessary to prescribe apheresis therapy for a certain disorder. These fact sheets were then reviewed by two additional members of the committee and underwent revision. Following this, selected fact sheets were reviewed by an external, independent experts with feedback incorporated into a third draft. Finally, this third draft was reviewed by the entire committee, incorporating their suggestions, and an ASFA category and recommendation grade were assigned to each disease/disorder by consensus. The individual fact sheets were then published as the ASFA guidelines.

J. L. Winters (✉)
Division of Transfusion Medicine, Department of Laboratory Medicine and Pathology, Mayo Clinic, Rochester, MN, USA
e-mail: winters.jeffrey@mayo.edu

I. Kozanoglu (ed.), *Problem Solving in Apheresis Medicine*,
https://doi.org/10.1007/978-3-031-74081-7_6

6.2 ASFA Indication Categories

As described, the ASFA categories are assigned based on consensus of the ASFA guideline writing committee and are based upon the evidence in the published medical literature. The ASFA categories define the role of the specific apheresis procedure (e.g., plasma exchange, red cell exchange, etc.) in the treatment of the disease or disorder. Table 6.1 provides the definitions of the ASFA categories.

It is important to note that the ASFA category does not define the urgency with which the procedure should be performed. It is often assumed by those unfamiliar with the guidelines that all ASFA category I indications are emergencies, and the patient should be treated immediately, while an ASFA category III indication would not be an emergency and, therefore, would never need to be treated in the middle of the night or on weekends. This is not the case. Each patient, irrespective of the ASFA category assigned to their underlying disease process, requires an individual assessment of their medical condition to determine the urgency of the apheresis procedure. The ASFA category simply defines at what point in the treatment of the disease apheresis should be considered.

Table 6.1 ASFA categories [2]

ASFA category	Definition
I	Disorders for which apheresis is accepted as first-line therapy, either as a primary standalone treatment or in conjunction with other modes of treatment
II	Disorders for which apheresis is accepted as second-line therapy either as a primary standalone treatment or in conjunction with other modes of treatment
III	Optimum role for apheresis therapy is not established. Decision-making should be individualized
IV	Disorders in which published evidence demonstrates or suggests apheresis to be ineffective or harmful. IRB approval is desirable if apheresis treatment is undertaken in these circumstances

ASFA American Society for Apheresis, *IRB* Institutional Review Board
Modified with permission from: Padmanabhan A, Connelly-Smith L, Aqui N, et al. (2019) Guidelines on the use of therapeutic apheresis in clinical practice: evidence-based approach from the Apheresis Applications Committee of the American Society for Apheresis. The Eighth Special Issue, *J Clin Apher* 34:171–2354

Another important consideration when examining the ASFA categories is related to the definition of ASFA category III indication. It is frequently misinterpreted by many, especially by insurance companies and other third-party payors, that the assignment of an ASFA category III indicates that the apheresis treatment is "experimental" or that there is no evidence of efficacy. This is not the case with a category III assignment indicating the presence of published evidence of efficacy of the apheresis treatment but only in a subset of patients with the disease/disorder based upon the patient's presentation, disease characteristics, or comorbid conditions.

6.3 ASFA Recommendation Grades

The recommendation grades (Table 6.2) assigned to each disease is based upon the Grading of Recommendations, Assessment, Development, and Evaluation (GRADE) system [4]. The ASFA grade provides the committee's opinion of the strength of the evidence supporting the ASFA categorization as well as the quality of the evidence in the medical literature that was reviewed. A "1" recommendation is a strong recommendation, while a "2" recommendation is a weak recommendation that the apheresis procedure should be applied in the treatment of ASFA category I, II, and III indications. Of note, for category IV indications, a "1" recommendation is a strong

Table 6.2 ASFA recommendation grades [2]

Recommendation grade	Description
1A	Strong recommendation with high-quality evidence. Can apply to most patients in most circumstances without reservation
1B	Strong recommendation with moderate-quality evidence. Can apply to most patients in most circumstances without reservation
1C	Strong recommendation with low-quality or very-low-quality evidence. May change when higher-quality evidence becomes available
2A	Weak recommendation with high-quality evidence. Best action may differ depending on circumstances or patient or societal values
2B	Weak recommendation with moderate-quality evidence. Best action may differ depending on circumstances or patient or societal values
2C	Weak recommendation with low-quality or very-low-quality evidence. Other alternatives may be equally reasonable

Modified with permission from: Padmanabhan A, Connelly-Smith L, Aqui N, et al. (2019) Guidelines on the use of therapeutic apheresis in clinical practice: evidence-based approach from the Apheresis Applications Committee of the American Society for Apheresis. The Eighth Special Issue, *J Clin Apher* 34:171–2354

recommendation that the treatment should *not* be performed, while a "2" recommendation is a weak recommendation that the procedure should *not* be performed and implies some uncertainty, such as the presence of only poor-quality evidence in the literature indicating that the apheresis treatment is ineffective.

The quality of the evidence is indicated by "A," "B," or "C." "A" quality evidence is defined as high-quality evidence, randomized controlled clinical trials [2]. "B" quality evidence consists of controlled, but not randomized trials as well as flawed randomized trials, such as those randomized controlled trials which are under-powered [2]. Finally, "C" quality evidence is low- to very-low-quality evidence and consists of case series, case reports, and expert opinion [2].

6.4 2019 ASFA Indications

As described earlier, the ASFA guidelines consist of individual fact sheets that provide a concise description of disorders and the role of apheresis in the treatment of that disorder. For a fact sheet to be created by the committee, a sufficient body of published peer-reviewed literature must exist, at least with ten cases published within the last decade by more than one author or group [2]. Not all indications for which apheresis has been used or could potentially be used are included in the guidelines; only those for which a minimal amount of peer-reviewed publications have appeared are included. Recapitulation of the ASFA guidelines in this chapter is not possible, and the interested reader is referred to the most recently published guidelines for more information. It is also important to note that the ASFA categories and recommendation grades are not static and fixed and thus can change between guideline editions as new evidence is published in the peer-reviewed medical literature.

Table 6.3 provides a synopsis of the indications categorized in the 2019 ASFA guidelines but is not inclusive of all the information contained within the guidelines.

Table 6.3 Indications included in the 2019 ASFA guidelines [2, 5–7]

Disease	Indications for apheresis	ASFA category	ASFA recommendation grade	Apheresis treatment	Treatment notes
Acute disseminated encephalomyelitis (ADEM)	Steroid refractory	II	2C	TPE	1–1.5 PV, albumin replacement, every other day for 5–7 treatments
Acute inflammatory demyelination polyradiculopathy (Guillain-Barré syndrome)	Primary treatment	I	1A	TPE	1–1.5 PV, albumin replacement, daily or every other day for 5–6 treatments
		I	1B	IA	3 PV, daily or every other day for 5–7 treatments
Acute liver failure		I	1A	High volume TPE	8–12 L, albumin and plasma replacement, daily until liver transplant or hepatic regeneration
		III	2B	TPE	1–1.5 PV, albumin and plasma replacement, daily until liver transplant or hepatic regeneration
Age-related macular degeneration, dry	High risk	II	2B	Rheopheresis	1–1.5 PV, 8–10 treatments over 8–21 weeks
Amyloidosis, systemic	Dialysis-related amyloidosis	II	2B	β_2-microglobulin column	3 times per week with dialysis
	Other causes	IV	2C	TPE	NA
Amyotrophic lateral sclerosis		IV	1C	TPE	NA
Anti-glomerular basement membrane disease (Goodpasture syndrome)	Diffuse alveolar hemorrhage (DAH)	I	1C	TPE	1–1.5 PV, plasma replacement, daily or every other day until anti-GBM antibodies are undetectable and resolution of evidence of active glomerular or alveolar injury
	Dialysis-independent renal disease	I	1B	TPE	1–1.5 PV, albumin replacement, daily or every other day until anti-GBM antibodies are undetectable and resolution of evidence of active glomerular or alveolar injury
	Dialysis-dependent renal disease, no DAH	III	2B	TPE	1–1.5 PV, albumin replacement, daily or every other day until anti-GBM antibodies are undetectable and resolution of evidence of active glomerular or alveolar injury
Atopic dermatitis, recalcitrant		III	2A	ECP	1 cycle every 2 weeks for 12 weeks then taper
		III	2C	IA	3–5 daily every 4 weeks for 10–12 IA procedures
		III	2C	TPE	1–1.5 PV, albumin replacement, weekly
Autoimmune hemolytic anemia	Severe cold agglutinin disease	II	2C	TPE	1–1.5 PV, albumin replacement, daily or every other day until hemolysis decreases
	Severe warm autoimmune	III	2C	TPE	1–1.5 PV, albumin replacement, daily or every other day until hemolysis decreases

Babesiosis	Severe	II	2C	RBC exchange	1–2 RBC volumes, RBC replacement, single procedure or until parasitemia is <5% of red blood cells
Burn shock resuscitation		III	2B	TPE	1–1.5 PV, albumin and plasma replacement, once in the first 24 hours with additional procedures in patients who do not demonstrate increased mean arterial pressure or urine output or whose IV fluid requirements do not decline
Cardiac neonatal lupus		III	2C	TPE	1–1.5 PV, albumin replacement, 3 per week to weekly or monthly until antibody levels decline
Catastrophic antiphospholipid syndrome (CAPS)		I	1B	TPE	1–1.5 PV, plasma alone or with albumin replacement, daily or every other day with number of treatments determined by clinical response
Chronic focal encephalitis (Rasmussen encephalitis)		III	2C	TPE	1–1.5 PV, albumin replacement, 5–6 daily treatments
Chronic inflammatory demyelinating polyradiculopathy (CIDP)		I	1B	TPE/IA	1–1.5 PV, albumin replacement, 2–3 per week until improvement and then tapered
Coagulation factor inhibitors		III	2C	TPE	1–1.5 PV, plasma replacement, daily until bleeding is controlled
		III	2B	IA	Daily until bleeding is controlled
Complex regional pain syndrome	Chronic	III	2C	TPE	1–1.5 PV, albumin replacement, 5–7 over 2–3 weeks
Cryoglobulinemia	Severe/ symptomatic	II	2A	TPE	1–1.5 PV, albumin replacement, every 1–3 days for 3–8 procedures determined by clinical response
		II	2B	IA	Every 1–3 days for 3–8 procedures determined by clinical response
Cutaneous T-cell lymphoma (CTCL); Mycosis fungoides; Sézary syndrome	Erythrodermic	I	1B	ECP	Two consecutive days every 2–4 weeks with reduction to 2 consecutive days every 6–12 weeks once maximal response has been achieved median time to maximal response if 5–6 months
	Non-erythrodermic	III	2C	ECP	
Dermatomyositis/ polymyositis		IV	2B	TPE	NA
			2C	ECP	

(continued)

Table 6.3 (continued)

Disease	Indications for apheresis	ASFA category	ASFA recommendation grade	Apheresis treatment	Treatment notes
Dilated cardiomyopathy, idiopathic	NYHA II–IV	II	1B	IA	5 treatments daily to every other day
	NYHA II–IV	III	2C	TPE	1–1.5 PV, albumin replacement, 3–5 treatments
Erythropoietic protoporphyria, liver disease		III	2C	TPE	1–1.5 PV, albumin and/or plasma replacement, every 1–3 days
		III	2C	RBC exchange	3 times per week
Familial hypercholesterolemia	Homozygotes	I	1A	LA	Weekly or every other week until target LDL-C obtained
	Heterozygotes	II	1A	LA	
	Homozygotes/ heterozygotes	II	1B	TPE	1–1.5 PV, albumin replacement, weekly or every other week until target LDL-C obtained. TPE used predominantly in low-weight patients, primarily pediatric patients, who cannot tolerate extracorporeal volume of LA devices
Focal segmental glomerulosclerosis (FSGS)	Recurrent in kidney transplant	I	1B	TPE/IA	1–1.5 PV, albumin replacement, daily or every other day, duration determined by patient response
	Recurrent in kidney transplant/ Steroid resistant in native kidney	II	2C	LA	Twice per week for 3 weeks followed by once per week for 6 weeks for a total of 12 procedures
	Steroid resistant in native kidney	III	2C	TPE	1–1.5 PV, albumin replacement, daily or every other day, duration determined by patient response
Graft-versus-host disease	Acute	II	1C	ECP	2–3 treatments weekly tapering to 2 treatments on consecutive days every 2 weeks
	Chronic	II	1B	ECP	2 treatments on consecutive days every week for 4 weeks and then 2 treatments on consecutive days every 2 weeks for 8–12 weeks until maximal response and then taper
Hemolysis, elevated liver enzymes, and low platelets (HELLP) syndrome	Postpartum	III	2C	TPE	1–1.5 PV, plasma replacement, daily if no improvement 48–72 h after delivery
	Antepartum	IV	2C	TPE	NA

Hemophagocytic lymphohistiocytosis (HLH); Hemophagocytic syndrome; Macrophage activating syndrome		III	2C	TPE	1–1.5 PV, albumin or plasma replacement, daily number determined by patient response
Heparin-induced thrombocytopenia and thrombosis (HIT/HITT)	Pre-cardiopulmonary bypass	III	2C	TPE	1–1.5 PV, albumin or plasma replacement, daily or every other day, until HIT antibody titers become negative
	Thrombosis	III	2C	TPE	1–1.5 PV, albumin replacement, daily or every other day, duration determined by patient response
Hereditary hemochromatosis		I	1B	Erythrocytapheresis	Up to 800 mL of RBC. Every 2–3 weeks maintaining pre-procedure hematocrit >30–36% and post-procedure hematocrit >30%
Hyperleukocytosis	Symptomatic	II	2B	Leukocytapheresis	Daily as need to control symptoms
	Prophylactic or secondary	III	2C	Leukocytapheresis	For AML, until WBC is less than 50–100 × 10^9/L. For ALL, until WBC is less than 400 × 10^9/L
Hypertriglyceridemic pancreatitis	Severe	III	1C	TPE/LA	1–1.5 PV, albumin replacement, daily for 1–3 days determined by patient response and triglyceride levels
	Prevention of relapse	III	2C	TPE/LA	1–1.5 PV, albumin replacement, weekly to monthly to maintain triglyceride levels at moderate levels
Hyperviscosity in hypergammaglobulinemia	Symptomatic	I	1B	TPE	1–1.5 PV, albumin replacement, daily or every other day until resolution of symptoms
	Prophylaxis for rituximab	I	1C	TPE	1–1.5 PV, albumin replacement, daily or every other day
IgA nephropathy (Berger's disease)	Crescentic	III	2B	TPE	1–1.5 PV, albumin or plasma replacement, daily or every other day, duration determined by patient response
	Chronic progressive	III	2C	TPE	1–1.5 PV, albumin or plasma replacement, 6–9 over 3 weeks followed by 3–6 over 6 weeks
Inclusion body myositis		IV	2C	TPE/leukocytapheresis	NA
Immune thrombocytopenia (ITP)	Refractory	III	2C	TPE	1–1.5 PV, albumin or plasma replacement, daily or every other day, until platelet count >50 × 10^9/L or no improvement after 6 treatments
				IA	2–4 PV, daily or every other day, until platelet count >50 × 10^9/L or no improvement after 6 treatments

(continued)

Table 6.3 (continued)

Disease	Indications for apheresis	ASFA category	ASFA recommendation grade	Apheresis treatment	Treatment notes
Inflammatory bowel disease	Ulcerative colitis/ Crohn's disease	III	1B	Adsorptive cytapheresis	Once per week for 5–10 treatments
	Crohn's disease	III	2C	ECP	Recommendations not provided
Lambert-Eaton myasthenic syndrome		II	2C	TPE	1–1.5 PV, albumin, daily or every other day, course determined by clinical and electromyography response, at least 2–3 weeks
Lipoprotein(a) hyperlipoproteinemia	Progressive atherosclerotic cardiovascular disease	II	1B	LA	Weekly to every other week
Malaria	Severe	III	2B	RBC exchange	1–2 treatments until clinical improvement and parasitemia is less than 1%
Multiple sclerosis	Acute attack/ relapse	II	1A	TPE	1–1.5 PV, albumin replacement, 5–7 over 10–14 days
	Acute attack/ relapse	II	1B	IA	5–7 over 10–14 days
	Chronic	III	2B	TPE/IA	No recommendation
Myasthenia gravis	Acute, short-term treatment	I	1B	TPE/IA	1–1.5 PV, albumin replacement, 3–6 treatments over 10–14 days
	Long-term treatment	II	2B	TPE/IA	1–1.5 PV, albumin replacement, weekly or every other week adjusted for patient response
Myeloma cast nephropathy		II	2B	TPE	1–1.5 PV, albumin replacement, daily or every other day until free serum light chain reduced to 100 mg/dL or by 50%
Nephrogenic systemic sclerosis		III	2C	ECP	Various from 2 consecutive days every 2–4 weeks to 5 procedures every other day with increasing weeks between cycles
				TPE	1–1.5 PV, albumin replacement, various from 5 daily treatments to twice per week for 10–14 treatments

Neuromyelitis optica spectrum disorder (NMOSD)	Acute attack/relapse	II	1B	TPE	1–1.5 PV, albumin replacement, 5–7 over 10–14 days
	Acute attack/relapse	II	1C	IA	Up to 2.5 PV, 5–7 over 10–14 days
	Maintenance	III	2C	TPE	1–1.5 PV, albumin replacement, frequency adjusted to control relapse
N-methyl-D-aspartate receptor antibody encephalitis		I	1C	TPE/IA	1–1.5 PV, albumin replacement, 5–12 over 1–3 weeks
Overdose, envenomation, and poisoning	Mushroom poisoning	II	2C	TPE	1–1.5 PV, albumin or plasma replacement, daily until clinical symptoms abated
	Envenomation	III	2C	TPE	
	Drug overdose/poisoning	III	2C	TPE	
Paraneoplastic neurological syndromes		III	2C	TPE/IA	1–1.5 PV, albumin replacement, daily or every other day for 5–6 treatments
Paraproteinemic demyelinating neuropathies; Chronic acquired demyelinating polyneuropathies	IgG/IgA/IgM	I	1B	TPE	1–1.5 PV, albumin replacement, 5–6 over 10–14 days
	Anti-MAG	III	1C	TPE	
	Multiple myeloma	III	2C	TPE	
	Multifocal motor neuropathy	IV	1C	TPE	NA
Pediatric autoimmune neuropsychiatric disorders associated with streptococcal infections (PANDAS); Sydenham chorea	PANDAS, exacerbation	II	1B	TPE	1–1.5 PV, albumin replacement, daily or every other day for 6 procedures
	Sydenham chorea, severe	III	2B	TPE	
Pemphigus vulgaris	Severe	III	2B	TPE	1–1.5 PV, albumin or plasma replacement, daily or every other day monitoring antibody titers and clinical symptoms
	Severe	III	2C	ECP	Two consecutive days every 2–4 weeks
				IA	Daily or every-other-day monitoring antibody titers and clinical symptoms
Peripheral vascular disease		II	1B	LA	Once or twice per week for 10 treatments over 8 weeks

(continued)

Table 6.3 (continued)

Disease	Indications for apheresis	ASFA category	ASFA recommendation grade	Apheresis treatment	Treatment notes
Phytanic acid storage disease (Refsum's disease)		II	2C	TPE/LA	1–1.5 PV, albumin replacement, daily for acute exacerbations. Variable individualized course for chronic therapy
POEMS syndrome		IV	1C	TPE	NA
Polycythemia vera, erythrocytosis	Polycythemia vera	I	1B	Erythrocytosis	As needed for symptom relief or to maintain target hematocrit
	Secondary erythrocytosis	III	1C	Erythrocytosis	
Post-transfusion purpura (PTP)		III	2C	TPE	1–1.5 PV, albumin or plasma replacement, daily until platelet count >20 × 10^9/L and clinically significant bleeding improves
Progressive multifocal leukoencephalopathy (PML) associated with natalizumab		III	1C	TPE	1–1.5 PV, albumin replacement, every other day for 5 treatments with a goal to reduce natalizumab levels <1 μg/mL
Pruritus due to hepatobiliary diseases	Treatment resistant	III	1C	TPE	1–1.5 PV, albumin replacement, 3 procedures and then 2–4 times per month for maintenance
Psoriasis	Disseminated pustular	III	2B	ECP	Two consecutive days per week for 4 months followed by taper
	Disseminated pustular	III	2C	Adsorptive cytapheresis	Once per week for 5 weeks
	Disseminated pustular	IV	2C	TPE	NA
Red cell alloimmunization, prevention, and treatment	Exposure to RhD+ red cells	III	2C	RBC exchange	Target fraction of cells remaining based upon the volume of red cells transfused and what can be safely treated with Rh immunoglobulin
	Pregnancy, gestational age < 20 weeks	III	2C	TPE	1–1.5 PV, albumin replacement, 1–3 times per week until intrauterine transfusion can be safely performed (around 20 weeks gestation)
Rheumatoid arthritis		IV	NA	TPE	NA
Schizophrenia		IV	1A	TPE	NA
Scleroderma (Systemic sclerosis)		III	2C	TPE	1–1.5 PV, albumin replacement, 1–3 times per week
		III	2A	ECP	Two procedures on consecutive days every 4–6 weeks for 6–12 months
Sepsis with multiorgan failure		III	2B	TPE	1–1.5 PV, plasma replacement, daily for 1–14 days or symptom resolution

Sickle cell disease, acute	Acute stroke	I	1C	RBC exchange	One procedure with a goal to reduce HbS below 30% and a final hematocrit of less than 30–33%
	Acute chest syndrome, severe	II	1C	RBC exchange	
	Other complications	III	2C	RBC exchange	
Sickle cell disease, non-acute	Stroke prophylaxis	I	1A	RBC exchange	Frequency as needed to maintain HbS below 30% and a final hematocrit of less than 33–36%
	Pregnancy	II	2B	RBC exchange	
	Recurrent vaso-occlusive pain crisis	II	2B	RBC exchange	
	Pre-operative management	III	2A	RBC exchange	
Steroid-responsive encephalopathy associated with autoimmune thyroiditis (Hashimoto's encephalopathy)		II	2C	TPE	1–1.5 PV, albumin replacement, daily to every other day for 3–9 procedures
Stiff-person syndrome		III	2C	TPE	1–1.5 PV, albumin replacement, 4–5 procedures over 8–14 days
Sudden sensorineural hearing loss		III	2A	LA/Rheopheresis/TPE	1–1.5 PV, albumin replacement, daily or every other day for 1–3 treatments
Systemic lupus erythematosus (SLE)	Severe complications	II	2C	TPE	1–1.5 PV, albumin and/or plasma replacement, daily or every other day, 1–3 times per week
Thrombocytosis	Symptomatic	II	2C	Thrombocytapheresis	Daily or as indicated to reach or maintain platelet goal
	Prophylactic or secondary	III	2C	Thrombocytapheresis	
Thrombotic microangiopathy, coagulation mediated	*THBD*, *DKGE*, and *PLG* mutations	III	2C	TPE	1–1.5 PV, plasma replacement, daily to every other day utilizing clinical endpoints from TTP

(continued)

Table 6.3 (continued)

Disease	Indications for apheresis	ASFA category	ASFA recommendation grade	Apheresis treatment	Treatment notes
Thrombotic microangiopathy, complement mediated	Factor H autoantibody	I	2C	TPE	1–1.5 PV, plasma replacement, daily to every-other-day utilizing clinical endpoints from TTP
	Complement factor gene mutations	III	2C	TPE	
Thrombotic microangiopathy, drug associated	Ticlopidine	I	2B	TPE	1–1.5 PV, plasma replacement, daily to every-other-day utilizing clinical endpoints from TTP
	Clopidogrel	III	2B	TPE	1–1.5 PV, plasma replacement, daily to every-other-day utilizing clinical endpoints from TTP
	Gemcitabine/ Quinine	IV	2C	TPE	NA
Thrombotic microangiopathy, infection associated	STEC-HUS, severe	III	2C	TPE/IA	1–1.5 PV, plasma replacement, daily to every other day utilizing clinical endpoints from TTP
	pHUS	III	2C	TPE	1–1.5 PV, albumin replacement, daily to every other day utilizing clinical endpoints from TTP
Thrombotic microangiopathy, Thrombotic thrombocytopenic purpura		I	1A	TPE	1–1.5 PV, plasma replacement, daily until platelet count >150 × 10^9/L for 2 days, LDH near normal, and resolution of non-fixed neurologic symptoms
Thrombotic microangiopathy, transplantation associated		III	2C	TPE	1–1.5 PV, plasma or plasma/albumin replacement, daily or as indicated for chronic management
Thyroid storm		II	2C	TPE	1–1.5 PV, plasma or albumin replacement, daily to every 3 days guided by symptoms
Toxic epidermal necrolysis (TEN)	Refractory	III	2B	TPE	1–1.5 PV, albumin or plasma replacement, daily to every other day for 1–5+ procedures guided by clinical improvement

Transplantation, cardiac	Cellular/recurrent rejection	II	1B	ECP	Two consecutive days weekly or every 2–8 weeks for months
	Rejection prophylaxis	II	2A	ECP	
	Desensitization	II	1C	TPE	1–1.5 PV, albumin or plasma replacement, daily to every-other-day monitoring donor-specific antibody levels
	Antibody-mediated rejection	III	2C	TPE	1–1.5 PV, albumin or plasma replacement, daily to every-other-day monitoring cardiac function, biopsy findings, or donor-specific antibody levels
Transplantation, hematopoietic stem cell, ABO incompatible (ABOi)	Major ABOi HPC(M)	II	1B	TPE	1–1.5 PV, albumin or plasma (donor and recipient ABO compatible) replacement, daily until recipient's IgG and IgM titers <16
	Major ABOi HPC(A)	II	2B	TPE	1–1.5 PV, albumin or plasma (donor and recipient ABO compatible) replacement, daily until recipient's IgG and IgM titers <16
	Minor ABOi HPC(A)	III	2C	RBC exchange	Once using group O red blood cells
	Major/Minor ABOi with pure red cell aplasia	III	2C	TPE	1–1.5 PV, albumin or plasma (donor and recipient ABO compatible) replacement, daily or every other day following red cell production/red cell transfusion requirements
Transplantation, hematopoietic stem cell, HLA desensitization		III	2C	TPE	1–1.5 PV, albumin replacement, every other day following donor-specific antibody levels. Patients may require additional TPE post-transplant

(continued)

Table 6.3 (continued)

Disease	Indications for apheresis	ASFA category	ASFA recommendation grade	Apheresis treatment	Treatment notes
Transplantation, liver	Desensitization, ABOi living donor	I	1C	TPE	1–1.5 PV, albumin or plasma (donor and recipient ABO compatible) replacement, daily or every other day to reduce isoagglutinin titers below critical threshold
	Desensitization, ABOi deceases donor/ antibody-mediated rejection	III	2C	TPE	1–1.5 PV, albumin or plasma (donor and recipient ABO compatible) replacement, daily or every other day to reduce isoagglutinin titers below critical threshold
	Desensitization, ABOi	III	2C	ECP	Two consecutive days per week or every 2–8 weeks for months
	Acute rejection/ Immune suppression withdrawal	III	2B	ECP	Two consecutive days per week or every 2–8 weeks for months
Transplantation, lung	Bronchiolitis obliterans syndrome	II	1C	ECP	Two consecutive days per week for 4 weeks and then every other week for four treatment pairs, and then every 4 weeks for 3 months
	Antibody-mediated rejection/ desensitization	III	2C	TPE	1–1.5 PV, albumin or plasma replacement, daily or every other day to reduce donor-specific antibody levels
Transplantation, renal, ABO compatible	Antibody-mediated rejection	I	1B	TPE/IA	1–1.5 PV, albumin or plasma replacement, daily or every other day to reduce donor-specific antibody levels
	Desensitization, living donor	I	1B	TPE/IA	1–1.5 PV, albumin or plasma replacement, daily or every other day to reduce donor-specific antibody levels. Post-operatively, 3 or more procedures may be performed to maintain donor-specific antibody levels below a critical threshold.
	Desensitization, deceased donor	III	2C	TPE/IA	1–1.5 PV, albumin or plasma replacement, daily or every other day to reduce donor-specific antibody levels. Post-operatively, 3 or more procedures may be performed to maintain donor-specific antibody levels below a critical threshold

Transplantation, renal, ABO incompatible	Desensitization, living donor	I	1B	TPE/IA	1–1.5 PV, albumin or plasma replacement, daily or every other day to reduce isoagglutinin titers below a critical thresholds. Post-operatively, additional procedures are performed to maintain isoagglutinin titers.
	Antibody-mediated rejection	II	1B	TPE/IA	1–1.5 PV, albumin or plasma replacement, daily or every other day to reduce isoagglutinin titers
Vasculitis, ANCA-associated (AAV)	MPA/GPA/RLV: RPGN, Cr >5.7 mg/dL	II	1B	TPE	1–1.5 PV, albumin replacement, plasma replacement if DAH is present, daily or every other day for 7 procedures
	MPA/GPA/RLV: RPGN, Cr <5.7 mg/dL	III	2C	TPE	1–1.5 PV, albumin replacement, plasma replacement if DAH is present, daily or every other day for 7 procedures
	MPA/GPA/RLV: DAH	I	1C	TPE	1–1.5 PV, albumin replacement, plasma replacement if DAH is present, daily or every other day for 7 procedures
	EGPA	III	2C	TPE	1–1.5 PV, albumin replacement, plasma replacement if DAH is present, daily or every other day for 7 procedures
Vasculitis, IgA (Henoch-Schönlein purpura)	Crescentic RPGN	III	2C	TPE	1–1.5 PV, albumin replacement, daily for 4–11 procedures until resolution of symptoms
	Severe extrarenal manifestations	III	2C	TPE	1–1.5 PV, albumin replacement, daily for 4–11 procedures until resolution of symptoms
Vasculitis, other	Hepatitis B polyarteritis nodosa	II	2C	TPE	1 PV, albumin replacement, 9–12 procedures, 2 to 3 per week
	Idiopathic polyarteritis nodosa	IV	1B	TPE	NA
	Behçet's disease	II	1C	Adsorptive cytapheresis	1 procedure per week for 5 weeks
	Behçet's disease	III	2C	TPE	1 PV, albumin replacement, 9–12 procedures, 2–3 per week

(continued)

Table 6.3 (continued)

Disease	Indications for apheresis	ASFA category	ASFA recommendation grade	Apheresis treatment	Treatment notes
Voltage-gated potassium channel (VGKC) antibody related diseases		II	1B	TPE/IA	1–1.5 PV, albumin replacement, 5–10 treatments over 7–14 days adjusted to treat symptoms
Wilson disease, fulminant		I	1C	TPE	1–1.5 PV, albumin or plasma replacement, daily or every other day with number of procedures determined by clinical response and availability of liver transplantation

TPE plasma exchange, *PV* plasma volume, *IA* immunoadsorption, *NA* not applicable, *ECP* extracorporeal photopheresis, *RBC* red blood cell, *NYHA* New York Heart Association, *LA* lipid apheresis, *RBC* red blood cell, *AML* acute myelogenous leukemia, *ALL* acute lymphoblastic leukemia, *STEC* Shiga toxin-producing *Escherichia coli*, *HUS* hemolytic uremic syndrome, *pHUS* pneumococcal hemolytic uremic syndrome, *HPC(M)* hematopoietic progenitor cell marrow, *HPC(A)* hematopoietic progenitor cell apheresis, *MPA* microscopic polyangiitis, *GPA* granulomatosis with polyangiitis, *RLV* renal-limited vasculitis, *RPGN* rapidly progressive glomerulonephritis, *DAH* diffuse alveolar hemorrhage, *EGPA* eosinophilic granulomatosis with polyangiitis

Modified with permission from: Padmanabhan A, Connelly-Smith L, Aqui N, et al. (2019) Guidelines on the use of therapeutic apheresis in clinical practice: evidence-based approach from the Apheresis Applications Committee of the American Society for Apheresis. The Eighth Special Issue, *J Clin Apher* 34:171–2354

6.5 How to Use the ASFA Indication Categories in Clinical Practice

For all requests for therapeutic apheresis procedures, irrespective of the ASFA category for the disorder, the apheresis medicine practitioner must evaluate the diagnosis for which the procedure is being requested. The questions that must be first considered are listed in Table 6.4.

The answers to these questions guide the apheresis medicine practitioner concerning whether the requested apheresis procedure should be considered. In those circumstances where the evaluation indicates that the apheresis procedure should be considered, the next step is to examine the ASFA category for the disorder.

ASFA category I, II, and IV indications are those which are relatively straightforward to evaluate. For ASFA category I indications, given that this designation indicates a primary treatment modality, it would be appropriate if the patient had no contraindications for the procedure, to proceed with the apheresis therapy [8]. For ASFA category II indications, apheresis is considered a second-line therapy. It is therefore necessary to determine whether the appropriate first-line therapy has been applied or is currently being applied to the patient. In the instance where this is not the case, the apheresis medicine practitioner should decline performing the apheresis procedure until the first-line therapy has been initiated [8]. It is important to note that the ASFA recommendation grade also influences the decision in utilizing the apheresis treatment. Strong recommendations, especially if there is "A" or "B" quality evidence, indicate that there is published evidence supporting its use. A weak recommendation, especially in the presence of "C" quality evidence, indicates a degree of uncertainty and, therefore, alternate therapies may be as appropriate [8].

Table 6.4 Questions to be answered before considering performing a course of apheresis treatment [8]

• Is the patient's diagnosis the most likely diagnosis?
• Is the patient's presentation similar to other patients with the diagnosis which have been treated with apheresis and described in the medical literature?
• Have standard medical treatments for the disorder been attempted and failed or are contraindicated?
• Are there alternate treatments to the apheresis procedure that are equally efficacious but not as invasive, not as resource intensive, or have more published supporting evidence?
• What is the risk/benefit ratio of the apheresis procedure considering the patient's comorbid conditions and current therapy?

Modified with permission from: Shaz BH, Winters JL, Bandarenko N, Szczepiorkowski ZM. (2007) How we approach an apheresis request for a category III, category IV, or noncategorized indication. *Transfusion* 47:1963–1971

For ASFA category IV indications, as the published evidence indicates that the apheresis procedure is ineffective or harmful, the procedure should not be performed. The exception to this would be if the procedure was being performed in the context of an Institutional Review Board (IRB)-approved research protocol [8]. As with the ASFA category I and II indications, the recommendation grade should also be considered in the decision-making process for ASFA category IV indications. Here, a weak recommendation with low-quality evidence indicates that the category IV indication has the potential, should new higher-quality evidence be published, to move into a different ASFA category. It is important for indications with an ASFA category IV and an ASFA recommendation grade of 2C that literature published since the most recent ASFA guidelines were written and reviewed to ensure that newer, higher-quality evidence does not indicate that the procedure may be of benefit [8].

For ASFA category III indications, decision-making is more complex. The definition of this category indicates that "optimum role is not established" and "decision-making should be individualized" [2]. This means that the apheresis medicine practitioner must consider whether or not the apheresis procedure is appropriate for the individual patient based upon the patient's presentation, clinical symptoms, and comorbid conditions [8]. It is the greater detail provided in the full ASFA guidelines concerning what to consider for the various ASFA category III indications that should be reviewed when making decisions.

6.6 What About Uncategorized Indications?

As indicated earlier, it would be impossible for *all* potential indications to be described in the ASFA guidelines. A flowchart for evaluating a request to treat an uncategorized indication is given in Fig. 6.1. When confronted with such a request, the initial action should be to search for medical literature to determine if there has been literature published concerning the disease in question. It could be that substantial literature has been published since the guidelines were drafted or that there existed literature at the time the guidelines were drafted, but it was insufficient to generate a fact sheet. Even if new publications are not present, the literature may still inform the apheresis medicine practitioner.

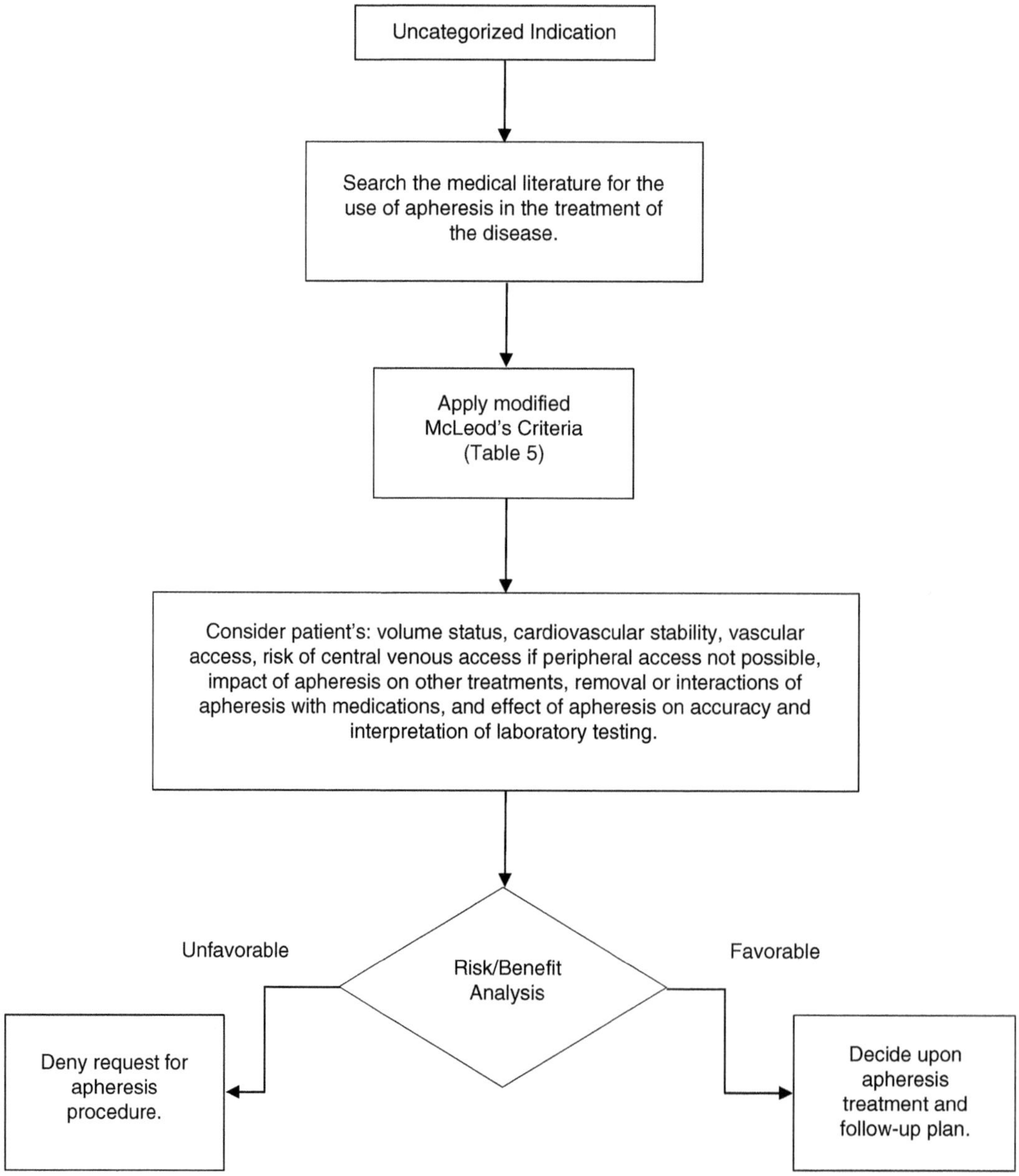

Fig. 6.1 Decision-making in uncategorized indications [8]. (Modified with permission from: Shaz BH, Winters JL, Bandarenko N, Szczepiorkowski ZM. (2007) How we approach an apheresis request for a category III, category IV, or noncategorized indication. *Transfusion* 47:1963–1971)

Table 6.5 McLeod's modified criteria [8, 9]

Mechanism	Current understanding of disease pathophysiology supports the use of the apheresis procedure
Correction	Abnormality involved in disease pathogenesis is corrected by the apheresis procedure
Clinical effect	Evidence the apheresis procedure confers clinical benefit and not simply statistically significant change in laboratory value

Modified with permission from: Shaz BH, Winters JL, Bandarenko N, Szczepiorkowski ZM. (2007) How we approach an apheresis request for a category III, category IV, or noncategorized indication. *Transfusion* 47:1963–1971

In the presence of insufficient literature or, potentially, no literature at all, McLeod's criteria (Table 6.5) can be used to help guide the decision-making process. The point of these criteria is to apply apheresis therapy to disorders in a rationale, evidence-based manner and not simply to do the procedure because "you can" or because "we have tried everything else." It requires a thoughtful consideration of the pathophysiology, or potential pathophysiology, of the disease and an understanding of how the apheresis treatment being considered could influence this pathology.

If it appears that apheresis may modify a disease process and produce a clinical benefit, not solely a laboratory value change, then the patient's clinical situation should be assessed to determine the risk of the procedure versus the potential benefit. If this analysis indicates a positive risk/benefit ratio, then the procedure can be performed.

6.7 Summary

In summary, the ASFA guidelines provide evidence-based clinical guidance on the use of apheresis to treat disease. The guidelines describe indications utilizing the ASFA categories to outline the role of apheresis procedures in the treatment of these diseases. Only those diseases and disorders for which a critical mass of peer-reviewed literature has been published are included as indicated in the guidelines.

References

1. Klein HG, Balow JE, Dau PC, et al. Clinical applications of apheresis. Report of the clinical applications Committee American Society for Apheresis. J Clin Apher. 1986;3:1–92.
2. Padmanabhan A, Connelly-Smith L, Aqui N, et al. Guidelines on the use of therapeutic apheresis in clinical practice: evidence-based approach from the Apheresis Applications Committee of the American Society for Apheresis. The eighth special issue. J Clin Apher. 2019;34:171–2354.
3. Winters JL. Randomized controlled trials in therapeutic apheresis. J Clin Apher. 2013;28:48–55.
4. Guyatt G, Gutterman D, Baumann MH, et al. Grading strength of recommendations and quality of evidence in clinical guidelines: report from an American College of Chest Physicians Task Force. Chest. 2006;129:174–81.
5. Balogun RA, Sanchez AP, Klingel R, et al. Update to the ASFA guidelines on the use of therapeutic apheresis in ANCA-associated vasculitis. J Clin Apher. 2020;35:493–9.
6. Schwartz J, Winters JL, Padmanabhan A, et al. Guidelines on the use of therapeutic apheresis in clinical practice: evidence-based approach from the Apheresis Applications Committee of the American Society for Apheresis. The sixth special issue. J Clin Apher. 2013;28:145–284.
7. Schwartz J, Padmanabhan A, Aqui N, et al. Guidelines on the use of therapeutic apheresis in clinical practice: evidence-based approach from the Apheresis Applications Committee of the American Society for Apheresis. The seventh special issue. J Clin Apher. 2016;31:149–338.
8. Shaz BH, Winters JL, Bandarenko N, et al. How we approach an apheresis request for a category III, category IV, or noncategorized indication. Transfusion. 2007;47:1963–71.
9. McLeod BC. An approach to evidence-based therapeutic apheresis. J Clin Apher. 2002;17:124–32.

Category IV Diseases for ASFA

7

Kaya Ali Hakan

7.1 Introduction

Therapeutic apheresis methods have been used for many years in the treatment of several diseases. Since it is a treatment method that requires a multidisciplinary approach, guidelines are utilized for its indications. The American Society for Apheresis (ASFA) Journal of Clinical Apheresis Special Issue Writing Committee has periodically published guidelines for the use of therapeutic apheresis since 1986. The most recent update is the eighth special issue published in 2019 and is available for clinical use. In this guideline, indications for use are categorized according to the level of disease-based benefit. The diseases are divided into a total of four categories. Category IV diseases in the guideline are defined as "Disorders in which published evidence demonstrates or suggests apheresis to be ineffective or harmful. Institutional Review Board (IRB) approval is desirable if apheresis treatment is undertaken in these circumstances" [1, 2]. Changes are made by evaluating the current literature on diseases in this category. The category IV diseases included in this latest guideline and previous guidelines are given in Table 7.1. Cynical data obtained with these diseases will be discussed, respectively.

K. A. Hakan (✉)
Division of Hematology, Department of Internal Medicine, Biruni University Faculty of Medicine, İstanbul, Turkey

Department of Hematology and Adult Bone Marrow Transplantation Center, Biruni University Hospital, İstanbul, Turkey
e-mail: alihakan.kaya@maltepe.edu.tr

I. Kozanoglu (ed.), *Problem Solving in Apheresis Medicine*,
https://doi.org/10.1007/978-3-031-74081-7_7

Table 7.1 Category definitions for therapeutic apheresis, category IV indications

Disease	Procedure	ASFA 2019	ASFA 2016	ASFA 2013
Amyloidosis, systemic	TPE	4	4	4
Amyotrophic lateral sclerosis	TPE	4[a]	4[a]	4
Coagulation factor inhibitors	TPE	3	4	4
Dermatomyositis or polymyositis	TPE Leukocytapheresis	4[a]	4	4 4
Hemolysis, elevated liver enzymes, and low platelets syndrome (HELLP syndrome-antepartum)	TPE	4	4	NC
Immune thrombocytopenia (refractory)	TPE	3	3	4
Inclusion body myositis	TPE Leukocytapheresis	4[a]	4[a]	4 4
Paraproteinemic demyelinating neuropathies; chronic acquired demyelinating polyneuropathies (multifocal motor neuropathy)	TPE	4	4	NC
POEMS syndrome	TPE	4[a]	4[a]	4
Psoriasis	TPE	4	4	4
Rheumatoid arthritis	TPE	4[a]	4[a]	NC
Schizophrenia	TPE	4[a]	4[a]	4
Thrombotic microangiopathy, drug associated (gemcitabine, quinine)	TPE	4	4	4
Vasculitis, others—idiopathic polyarteritis nodosa	TPE	4	4	NC

NC not categorized, *TPE* therapeutic plasma exchange
[a] Listed in separate table in ASFA 2019 guideline—no new evidence

7.2 Amyloidosis, Systemic: Procedure, TPE

Amyloidosis is a group of heterogeneous diseases characterized by extracellular accumulation of fibrillar proteins called "amyloid" in tissues and dysfunction in organs. More than 30 human protein precursors of amyloid fibrils are known [3]. Amyloid deposition limited to one area is classified as localized amyloidosis, which may spread to different organs via blood stream and may clinically lead to systemic amyloidosis [4]. There are three types of systemic amyloidosis commonly encountered in the clinic. These are AL amyloidosis, AA amyloidosis, and hereditary ATTR amyloidosis. Amyloid deposition leads to a clinical picture of organ failure (heart failure, renal failure, hepatosplenomegaly, pancytopenia, or gastrointestinal malabsorption). Treatment in type AL is usually the same as for plasma cell diseases, such as chemotherapy and stem cell transplantation. In AA type, controlling the primary disease causing the underlying inflammation is important.

In systemic amyloidosis, TPE has been used in clinical practice, with the hypothesis that amyloid fibrils in plasma can be removed by plasma exchange therapy and thus the progression of the disease can be stopped. In a study investigating the effect of combined chemotherapy and TPE treatment in AL amyloidosis, it was found to have a limited positive effect in terms of reducing skin lesions and IL-6 levels [5]. Two studies on this subject have contradictory findings. One study reported that AL amyloidosis may lead to factor X deficiency, while the other concluded that there is no such effect [6, 7]. Considering the results of the few case series presented in the literature, TPE treatment was classified as category IV because it did not have any significant positive effect in systemic amyloidosis.

7.3 Amyotrophic Lateral Sclerosis: Procedure, TPE

Amyotrophic lateral sclerosis (ALS), which is a typical upper and lower motor neuron disease, is a fatal disease with a progressive and degenerative process that is explained by not one but many causes in the first and second motor neurons. Immunosuppressant and immunomodulatory treatments are mainly used.

There is very little literature data supporting the effect of TPE in the treatment of ALS. In two case-based studies presented in the literature about 30 years ago, it was concluded that there was no positive effect of TPE treatment in patients with ALS [8, 9]. It was then classified as category IV due to lacking literature support.

7.4 Dermatomyositis or Polymyositis: Procedure, TPE—Leukocytapheresis

Idiopathic inflammatory myopathies are a heterogeneous and rare group of diseases characterized by muscle damage due to inflammation of proximal skeletal muscles that develop on an autoimmune background. Physical exercise and immunosuppressive drugs are used in treatment. There are very few studies using TPE in treatment. In 39 prospectively designed steroid-resistant patients from these studies, it was concluded that there was no clinical change in muscle strength despite regression in muscle enzymes after 1 month of TPE treatment [10, 11]. It was then classified as category IV due to lack of clinical support.

7.5 Hemolysis, Elevated Liver Enzymes, and Low Platelets Syndrome (HELLP Syndrome-Antepartum): Procedure, TPE

HELLP is one of the thrombotic microangiopathy syndromes that occurs during pregnancy along with hemolysis, thrombocytopenia, and liver dysfunction. Although HELLP typically occurs in the third trimester of pregnancy, it may also occur during postpartum in up to 25% of patients [12]. Treatment is generally supportive therapy; meanwhile, the definitive treatment in antepartum cases is termination of pregnancy, i.e., delivery. Although there are studies showing the benefit of TPE treatment mostly in postpartum cases, there is no clinical study supporting its benefit in the antepartum period. Therefore, TPE treatment for HELLP syndrome in the antepartum period is classified as category IV.

7.6 Inclusion Body Myositis: Procedure, TPE—Leukocytapheresis

It is a rare inflammatory disease of the skeletal muscle, especially involving the muscles of the upper and lower extremities and causing muscle atrophy. In these cases where there is no effective treatment, treatment is usually supportive care. In two studies conducted for the efficacy of TPE treatment, it was concluded that TPE application in addition to immunosuppressive therapies did not add any additional benefit to the clinical course of the disease [13, 14]. It is therefore a category IV disease.

7.7 Paraproteinemic Demyelinating Neuropathies, Chronic Acquired Demyelinating Polyneuropathies (Multifocal Motor Neuropathy): Procedure, TPE

TPE may be effective in the treatment of paraproteinemic demyelinating neuropathies excluding multifocal motor neuropathy. With regard to the treatment of multifocal motor neuropathy, TPE treatment is not recommended in these cases since there are highly effective treatments (category IV).

7.8 POEMS Syndrome: Procedure, TPE

POEMS syndrome is a rare clonal plasma cell disorder characterized by polyneuropathy, organomegaly, endocrinopathy, M-protein, and skin changes. Treatment includes therapies such as chemotherapy, immunotherapy, radiotherapy, and stem cell transplantation, usually targeting the plasma cell clone. These patients may receive TPE treatment because chronic inflammatory demyelinating neuropathy is included in the differential diagnosis. In a study investigating the effect of TPE treatment on POEMS cases, 16 of 30 patients with POEMS were given isolated TPE treatment, while 14 were given TPE treatment combined with steroids. While there was no clinical improvement in patients receiving isolated TPE treatment, responses in the steroid-combined arm were similar to the response rates of isolated steroid treatment [15, 16]. According to literature data, TPE treatment, which has no additional contribution to POEMS treatment, is positioned in category IV in these cases.

7.9 Psoriasis: Procedure, TPE

Psoriasis is a chronic, inflammatory disease characterized by sharply circumscribed erythematous-squamous plaques. TPE treatment in these cases was applied in a very limited number of studies. Since no results supporting the effect of TPE could be obtained in these series of cases, it is classified as category IV [17].

7.10 Rheumatoid Arthritis: Procedure, TPE

Rheumatoid arthritis (RA) is an autoimmune disease of unknown etiology characterized by symmetrical, erosive synovitis and sometimes multisystem organ involvement. There are very few studies investigating the efficacy of TPE. In two studies of 26 and 20 patients respectively, patients were divided into two arms. One arm received standard rheumatoid arthritis treatment, while the other arm received TPE treatment in addition to other drugs. As a result of these studies, no change was observed in treatment responses in the TPE-added arm [18, 19]. This disease is therefore classified as category IV.

7.11 Schizophrenia: Procedure, TPE

Schizophrenia is a psychiatric disorder that occurs in 1% of the population, which affects emotion, thought, perception, and behavior. It comes along with positive symptoms such as delusions and hallucinations; negative symptoms such as shallow affect, social withdrawal, decrease in speech, and impoverishment in thought content; and cognitive symptoms such as impairment in attention, memory, and executive functions; it may also present with different clinical pictures. In a study investigating the effect of TPE in the treatment of schizophrenia, wherein it was applied in ten patients, it was concluded that it had no effect [20]. This disease is therefore classified as category IV.

7.12 Thrombotic Microangiopathy, Drug Associated (Gemcitabine, Quinine): Procedure, TPE

Many drugs are known to cause secondary thrombotic microangiopathy (TMA). Secondary TMA may develop due to gemcitabine and quinine use. In many cases of drug-associated TMA, TPE treatment may be effective, albeit limited. In a 29-patient study on gemcitabine-associated TMA, it was improved with clinical supportive treatment in 56% of the group without TPE treatment [21]. In another study of 18 patients, only 30% of TMA findings regressed in patients who received TPE [22]. Likewise, it has been revealed in clinical studies that adding TPE to treatment in quinine-associated TMA cases is of no benefit [23]. Therefore, in the case of both drug-associated TMA, TPE treatment is classified as category IV.

7.13 Vasculitis, Others: Idiopathic Polyarteritis Nodosa: Procedure, TPE

Polyarteritis nodosa (PAN) is a systemic vasculitis involving small- and medium-sized arteries. The skin, joints, kidneys, peripheral nerves, and gastrointestinal tract are mainly affected. In a study of 60 patients investigating the efficacy of TPE in treatment, it was shown that the addition of TPE to steroid treatment did not contribute to the treatment [24]. It was therefore classified as category IV.

References

1. Padmanabhan A, Connelly-Smith L, Aqui N, Balogun RA, Klingel R, Meyer E, et al. Guidelines on the use of therapeutic apheresis in clinical practice—Evidence-based approach from the Writing Committee of the American Society for Apheresis: the eighth special issue. J Clin Apher. 2019;34(3):171–354.
2. Schwartz J, Padmanabhan A, Aqui N, Balogun RA, Connelly-Smith L, Delaney M, et al. Guidelines on the use of therapeutic apheresis in clinical practice—Evidence-based approach from the Writing Committee of the American Society for Apheresis: the seventh special issue. J Clin Apher. 2016;31(3):149–62.
3. Ke PC, Zhou R, Serpell LC, Riek R, Knowles TPJ, Lashuel HA, et al. Half a century of amyloids: past, present and future. Chem Soc Rev. 2020;49:5473.
4. Benson MD, Buxbaum JN, Eisenberg DS, Merlini G, Saraiva MJM, Sekijima Y, et al. Amyloid nomenclature 2020: update and recommendations by the International Society of Amyloidosis (ISA) Nomenclature Committee. Amyloid. 2020;27:217.
5. Katayama I, Sawada Y, Yokozeki H, Nishioka K, Akiba T. Successful treatment of systemic amyloidosis by combination chemotherapy and plasmapheresis. Effect on plasma IL6 and serum amyloid protein A. Int J Dermatol. 1994;33:672–3.
6. Barker B, Altuntas F, Paranjape G, Sarode R. Presurgical plasma exchange is ineffective in correcting amyloid associated factor X deficiency. J Clin Apher. 2004;19:208–10.
7. Beardell FV, Varma M, Martinez J. Normalization of plasma factor X levels in amyloidosis after plasma exchange. Am J Hematol. 1997;54:68–71.
8. Olarte MR, Schoenfeldt RS, McKiernan G, Rowland LP. Plasmapheresis in amyotrophic lateral sclerosis. Ann Neurol. 1980;8(6):644–5.
9. Kelemen J, Hedlund W, Orlin JB, Berkman EM, Munsat TL. Plasmapheresis with immunosuppression in amyotrophic lateral sclerosis. Arch Neurol. 1983;40(12):752–3.
10. Miller FW, Leitman SF, Cronin ME, Hicks JE, Leff RL, Wesley R, et al. Controlled trial of plasma exchange and leukapheresis in polymyositis and dermatomyositis. N Engl J Med. 1992;326(21):1380–4.
11. Gordon PA, Winer JB, Hoogendijk JE, Choy EH. Immunosuppressant and immunomodulatory treatment for dermatomyositis and polymyositis. Cochrane Database Syst Rev. 2012;2012(8):CD003643.
12. Abildgaard U, Heimdal K. Pathogenesis of the syndrome of hemolysis, elevated liver enzymes, and low platelet count (HELLP): a review. Eur J Obstet Gynecol Reprod Biol. 2013;166:117.
13. Steven A, Greenberg SA. Inclusion body myositis. Opin Rheumatol. 2011;23:574–8.
14. Dau PC. Leukocytapheresis in inclusion body myositis. J Clin Apher. 1987;3:167–70.
15. Dispenzieri A, Kyle RA, Lacy MQ, Rajkumar SV, Therneau TM, Larson DR. POEMS syndrome: definitions and longterm outcome. Blood. 2003;101:2496–506.
16. Dispenzieri A. POEMS Syndrome. Hematology Am Soc Hematol Educ Program. 2005;2005:360–7.
17. Clemmensen OJ, Andresen R, Andersen E. Plasmapheresis in the treatment of psoriasis. A controlled clinical study. J Am Acad Dermatol. 1983;8:190–2.
18. Rothwell RS, Davis P, Gordon PA, Dasgupta MK, Johny KV, Russell AS, et al. A controlled study of plasma exchange in the treatment of severe rheumatoid arthritis. Arthritis Rheum. 1980;23:785–90.
19. Dwosh IL, Giles AR, Ford PM, Pater JL, Anastassiades TP. Plasmapheresis therapy in rheumatoid arthritis. A controlled, double-blind, crossover trial. N Engl J Med. 1983;308:1124–9.
20. Schulz SC, van Kammen DP, Waters R, Klein HG, Balow JE, Bunney WE Jr. Double-blind evaluation of plasmapheresis in schizophrenic patients: a pilot study. Artif Organs. 1983;7:317–21.
21. Glezerman I, Kris MG, Miller V, Seshan S, Flombaum CD. Gemcitabine nephrotoxicity and haemolytic uremic syndrome: a report of 29 cases from a single institution. Clin Nephrol. 2009;71:130–9.
22. Gore EM, Jones BS, Marques MB. Is therapeutic plasma exchange indicated for patients with gemcitabine-induced hemolytic uremic syndrome? J Clin Apher. 2009;24:209–14.
23. Park YA, Hay SN, King KE, Matevosyan K, Poisson J, Powers A, et al. Is it quinine TTP/HUS or quinine TMA? ADAMTS 13 levels and implications for therapy. J Clin Apher. 2009;24:115–9.
24. Guillevin L, Fain O, Lhote F, Jarrousse B, Le Thi Huong D, Bussel A, et al. Lack of superiority of steroids plus plasma exchange to steroids alone in the treatment of polyarteritis nodosa and Churg-Strauss syndrome. A prospective, randomized trial in 78 patients. Arthritis Rheum. 1992;35:208–15.

Part III

Top Problems and Solutions in Apheresis

8 Vascular Access Problems During Apheresis

David Barth

8.1 Background

One of the most important decisions prior to the start of an apheresis treatment is deciding on what type of vascular access will be chosen for the treatment. This decision has impact on the timing of the start of the procedure, how stable and successful it will be, how long it will take, how efficient the process will be, and what potential adverse events the patient will be exposed to. Good vascular access will allow for stable and adequate blood flow rates, which are deemed critical for a successful apheresis treatment. Most centrifugal apheresis procedures require flow rates of 50–120 mL/min, and membrane apheresis procedures require flow rates of 150–200 mL/min [1, 2]. Poor blood flow rates or unstable rates, which may cause multiple stoppages during the procedure due to obstruction of vascular access or pressure alarms, can result in excessively prolonged procedures, which can lead to complications including increased citrate accumulation and toxicity, decreased efficiency of procedure, or premature discontinuation of the procedure before target volumes or therapeutic endpoints have been met. Regardless of the various modalities of vascular access that may be available to the apheresis provider, the decision on the type of vascular access should primarily be driven by the status of the patient being treated and the clinical issues that are specific for that individual patient, ensuring that stable and adequate blood flow rates can be provided for the apheresis treatment while being done in the safest way possible.

8.2 Considerations

The first decision point is whether the patient already has an existing viable central vascular access (CVA) for another medical reason that could be used for the proposed apheresis procedure. This situation may occur in patients with renal disorders that have existing dialysis-compatible CVA or arteriovenous fistulas or grafts. It may also occur in intensive care unit patients on a cardiopulmonary bypass circuit (i.e., extracorporeal membrane oxygenation, ECMO). In these cases, using the existing central vascular access reduces any wait time needed to obtain vascular access and prevents further interventions on the patient to obtain other vascular access [3].

If no preexisting viable central vascular access exists, the next decision point is whether the patient is clinically stable to have this apheresis procedure performed using peripheral venous

D. Barth (✉)
Departments of Laboratory Medicine and Pathobiology and Medicine, University Health Network and University of Toronto, Toronto General Hospital, Toronto, ON, Canada
e-mail: david.barth@uhn.ca

I. Kozanoglu (ed.), *Problem Solving in Apheresis Medicine*,
https://doi.org/10.1007/978-3-031-74081-7_8

access (PVA). PVA, in the appropriate clinical situation, may be the most ideal choice for vascular access due to ease and speed of insertion and low risk of complications. PVA will be discussed in more depth later in this chapter. In this situation, clinical instability refers to a patient with decreased level of consciousness, confusion, severe developmental or cognitive impairment, or having prolonged seizures. In these situations, even if the patient has PVA, they will not be able to maintain muscle tone in their arms due to decreased level of consciousness or are not able to keep still while intravenous lines are in their arms, risking venous damage or dislodging of PVA, or they may even try to pull out the PVA. Also, patients with hypotension or autonomic neuropathies may not be able to maintain adequate blood flow with PVA. This group of patients will require CVA for the apheresis procedure.

Clinical instability is not the only reason for choosing CVA for apheresis procedures. Stable patients may require CVA if they do not have adequate veins for PVA. Individuals with significant previous venipunctures, both acute and chronically, may have damaged or sclerotic peripheral veins. Patients may have significant edema in their arms, a history of lymphedema, severe bruising, or hematomas from recent venipunctures, which then decrease the ability to access the peripheral veins. Autonomic insufficiency, tortuous veins, small veins that rupture easily, and veins close to the arteries may prevent peripheral venous access even with assistant imaging techniques (i.e., ultrasound). Individuals with needle phobia may refuse peripheral access even when they have good peripheral veins.

The group of patients with clinical instability usually needs apheresis procedures urgently; moreover, even individuals without clinical instability but poor venous access may have urgent needs for apheresis. A hemodialysis-compatible catheter may be required. CVA devices for apheresis procedures generally have diameters of at least 11.5 French and are required to have two lumens, a shorter and sometimes larger lumen for drawing (red port) and a longer lumen for returning blood (blue port). Some hemodialysis-compatible catheters have a smaller third lumen, which can be used for additional intravenous therapies or blood drawing for laboratory testing [2, 4, 5].

This type of catheter can be placed as a non-tunneled (NTCVA) or tunneled CVA (TCVA). Non-tunneled CVA allows for fast direct insertion by a physician, which can also be done at the bedside or in interventional radiology. It can be immediately used post insertion after confirming placement on radiographic imaging in internal jugular placement; it is generally designed to stay in up to 10–14 days, does not require as tight coagulation parameters as TCVA insertion, and can be removed easily at the end of the treatment. These catheters are placed in the internal jugular or femoral veins. NTCVA have a local and systemic blood infection risk which increases the longer the CVA remains in place. The entry site needs to be kept clean and dry to decrease infection risk. Other risks include: risk of venous thrombosis, bleeding or pneumothorax during insertion, possibility of becoming dislodged more easily as they are held in placed by sutures and dressings at the insertion site on the skin which can lead to loss of access and potentially significant bleeding from the site if not controlled quickly. NTCVA can be a cause of air embolism, and may be uncomfortable for the patient because of pain, restriction on showering and can be difficult to lie down with a NTCVA sticking out of their neck. Femoral vein access may limit a patient's ability to ambulate due to increased risk of kinking and dislodging of the CVA with ambulation and can have an increased infection risk due to the less hygienic situation at this location. Moreover, major bleeding can occur if a NTCVA falls out and is not dealt with quickly by applying pressure. This risk increases especially in a femoral line in a patient that may not be able to recognize the NTCVA dislodging or may lack strength or awareness to alert someone to help or to compress the bleed site themselves. Many institutions will require a patient to remain admitted in hospital while NTCVA is in place. NTCVA is ideal for a patient needing urgent apheresis or needing a short course of apheresis (i.e., daily apheresis treatment for 5–10 days). NTCVAs should be removed as soon as the planned apheresis course is completed. If a NTCVA is in place after 10–14 days and further apheresis is required, removal of NTCVA and replacement with a more durable CVA should be considered in an effort to decrease infection risk [2, 4, 5].

For patients requiring a CVA, and apheresis procedures are expected to continue past 10–14 days, a tunneled CVA can be used. A surgically created channel/tunnel between the skin and central vein is created. The TCVA has a cuff of polyester on the catheter with an imbedded antimicrobial product. The cuff results in the growth of fibroblasts around it inside the tunnel, which reduces dislodging and infection risk. A TCVA allows for immediate use post insertion, is generally designed to stay in for months to years, has a lower risk of infection compared to NTCVA, and allows for outpatient use and less risk of being dislodged than NTCVA. These catheters are most commonly placed in the internal jugular or subclavian veins but can also be placed in femoral veins. TCVA requires interventional radiology or surgical services to insert, which can delay insertion in some cases, requires more normal coagulation parameter for insertion than non-tunneled CVA, has risk of venous thrombosis, and needs entry site remain dry to decrease infection risk. Moreover, it is more difficult to remove once apheresis treatment is no longer required or in the event of infection or CVA complication. Both NTCVA and TCVA require rigorous sterile conditions when being accessed to decrease risk of systemic blood infections [5, 6].

In the event that CVA is required, but the onset of treatment is not urgent and a prolonged course of apheresis therapy (i.e., greater than 3 months) is expected, an apheresis-compatible portacath (ACP) can be used. Regular portacaths are not able to handle the pressures of an apheresis procedure. A surgical procedure is done to create a subcutaneous pocket under the anterior chest wall. A portacath, which is described as a chamber that is attached to a catheter, is inserted into the pocket, and the catheter is then inserted into the subclavian or intrajugular vein. The skin is then closed over the ACP. ACPs can have a double or single chamber. Double-chamber ACP is more ideal for apheresis treatments, as they allow for separate draw and return access at the same time [7]. Other configurations of ACPs could include two single-chamber ACPs inserted side by side to allow for one ACP to be used for draw access and the other ACP to be used for return access, or one single-chamber ACP could be inserted for apheresis procedures that can be performed with a single needle technique; also, the single-chamber ACP could be used for the draw access, while peripheral venous access could be used for the return. The ACP chamber has a silicone dome to which special access needles are inserted only during the time of each apheresis procedure and then removed in between treatments. ACPs are generally designed to stay in for months to years (depending on the frequency of dome puncture), have a decreased risk of infection compared to NTCVA and TCVA, have no external dislodging risk, and do not have to be kept dry as they are completely internalized under the patient's skin. This allows a patient with ACP to shower, swim, and do more activities without a NTCVA protruding from their chest wall. However, ACP requires interventional radiology or surgery to insert, requires more normal coagulation parameter for insertion than NTCVA, cannot be accessed for apheresis for a few days to weeks after insertion to allow for healing at site, may have some local pain with needle insertion for access, requires thrombolytic medications in some cases to clear local clotting inside the ACP chamber, has risk of venous thrombosis, and are more difficult to remove once apheresis treatment is no longer required or in the event of infection or CVA complication. ACP require rigorous sterile conditions when being accessed to decrease risk of systemic blood infections [8, 9].

The risk of venous thrombosis in patients with NTCVA, TCVA, and ACP needs to be watched closely. This should be considered in patients with malfunctioning access, pain at site of access, swelling in arms and neck or legs (if femoral placement), unexplained tachycardia, shortness of breath, chest discomfort, or even headaches or feeling fullness in face. Symptoms can be subtle in presentation. In patients with thrombotic thrombocytopenic purpura, a rising LDH with otherwise stable platelets, hemoglobin, and even ADAMTS13 level can be an early sign of venous thrombosis. Prophylactic anticoagulation could be considered depending on the patient's thrombosis and bleeding risk. Patients with previous venous thrombosis due to central vascular access and those with sickling disorders and known thrombophilic states should be considered for prophylactic anticoagulation.

There are situations where poor or absent flow rates or frequent pressure alarms may occur when using a NTCVA, TCVA, or ACP for an apheresis procedure. This could be due to poor placement of the catheter (i.e., distal opening port is up against the vessel wall), kinking of the catheter, a clot within the lumen or at the distal opening port, a fibrin sheath covering the exterior of the catheter, or a deep vein thrombosis at the site of the catheter. To address these issues, thrombolytic agents into the lumen of the catheter may clear intraluminal or line tip clots. Radiographic imaging may be required to see if catheter placement needs to be readjusted or replaced, if angioplasty is required for fibrin sheath, or if systemic anticoagulation is required for deep vein thrombosis. Reversing catheter ports (i.e., using the proximal-red port for return and the distal-blue port for draw) can sometimes allow a poor or absent flow rate procedure to be continued in the immediate situation. However, this will result in some recirculation of blood flow that could represent up to 20% of the total blood flow, which will then decrease the efficiency of the procedure [10]. This should not be used as a long-term solution and should be followed up after the immediate apheresis procedure with more definite addressing of the root cause of the catheter problem.

For situations where chronic apheresis treatments are expected without clear endpoint and risks of TCVA or ACP are seen to be significant, an AV fistula or graft could be used. A surgical procedure is required to create an anastomosis between an artery and vein. These can be created in the arm as a brachiocephalic or radiocephalic anastomosis or in the leg as a femoral vein transposition, femoral artery-great saphenous vein looped transposition, or posterior tibial artery-greater saphenous vein. A surgical procedure is required to place a prosthetic graft between an artery and vein for an AV graft. AV fistula/graft has a lower risk of infection or venous thrombosis than CVA devices. However, they require a surgical procedure to create and require weeks (for AV graft) to months (for AV fistula) before they can be used for apheresis; have risks of failure of patency, local clotting or stenosis, reduced peripheral circulation and steal phenomenon; can have post-apheresis procedure bleeding; require specific operator skills to assess and access for each apheresis procedure, and can be a cosmetic issue [11, 12].

Peripherally inserted central catheter (PICC) [13], soft plastic CVA catheters, and non-apheresis-compatible portacaths are not compatible in general for apheresis procedures. These catheters will collapse from negative pressure developed during the apheresis procedure. Some soft plastic CVA catheters and special hard plastic PICC lines used for high-flow infusions of medications or radiographic dye (power PICCs) can be used for extracorporeal photopheresis procedures that can run with lower-flow rates and pressures other than apheresis procedures.

If there is no other clinical reason to use CVA for the apheresis procedure, then assessment for peripheral veins that will allow for adequate apheresis treatment should be made. Median cubital veins are required for the draw access and require 16–19 gauge steel or hard plastic needles that will tolerate the flow rates and negative pressure developed during an apheresis procedure. In fact, hard plastic needles are preferred over steel as they have decreased risk of doing venous damage at the elbow in the event the patient bends their arm significantly during the procedure. The blood flow rate for a 17-gauge needle is approximately 80 mL/min or greater. Smaller-gauge needles have greater resistance to flow as a 19–20 gauge needle provides blood flows around 60 mL/min [11, 14]. The larger gauge will generally allow for faster flow rates. Patients with higher hematocrits, generally above 0.4 or with hyperviscosity, will require draw needles with larger gauges (i.e., 16 gauge) to prevent clotting and poor or stoppage of flow rates during the apheresis procedure. Veins above the elbow (i.e., basilic and cephalic veins) can be used for draw access but require ultrasound guidance to safely access these areas [15]. Return access generally requires 17–19 gauge hard plastic needles, and hand (superficial palmar), forearm (radial), elbow (median cubital) and above elbow (basilic and cephalic) veins can be used. Ideally, separate arms should be used for draw and return access to reduce recirculation, which could decrease the efficiency of the apheresis procedure [11, 14].

While most apheresis procedures require a separate draw and return access, there are a few procedures that can be performed with a single needle access. Some extracorporeal photopheresis procedures, therapeutic apheresis, and red blood cell exchanges can be performed with single needle access. This will prolong the apheresis treatment but does decrease the need for a second peripheral access if that is difficult to achieve [16, 17].

The benefit of PVA is that it is quick to insert; can be done by a trained operator (usually a nurse); supports flow rates required for centrifugal apheresis procedures; has a low complication rate with reduced infection, thrombosis, and bleeding risks; is inexpensive; and can be removed between apheresis treatments. The drawbacks of PVA may include local bruising or hematoma, superficial thrombophlebitis, vasospasm, local nerve injury, and potential to lose access during the apheresis procedure. Recurrent venipuncture may cause patient discomfort, and some patients have difficult peripheral veins to access, which requires an operator who is skilled in venous access [2, 4, 5].

If patient characteristics allow for its use, PVA has a lower risk of all complications and serious complications compared to CVA and thus should always be considered to see if it is a reasonable approach to venous access for apheresis treatment. Even when starting a course of apheresis treatment using PVA, there could be situations that require consideration of switching to CVA. Patients requiring high frequency (i.e., daily) of apheresis treatment especially over extended periods may develop bruising, pain, and swelling at the PVA sites, making this approach more difficult as treatment progresses. Patients with small, fragile, and tortuous veins with few borderline adequate sites may have their limited borderline venous sites blown and damaged with a few PVA attempts and thus lose the ability for further PVA. However, for many patients with adequate peripheral veins, a common course of therapeutic apheresis treatment of 5–7 days can be generally done using PVA [3]. Chronic PVA can lead to sclerosis and thrombosis of the peripheral veins over multiple catheterizations and eventual loss of PVA. Patient preference should also be taken into account [18].

Patient-related non-modifiable factors that increase the difficulty of successful PVA include older age, female gender, previous history of failed venipuncture attempts, recurrent venipunctures, cancer diagnosis, chemotherapy, diabetes, intravenous drug use, limited number of suitable veins, and patient anxiety about venipunctures [19, 20].

Patient-related and modifiable factors to increase the chances of a successful PVA include making sure the patient is adequately hydrated and warmed before access. Techniques or medications to relax the patients as well as educating them in advance as to what to expect can be helpful. Proper pretreatment venous assessment to find the best vein appropriate for the procedure with the least risk of complication and use the smallest gauge needle to allow for the required blood flows can be of help. Topical anesthetics applied to the skin over the planned site of PVA for 45–60 min before venous access can decrease patient experience of pain. Applying cold and compression bandages after the removal of the PVA can decrease bruising, swelling, and pain. Rotation of venipuncture sites to prevent frequent and recurrent access of the same vein can decrease the risk of damage to veins if multiple adequate venous access sites are available on the patient. If clinically possible, spreading out treatments from daily to every second day will decrease repetitive trauma to the vein especially if there are limited good venous locations to use for PVA [21].

Two of the most important modifiable factors to increase the chances of a successful PVA are the skill and experience of the operator performing the PVA and the operator being trained and having access to the technology that will improve the success of PVA attempts.

PVA generally involves visualization and palpation of the vessels of the arms. A successful PVA takes into account the skill of the individual performing the access and their knowledge of the anatomy of the peripheral venous system. Operators with proper training and more experience in PVA will increase the success rates of PVA. Moreover, operators working in teams will allow for second assessments or opinions from other team members prior to a potentially difficult PVA, or the ability to call for backup to assist or take over in PVA if early attempts fail. This can be helpful in reducing the number of unsuccessful PVA attempts, which, in turn, will decrease the risk of damaged vessels rendered temporarily or permanently inaccessible, lessen hematomas which will hinder further PVA success, and lastly, decrease the pain, stress, and frustration to the patient [22, 23].

Regardless of an operator's skill and experience, ultrasound assessment allows for visualization of the location, size, depth, patency, pathway of the peripheral veins, and presence of any venous valves in that location and can differentiate arteries from venous structure. Even veins that appear to be good candidates for PVA by manual inspection and palpation may be demonstrated to be unsuitable for PVA by ultrasound by revealing underlying thrombosis, valves, a tortuous path, or significant proximity to an artery. Ultrasound can be used in this manner to identify the best candidate vein, mark the potential access site on the skin, and then use the marking to cannulate the vein without direct ultrasound visualization. Ultrasound can also be used to identify the target peripheral vein and then keep the ultrasound probe in place to provide continued visual guidance of the needle directly into the vein. This is known as the dynamic needle tip positioning placement technique [15, 24, 25]. Also, ultrasound allows for peripheral access of deeper veins above the elbow (basilic and cephalic) that would otherwise be inaccessible by visualization and palpation techniques alone. Longer needles are required for this type of access, for example, 1.88″ catheters compared to standard 1–1.25″ catheters. Topical anesthetic should be used in advance for this type of access, as there can be more pain associated with this deeper approach and more prolonged pressure above the access site on the skin required after the removal of the peripheral catheter because the site of the venous puncture does not line up with the superficial skin access site [15]. Ultrasound-guided PVA has been shown to decrease the need for CVC access; improve ease and decrease the time to establish access; reduce rates of infection, thrombosis, and bleeding; and decrease the costs compared to CVC insertion [15, 24, 25].

Near-infrared (NIR) imaging devices can be used to assist in the visual mapping of superficial veins to assist in PVA. These devices project NIR light onto the skin, which is then absorbed by deoxygenated hemoglobin, and the vascular image is projected back onto the patient's skin using visible green light. This technique has also shown to increase the ability to gain PVA [26].

In summary, good vascular access is critical for a successful apheresis therapy. Proper assessment of the clinical status of the patient, having a clear plan for the duration and frequency of apheresis treatments, understanding the benefits and risks of different vascular access modalities and taking into account patient preference will improve the success and safety of the treatment. Moreover, keeping an open mind to PVA and methods to increase success of PVA should always be strongly considered when appropriate.

References

1. Kaplan AA. Therapeutic plasma exchange: a technical and operational review. J Clin Apher. 2013;28:3–10.
2. Golestaneh L. Vascular access in therapeutic apheresis: update 2013. J Clin Apher. 2013;28:64–72.
3. Barth D. Peripheral vascular access for therapeutic plasma exchange: a practical approach to increased utilization and selecting the most appropriate vascular access. J Clin Apher. 2020;35:178.
4. Michaud D. Therapeutic plasma exchange. Dynamics. 2001;12:18–24.

5. Kelly L. The family of vascular access devices. J Infect Prev. 2009;10(suppl 1):s7–s12.
6. Gallieni M. Dialysis central venous catheter types and performance. J Vasc Access. 2014;15(Suppl 7):S140–6.
7. Walser E. Venous access ports: Indications, implantation technique, follow-up and complications. Cardiovasc Interv Radiol. 2012;35:751–64.
8. DeSimone N. A tale of two ports: an in vitro comparison of flow characteristics for therapeutic plasma exchange. Transfusion. 2018;58(suppl 1):605–8.
9. Ma L. Totally implantable venous access port systems and associated complications: a single-institution retrospective analysis of 2,996 breast cancer patients. Mol Clin Oncol. 2016;4:456–60.
10. Jones H. Chapter 13. Management of therapeutic apheresis patient. In: McLeod B, editor. Apheresis principles and practice. Vascular access. AABB Press. 2003. pp. 260–264.
11. Kalantari K. The choice of vascular access for therapeutic apheresis. J Clin Apher. 2012;27:153–9.
12. Maya ID. Outcomes of brachiocephalic fistulas, transposed brachiobasilic fistulas and upper arm grafts. Clin J Am Soc Nephrol. 2009;4:86–92.
13. Johansson E. Advantages and disadvantages of peripherally inserted central venous catheters (PICC) compared to other central venous lines; a systematic review of the literature. Acta Oncol. 2013;52:886–92.
14. Ipe TS. Vascular access for therapeutic plasma exchange. Transfusion. 2018;58(suppl 1):580–9.
15. Barth D. The practical integration of a hybrid model of ultrasound guided peripheral venous access in a large apheresis centre. J Clin Apher. 2020;35:328–34.
16. Doggett BM. Single needle: an effective alternative to dual needle peripheral access in therapeutic plasma exchange. J Clin Apher. 2019;34:21–5.
17. Bisaccia E. Safety of a new single integrated closed photopheresis system in patients with cutaneous T cell lymphoma. Br J Dermatol. 2009;161:167–9.
18. Mokrzycki MH. Therapeutic apheresis: a review of complications and recommendations for prevention and management. J Clin Apher. 2011;26:243–8.
19. Carr PJ. Development of a clinical prediction rule to improve peripheral intravenous cannulae first attempt success in the emergency department and reduce post insertion failure rates: the vascular access decisions in the emergency room (VADER) study protocol. BMJ Open. 2016;6:e009196.
20. Armenteros-Yeguas V. Prevalence of difficult venous access and associated risk factors in highly complex hospitalized patients. J Clin Nurs. 2017;26:4267–75.
21. Curtis SJ. Ultrasound or near-infrared vascular imaging to guide peripheral intravenous catheterization in children: a pragmatic randomized control trial. CMAJ. 2015;187:563–70.
22. Sou V. A clinical pathway for the management of difficult venous access. BMC Nurs. 2017;16:64.
23. Gerogianni SK. The role of nurses in therapeutic plasma exchange procedure. Int J Caring Sci. 2015;8:194–200.
24. Hanafusa N. Deep vein puncture under ultrasonographic guidance-an alternative approach for vascular access of apheresis therapies. J Clin Apher. 2015;30:380–1.
25. Gopalasingam N. A successful model to learn and implement ultrasound guided venous catheterization in apheresis. J Clin Apher. 2017;32:437–43.
26. Juric S. An innovative approach to near-infrared spectroscopy using a standard mobile device and its clinical application in the real time visualization of peripheral veins. BMC Med Inform Decis Mak. 2014;14:100.

Problems During Apheresis in Children

9

İkbal Ok Bozkaya and Namık Yaşar Özbek

9.1 Introduction

Childhood is defined as the period from birth to 18 years of age and is divided into infancy, preadolescence, adolescence, and post-adolescence according to the developmental stages. A newborn whose weight is 3–4 kg puts on a considerable weight and typically reaches to 50–70 kg at the end of this period [1]. Since apheresis devices are made for adults, the use of the devices adjusted for adults poses problems, most prominently in infants who have a lower weight and body mass. Therefore, the procedure sometimes requires modifications and should be used cautiously in pediatric patients. Furthermore, the pathophysiology of some diseases in pediatric patients can differ from that in adults, and their response to apheresis treatment may vary considerably. No randomized controlled studies in children were included in the Eighth Guideline of the American Society for Apheresis, which was published in 2019 [2]. Rather, the guideline included only case series of children: 21 publications on therapeutic plasma exchange (TPE) for the diagnosis of acute disseminated encephalomyelitis, acute liver failure, encephalitis, thrombocytopenia-associated multiple organ failure, sepsis, and focal segmental glomerulosclerosis; 3 publications on leukapheresis; and 7 publications on erythrocyte exchange for sickle cell anemia [2–35].

The use of TPE constitutes 70–80% of pediatric apheresis and is becoming widespread as the first treatment option in a broad range of diseases [2]. Disorders in which TPE is used as therapeutic approaches include neurologic, nephrologic, hematologic, rheumatologic, and organ transplantation disorders [2]. In this procedure, pathological substances such as cytokines, antibodies, immune complexes, and endotoxins are removed, and, at the same time, some deficient factors are replaced [1, 2]. However, the use of TPE in pediatric patients is not as common as in adult patients. In addition, due to peculiarities of the procedure and the difficulties arising from the low body mass of children, it is generally implemented only in the specialized centers with an experienced team.

9.2 Difficulties Related to TPE Use in Pediatric Age Groups

Although the pediatric TPE is similar to that in adults in terms of the application of the technique, the procedure has its own difficulties, which are mainly attributable to low body mass.

İ. Ok Bozkaya (✉) · N. Y. Özbek
Pediatric Hematology/Oncology and Pediatric Bone Marrow Transplantation Units and Therapeutic Apheresis Center of The Children Hospital, University of Health Sciences, Ankara Bilkent City Hospital, Ankara, Turkey
e-mail: ikbal.okbozkaya@saglik.gov.tr

I. Kozanoglu (ed.), *Problem Solving in Apheresis Medicine*,
https://doi.org/10.1007/978-3-031-74081-7_9

Another drawback is the lack of knowledge concerning pediatric TPE compared to adults. Accepted guidelines for the use of TPE in adult patients generally indicate at which stage of the disease the procedure should be used. On the other hand, the difference concerning the response to treatment in children treated with TPE is the main obstacle to deciding on its widespread use. Despite recent technological developments, apheresis equipment must still be adapted for children, which increases the likelihood of complications during the procedure [36, 37].

9.3 Problems in Providing Vascular Pathways

According to the guidelines, apheresis procedure usually needs to be repeated more than once. Therefore, adequate vascular access that draws with a high flow rate during apheresis is necessary to achieve and maintain a successful apheresis procedure. To accomplish this goal, a rigid hemodialysis catheter appropriate to the small caliber of the children's vasculature should be placed in the central veins. For this, internal jugular veins, subclavian veins, or femoral veins are most frequently preferred. The smallest catheter that can be used for the procedure is 7 Fr. According to the patient's weight, a hard dialysis catheter of 7 Fr is recommended for children at <10 kg, 8 Fr at 10–20 kg, 9 Fr at 20–50 kg, and more than 9 Fr at >50 kg [38]. In addition to the complications related to sedation or, in some instances, use of anesthesia for catheter insertion, catheter-related thrombosis, infections, and vessel rupture are the most common catheter-related complications in children. Therefore, before making the decision to treat a child using apheresis, the potential benefits and possible complications related to the interventions should be evaluated with the active involvement of the apheresis team, rather than leaving the choice of the most appropriate vascular access and catheter type to the radiologist or surgeon.

9.4 Volume

9.4.1 Extracorporeal Volume

Extracorporeal volume (ECV) represents the volume of blood that leaves the body during the apheresis procedure, which is equal to the sum of whole blood volumes in all disposable sets in the ECV system. Apheresis works in cycles by taking blood, spinning and processing it, and then giving back the unused parts to the donor in a bolus. The effect of the ECV on a patient's homeostasis depends on both the type of apheresis equipment used (filtration or membrane size) and the type of centrifugation, which may be intermittent flow (IF) or continuous flow (CF). In IF, the collection of whole blood, separation of necessary cells, and re-infusion of the unused portion to the patient are conducted at intervals. Meanwhile, in CF, withdrawal, separation, and re-infusion to the patient are performed without interruption. Therefore, a large ECV in the IF method causes hemodynamic fluctuations and a longer duration of the procedure, especially in low-weight children. In CF, the simultaneous collection of blood and the process of re-infusion of the unused parts to the patient by centrifugation makes this procedure a better choice in children [38–40]. Further, CF requires a lower ECV that is more suitable in children with low body weight. Since ECV changes during the procedure will cause hemodynamic changes in patients, it is important to determine the maximum ECV for each patient to ensure procedure safety. If the ECV is greater than 15% of the total blood volume (TBV), the procedure may become symptomatic (e.g., hypotension, tachycardia, circulatory disorders, or dyspnea). In case of severe hypotension developed in a child, the procedure should be temporarily stopped until the vital signs become pre-procedure. When more than 25% of TBV is lost, significant hypotension occurs. Hypotension has been defined as systolic blood pressure <45 mmHg in children under 4 years of age, <75 mmHg in children aged

5–8 years, <85 mmHg in children aged 9–12 years, and <95 mmHg in adolescents. Hypotension caused by hypovolemia should be treated by applying bolus saline or colloid solutions. In this case, the apheresis operating procedure should be changed, or additional measures should be taken. One of the measures to prevent hypovolemia in children is to prime the apheresis set with erythrocyte suspension [38]. The solution of choice for priming is usually saline. If ECV is more than 15% of the TBV, then apheresis sets can be primed with 5% albumin, fresh frozen plasma, or erythrocyte suspension. If red cell prime is used, the packed red blood cell (PRBC) volume needs to be diluted with saline to achieve a hematocrit equal to that of the patients. If the patient is anemic, then the PRBCs can be diluted to a hematocrit higher than the patient's initial hematocrit. Re-infusion should not be more than 15% of the TBV if the rinse-back volume is greater than 15% of the TBV or above the safety limits. The balance of change depends on whether the patient is normo-, hypo-, or hypervolemic [41].

9.4.2 Corporeal Volume

9.4.2.1 Red Blood Cell Volume

Providing sufficient red blood cell (RBC) volume for adequate tissue oxygenation is utmost important for the safety and continuation of the TPE procedure. After the initiation of the apheresis procedure, the ECV fills with the patient's blood, which causes a considerable deficit in the total body volume and continues until blood is returned to the patient [41]. In children who are hemodynamically stable and in whom TBV is sufficiently high, a decrease in RBC volume by the TPE procedure should be well tolerated; however, a reduction in RBC volume can be life-threatening in patients with cardiovascular or pulmonary disorders or in patients at risk for developing organ ischemia and in children with low TBV. It is quite important to determine a safe minimum hematocrit level before this procedure, depending on the clinical condition of the patient. The lower limit of hemoglobin is accepted as 8 g/dL in patients who have stable hemodynamics and sufficient respiratory function; however, in patients who are intubated or experiencing respiratory distress or heart failure, the lower limit of hemoglobin should be increased to 10 g/dL [38]. Therefore, as a general rule, in cases where the ECV is more than 10–15% of TBV, priming with erythrocyte suspension (filling the disposable membrane attached to the apheresis device and the set before the procedure) is recommended. Re-infusion of blood in the apheresis system after the procedure will prevent the decrease in RBC volume and reduce the possible complications in children who have hypotension, cardiac insufficiency, or low hemoglobin values.

9.4.2.2 Intravascular Volume

Continuing the apheresis procedure safely in a child depends on keeping the intravascular volume constant. Volume deficit or excessive volume loading during the procedure may cause undesirable hemodynamic changes, especially in children with cardiac, renal, or hepatic insufficiency, anemia, or dehydration. The hemodynamic effects of blood loss during the apheresis procedure depend on the patient weight, clinical condition, and rate of volume loss. For example, a 15% loss of TBV in a hemodynamically stable children can be tolerated by compensation mechanisms [8]. In cases of more than 15% TBV loss, hypovolemia can be partially tolerated by the activation of metabolic and endocrine mechanisms, for example, increasing cardiac output and vascular tone and decreasing blood flow to the muscles. Conversely, a loss of more than 30% of TBV causes circulatory shock in patients [8–10]. Due to poor hemodynamic adaptation, patients with cardiovascular or multiple organ disease may not tolerate acute hemodilution, even at less than 30% TBV loss [11–14]. Intravascular volume loss during the procedure is primarily dependent on the ECV of the apheresis system. Therefore, before the procedure, the extent of ECV in relation to TBV should be estimated. If apheresis is performed on a child who is hemodynamically or clinically unstable, it is not possible to clinically distinguish hypovolemia that may occur from circulatory disorders. Any procedures for such patients should be carried out under intensive care conditions.

9.4.2.3 Total Blood Volume

An accurate TBV is difficult to determine in children. Many factors, such as health and disease states, physiological states, and body composition, may cause changes in TBV. The TBV can be calculated using several formulas. It is preferred to use mL/kg in accordance with the age group. Average TBVs in young children are 82–86 mL/kg in term newborns, 89–105 mL/kg in premature infants, and 73–82 mL/kg in infants and preschool children [15]. The total body volume is calculated automatically by using automatic cell sorters when the patient's gender, weight, and height are entered into the device. Different devices use different formulas to calculate the TBV, which can cause significant inconsistencies between the TBVs calculated by various devices. It has also been shown that the difference in TBV calculated by the devices in the prepubertal period is less than 1% for women and more than 17% for men. Especially in prepubertal male patients, this difference decreases when their sex is entered as a female [42]. Therefore, the TBV displayed by the equipment should be verified with the formula appropriate for the patient's age group.

9.4.2.4 Volume Shifts

There may be a change in the volume of blood drawn from the patient by the device during the apheresis procedure and returned to the patient after the procedure. Considering the patient's weight and hemodynamic status, volume shifts should be less than or equal to 15% of TBV both during and after the procedure. The extent of the volume shift should be reassessed frequently in small patients, particularly when unexpected intravenous infusions are given or a substantial volume of blood is drawn during the procedure [43].

9.5 Problems with Anticoagulation

Anticoagulation treatment may be needed to ensure extravascular blood flow during the apheresis procedure. Usually, citrate or heparin is used as an anticoagulant. A well-known complication of apheresis in children is citrate toxicity. Young infants or children with liver disease, kidney disease, or shock may experience impaired citrate metabolism and/or delay in citrate excretion. Excess amount of citrate causes hypocalcemia by chelating with calcium. Hypocalcemia can occur when citrate is infused long term or very quickly. It may cause hypotension, arrhythmia, and prolonged QTc and hemodynamic and myocardial depression. The first symptoms of citrate toxicity in adults are perioral numbness and paresthesia of the hands and foots. Children may also feel tingling in the mouth or fingers due to citrate. However, they more often present hypocalcemia with acute abdominal pain and/or vomiting, agitation/irritability, anxiety, pallor, and hypotension attacks. Very young children may not complain of mild symptoms. Thus, mild reactions may not be detected and progress to more serious complications. Finally, babies and children who cannot yet speak may show lip smacking and sucking movements. This may indicate numbness and paresthesia on the lips. In order to determine hypocalcemia in young children, the initial phase of apheresis should be observed carefully; vital signs should be monitored frequently, and ionized calcium levels should be measured periodically. If the plasma ionized calcium level is <0.75 mmol/L, emergency replacement is required. In the presence of "severe" symptoms, or in the presence of ionized calcium level <0.9 mmol/L, intravenous calcium should be given at a dose and rate appropriate to the patient's body size. When infants and children develop serious reactions such as tetany, 0.5–1 mL/kg 10% calcium gluconate should be infused in a period of more than 10 min at a maximum of 10 mL per dose by carefully observing heart rates. Moreover, 10% calcium gluconate can be administered through a large peripheral vein at a maximum rate of 0.6–1.2 mEq/kg/h, at a maximum rate of 0.23 mEq/mL. Since extravasation can cause skin necrosis and peeling, skin veins and tiny hand-foot veins should not be used. In critically ill children, the bioavailability of calcium chloride appears to be superior to calcium gluconate. Also, 10% calcium chloride should be administered centrally because it carries the risk of periphery venous infiltration. According to the level of ionized calcium, 10% calcium chloride should be given as an infusion at a dose of 20 mg/kg (0.2 mL/kg) in more than 10 min. Citrate also chelates with ionized magnesium (Mg++), causing ionized hypomagnesemia. It may cause various cardiovascular abnormalities such as arrhythmias, hypertension, and changes in the electrocardiogram. Therefore, the Mg++ level should also be monitored to ensure that magnesium replacement is also performed when cardiac symptoms do not improve with calcium replacement [38, 41].

9.6 Hypothermia

One of the most important problems during the apheresis procedure is hypothermia due to ECV, which is more frequently seen in patients with low body weight. Especially in children with an ECV of more than 15% TBV, the possibility of developing hypothermia is high. To prevent this, a blood warmer, parent's lap, or a bed warmer can be used. Volume changes in heaters connected to the apheresis set, which cause an increase in ECV, should be closely monitored [38, 41].

Blood warming devices should be equipped with temperature-sensing devices and warning systems to detect malfunctions and prevent hemolysis or other damage to blood or blood components. Heating blood to less than or equal to 43 °C appears to be safe without significant hemolysis. Hemolysis increases as blood is warmed to greater than 46 °C. Other factors that contribute to hemolysis during warming are duration of storage, anticoagulant, duration of exposure to heat, and elements of the warming system. Blood warmers have several limitations in that the rate of infusion can be impeded by the additional tubing and blood warming bags, and they require substantial priming volumes that may make them unsuitable for small-volume transfusions [1, 44].

9.7 Psychological Considerations

The apheresis procedure takes approximately 2–3 h and may be repeated in some patients. Being immobile during this period and interventions may cause anxiety in children. Therefore, an individual approach to each patient is very important. Information should also be established by considering the developmental age of the patient, rather than the chronological age.

Infants (newborn to 12 months): The apheresis specialist should try to lower parental anxiety, thereby reducing the child's anxiety by explaining the need, benefits, and risks of the procedure to the parent. The baby should be surrounded by familiar home objects and familiar caregivers during the procedure. When possible, the baby's hands should be free to explore, and restraints should only be used to avoid self-induced injury and/or trauma to the intravenous or access site.

Toddler years (1–3 years): The specialist should also try to minimize parental anxiety and consequent child anxiety at this age group by explaining the need, benefits, and risks of the procedure. Dolls and toys may be used to depersonalize the illness. The child should be reassured that the illness is not a punishment, and any extraneous information including mention of internal organs should be avoided. The procedure should be described to the toddler just before starting, focusing on the reason for the procedure (i.e., relief of symptoms).

Preschool age (3–6 years): The apheresis specialist should again prepare the parents, use concrete terms with the child, describe all objects in terms of function, use body image outline and dolls if appropriate, focus on relief of symptoms, and teach the child signs of possible reaction and when to call the nurse (i.e., “I feel funny,” “I feel cold,” etc.).

School age (7–10 years): The specialist should use body outlines and technical names for body parts and equipment, inform the child of benefits and hazards of the procedure, teach signs and symptoms of a reaction, and emphasize the need to notify the nurse or apheresis specialist for any symptoms.

Preadolescent age (10–13 years): The apheresis specialist should prepare the child as in the school age period, allow sufficient time for questions, and clarify any misconceptions.

Adolescent age (13 and older): It is important to prepare the child as in the preadolescent age and, additionally, allow the adolescent to have control of scheduling if possible. Instrument and processes should be described in scientific terms. In addition, the adolescent should be included in all discussions, and there should be a discussion as to why the procedure is required. The incorporation of threats to body image should occur at an acceptable pace. Use of distraction, involvement of child life specialists, and parental/familial involvement are also important in lowering a child's anxiety, especially for younger patients. Regardless of patient agitation or cooperation, sedation is recommended in the presence of medically indicated symptoms, such as frequent seizures or neuromuscular instability [45].

To summarize, it is recommended that individuals involved in conducting the procedure do the following:

- Give detailed information to the patient and patient relatives before the procedure.
- Introduce the apheresis device.
- Arrange the apheresis environment in such a way that the patient can relax.
- Let the child and their parents be present in the same environment, if necessary.
- Give small gifts and prizes to the patient when the procedure is finished.
- Demonstrate to older children how the machines work to help them adapt to the process more easily [38].

References

1. Paglialonga F, Schmitt CP, Shroff R, Vondrak K, Aufricht C, Watson AR, et al. Indications, technique, and outcome of therapeutic apheresis in European pediatric nephrology units. Pediatr Nephrol. 2015;30(1):103–11.
2. Padmanabhan A, Connelly-Smith L, Aqui N, Balogun RA, Klingel R, Meyer E, et al. Guidelines on the use of therapeutic apheresis in clinical practice—Evidence-based approach from the Writing Committee of the American Society for Apheresis: the eighth special issue. J Clin Apher. 2019;34(3):171–354.
3. DeSena AD, Greenberg BM, Graves D. Three phenotypes of anti-N-methyl-D-aspartate receptor antibody encephalitis in children: prevalence of symptoms and prognosis. Pediatr Neurol. 2014;51(4):542–9.
4. Khurana DS, Melvin JJ, Kothare SV, Valencia I, Hardison HH, Yum S, et al. Acute disseminated encephalomyelitis in children: discordant neurologic and neuroimaging abnormalities and response to plasmapheresis. Pediatrics. 2005;116(2):431–6.
5. Huang Q, Wu Y, Qin R, Wei X, Ma M. Clinical characteristics and outcomes between children and adults with anti-N-methyl-D-aspartate receptor encephalitis. J Neurol. 2016;263(12):2446–55.
6. Hattori M, Chikamoto H, Akioka Y, Nakakura H, Ogino D, Matsunaga A, et al. A combined low-density lipoprotein apheresis and prednisone therapy for steroid-resistant primary focal segmental glomerulosclerosis in children. Am J Kidney Dis. 2003;42(6):1121–30.
7. Saylors RL, Watkins B, Saccente S, Tang X. Comparison of automated red cell exchange transfusion and simple transfusion for the treatment of children with sickle cell disease acute chest syndrome. Pediatr Blood Cancer. 2013;60(12):1952–6.
8. Schaefer B, Schaefer F, Engelmann G, Meyburg J, Heckert KH, Zorn M, et al. Comparison of molecular adsorbents recirculating system (MARS) dialysis with combined plasma exchange and hemodialysis in children with acute liver failure. Nephrol Dial Transplant. 2011;26(11):3633–9.
9. Eguiguren JM, Schell MJ, Crist WM, Kunkel K, Rivera GK. Complications and outcome in childhood acute lymphoblastic leukemia with hyperleukocytosis. Blood. 1992;79(4):871–5.
10. Byrne S, Walsh C, Hacohen Y, Muscal E, Jankovic J, Stocco A, et al. Earlier treatment of NMDAR antibody encephalitis in children results in a better outcome. Neurol Neuroimmunol Neuroinflamm. 2015;2(4):e130.
11. Lowe EJ, Pui CH, Hancock ML, Geiger TL, Khan RB, Sandlund JT. Early complications in children with acute lymphoblastic leukemia presenting with hyperleukocytosis. Pediatr Blood Cancer. 2005;45(1):10–5.
12. Wang CF, Nie XJ, Chen GM, Yu ZH, Li Z, Sun ZW, et al. Early plasma exchange for treating ricin toxicity

in children after castor bean ingestion. J Clin Apher. 2015;30(3):141–6.
13. Maurer HS, Steinherz PG, Gaynon PS, Finklestein JZ, Sather HN, Reaman GH, et al. The effect of initial management of hyperleukocytosis on early complications and outcome of children with acute lymphoblastic leukemia. J Clin Oncol. 1988;6(9):1425–32.
14. Velasquez MP, Mariscalco MM, Goldstein SL, Airewele GE. Erythrocytapheresis in children with sickle cell disease and acute chest syndrome. Pediatr Blood Cancer. 2009;53(6):1060–3.
15. Hulbert ML, Scothorn DJ, Panepinto JA, Scott JP, Buchanan GR, Sarnaik S, et al. Exchange blood transfusion compared with simple transfusion for first overt stroke is associated with a lower risk of subsequent stroke: a retrospective cohort study of 137 children with sickle cell anemia. J Pediatr. 2006;149(5):710–2.
16. Valavi E, Ahmadzadeh A, Amoori P, Daneshgar A. High frequency of acquired ADAMTS13 deficiency after hemolysis in Hemiscorpius Lepturus (scorpion) stung children. Indian J Pediatr. 2014;81(7):665–9.
17. Sharma R, Woods GM, Creary S, O'Brien S, Stanek J, Hor K, et al. Impact of erythrocytapheresis on natural anticoagulant levels in children with sickle cell disease: a pilot study. Pediatr Blood Cancer. 2019;66(4):e27588.
18. Bavle A, Raj A, Kong M, Bertolone S. Impact of long-term erythrocytapheresis on growth and peak height velocity of children with sickle cell disease. Pediatr Blood Cancer. 2014;61(11):2024–30.
19. Nguyen TC, Han YY, Kiss JE, Hall MW, Hassett AC, Jaffe R, et al. Intensive plasma exchange increases a disintegrin and metalloprotease with thrombospondin motifs-13 activity and reverses organ dysfunction in children with thrombocytopenia-associated multiple organ failure. Crit Care Med. 2008;36(10):2878–87.
20. Duclos C, Merlin E, Paillard C, Thuret I, Demeocq F, Michel G, et al. Long-term red blood cell exchange in children with sickle cell disease: manual or automatic? Transfus Apher Sci. 2013;48(2):219–22.
21. Gregorowski C, Lochner C, Martin L, Simmons C, Kidd M, Walker K, et al. Neuropsychological manifestations in children with Sydenham's chorea after adjunct intravenous immunoglobulin and standard treatment. Metab Brain Dis. 2016;31(1):205–12.
22. Koizumi K, Hoshiai M, Toda T, Katsumata N, Kise H, Hasebe Y, et al. Outcomes of plasma exchange for severe dilated cardiomyopathy in children. Heart Vessels. 2017;32(1):61–7.
23. Moriguchi T, Koizumi K, Matsuda K, Harii N, Goto J, Harada D, et al. Plasma exchange for the patients with dilated cardiomyopathy in children is safe and effective in improving both cardiac function and daily activities. J Artif Organs. 2017;20(3):236–43.
24. Basaran O, Cakar N, Uncu N, Celikel BA, Kara A, Cayci FS, et al. Plasma exchange therapy for severe gastrointestinal involvement of Henoch Schonlein purpura in children. Clin Exp Rheumatol. 2015;33(2 Suppl 89):S176–80.
25. Hattori M, Ito K, Konomoto T, Kawaguchi H, Yoshioka T, Khono M. Plasmapheresis as the sole therapy for rapidly progressive Henoch-Schonlein purpura nephritis in children. Am J Kidney Dis. 1999;33(3):427–33.
26. Sinha A, Gulati A, Saini S, Blanc C, Gupta A, Gurjar BS, et al. Prompt plasma exchanges and immunosuppressive treatment improves the outcomes of anti-factor H autoantibody-associated hemolytic uremic syndrome in children. Kidney Int. 2014;85(5):1151–60.
27. Suleiman J, Dale RC. The recognition and treatment of autoimmune epilepsy in children. Dev Med Child Neurol. 2015;57(5):431–40.
28. Fencl F, Vondrak K, Rosik T, Zieg J, Chadimova M, Hacek J, et al. Recurrence of nephrotic proteinuria in children with focal segmental glomerulosclerosis: early treatment with plasmapheresis and immunoadsorption should be associated with better prognosis. Minerva Pediatr. 2016;68(5):348–54.
29. Singer AL, Olthoff KM, Kim H, Rand E, Zamir G, Shaked A. Role of plasmapheresis in the management of acute hepatic failure in children. Ann Surg. 2001;234(3):418–24.
30. Latimer ME, L'Etoile N, Seidlitz J, Swedo SE. Therapeutic plasma apheresis as a treatment for 35 severely ill children and adolescents with pediatric autoimmune neuropsychiatric disorders associated with streptococcal infections. J Child Adolesc Psychopharmacol. 2015;25(1):70–5.
31. Borras-Novell C, Garcia Rey E, Perez Baena LF, Jordan Garcia I, Catella Cahiz D, Cambra F. Therapeutic plasma exchange in acute disseminated encephalomyelitis in children. J Clin Apher. 2015;30(6):335–9.
32. Fortenberry JD, Nguyen T, Grunwell JR, Aneja RK, Wheeler D, Hall M, et al. Therapeutic plasma exchange in children with thrombocytopenia-associated multiple organ failure: the thrombocytopenia-associated multiple organ failure network prospective experience. Crit Care Med. 2019;47(3):e173–e81.
33. Zekeridou A, Karantoni E, Viaccoz A, Ducray F, Gitiaux C, Villega F, et al. Treatment and outcome of children and adolescents with N-methyl-D-aspartate receptor encephalitis. J Neurol. 2015;262(8):1859–66.
34. Lima LM, McCracken CE, Fortenberry JD, Hebbar KB. Use of plasma exchange in pediatric severe sepsis in children's hospitals. J Crit Care. 2018;45:114–20.
35. Sevketoglu E, Yildizdas D, Horoz OO, Kihtir HS, Kendirli T, Bayraktar S, et al. Use of therapeutic plasma exchange in children with thrombocytopenia-associated multiple organ failure in the Turkish thrombocytopenia-associated multiple organ failure network. Pediatr Crit Care Med. 2014;15(8):e354–9.
36. Fosburg M, Dolan M, Propper R, Wolfe L, Kevy S. Intensive plasma exchange in small and critically ill pediatric patients: techniques and clinical outcome. J Clin Apher. 1983;1(4):215–24.
37. Stefanutti C, Lanti A, Di Giacomo S, Mareri M, De Lorenzo F, Landolfo A, et al. Therapeutic apheresis

in low weight patients: technical feasibility, tolerance, compliance, and risks. Transfus Apher Sci. 2004;31(1):3–10.
38. Kim HC. Therapeutic pediatric apheresis. J Clin Apher. 2000;15(1–2):129–57.
39. Vidal E, Garzotto F, Parolin M, Manenti C, Zanin A, Bellettato M, et al. Therapeutic plasma exchange in neonates and infants: successful use of a miniaturized machine. Blood Purif. 2017;44(2):100–5.
40. Greze V, Rouel N, Rochette E, Merlin E, Halle P, Plantaz D, et al. Peripheral blood stem cell collection in children with extremely low body weight (</=8 kg). What have we learned over the past 25 years and where are the limits? J Clin Apher. 2021;36(3):322–31.
41. Goldstein SL. Therapeutic apheresis in children: special considerations. Semin Dial. 2012;25(2):165–70.
42. Colavita D, Kim HC, Friedman DF. The sex parameter in estimation of total blood volume for pediatric erythrocytapheresis. J Clin Apher. 2019;34(6):692–9.
43. Meyer EK, Wong EC. Pediatric therapeutic apheresis: a critical appraisal of evidence. Transfus Med Rev. 2016;30(4):217–22.
44. McCullough J. Transfusion medicine. Hoboken: Wiley; 2021.
45. Wong EC, Balogun RA. Therapeutic apheresis in pediatrics: technique adjustments, indications and nonindications, a plasma exchange focus. J Clin Apher. 2012;27(3):132–7.

Problems During the Usage and Dosage of Anticoagulants

10

Eylem Eliacik

10.1 Background

Anticoagulation is necessary to prevent blood clotting in the extracorporeal circulation during the apheresis procedure. Citrate is the most commonly preferred anticoagulant worldwide due to its efficacy and safety for apheresis, while unfractionated heparin (UH) is the second most preferred. Administration of an anticoagulant during apheresis is necessary to avoid circuit clotting and impaired treatment effectiveness. However, anticoagulation has also been associated with electrolyte imbalances and bleeding. The frequency and types of complications demonstrate the differences based on the patient's general conditions, the number of procedures, and replacement fluids. More than 20,000 therapeutic apheresis procedures were reported by the Swedish Apheresis Group. The results showed that the incidence of adverse events was low (Grade I: mild 1.5%, Grade II: moderate 2.8%, Grade III: severe 0.8%, and Grade IV: fatal events 0%) [1].

The Canadian Apheresis Study Group reported 403 (7.7%) complications of using citrate (muscle cramps, paresthesias, nausea, vomiting, abdominal pain, chills, and fever) during 5235 plasma exchanges of procedures [2].

E. Eliacik (✉)
Hematology Department, Kahramanmaras Sutcu Imam University School of Medicine, Kahramanmaras, Turkey
e-mail: eylemeliacik@ksu.edu.tr

Citrate-related complications have been reported to occur in the following: 1.2% of donors during voluntary donation, 7.8% of patients undergoing therapeutic plasma exchange procedures, and 48% of patients undergoing large-volume leukapheresis during peripheral blood progenitor cell collection [3, 4]. Although extremely rare, severe hypocalcemia may develop during apheresis, particularly during large-volume exchanges.

Thus, the major complication of UH therapy is bleeding (major bleeding 0–7%, fatal bleeding 0–3%). Other complications include heparin-induced thrombocytopenia (HIT 1–5%) and osteoporosis (2–3% risk of vertebral fracture with >1 month treatment) [5].

10.2 Citrate Anticoagulation

Citrate has many characteristics of the ideal anticoagulant for apheresis. Citrate is a regional anticoagulant, effective in the extracorporeal area, and is neutralized as soon as it enters the body and does not increase the risk of systemic bleeding. Citrate ions chelate calcium ions and block many steps in the clotting of cascade-dependent $Ca+2$. The conformational changes of the coagulation factors V and VIII are triggered by the chelation of calcium [6].

I. Kozanoglu (ed.), *Problem Solving in Apheresis Medicine*,
https://doi.org/10.1007/978-3-031-74081-7_10

10.2.1 Citrate Metabolism

Citrate is metabolized in the Krebs cycle in the liver, muscles, and kidneys. The metabolism of one citrate molecule results in the release of three molecules of bicarbonate, which then contributes to blood alkalinity [7]. Approximately 18–20% of infused citrate remains unmetabolized and is excreted by the kidneys [8, 9]. In the presence of normal liver function, citrate is generally metabolized within approximately 1.5 h [10].

10.2.2 Citrate Formulas and Doses

Two citrate solutions, that is, acid-citrate-dextrose (ACD) A (ACD-A) and ACD-B, are used in apheresis [11]. These solutions have different citrate proportions. ACD-A contains 3% citrate, whereas ACD-B has 2% citrate [12, 13]. In order to have sufficient anticoagulation, the citrate infusion ratio is determined as higher than its removal. This is applied because donors can generally tolerate up to a 20% decline in ionized calcium levels, and higher infusion rates permit shorter runs [13]. However, the effect of infused citrate on plasma levels of Ca+2 depends on the rate of citrate infusion, redistribution into extravascular fluids, diffusion into cells, renal excretion, and intracellular metabolism to other organic compounds that do not chelate Ca+2 [14, 15]. Dilution and redistribution throughout the total extracellular fluid provide the first line of defense against high levels of citrate ions.

For effective apheresis procedures, the dose of anticoagulation should be adjusted according to the patient's defined conditions. Anticoagulant (AC) infusion rate (mL/min/L TBV) is calculated by using total blood volume (TBV) by instruments automatically.

To stabilize ionized calcium levels, citrate delivery rates are arranged between 1.0 and 1.8 mg/kg/min [16]. According to studies, ionized calcium values show decreases of 10–15%, 15–25%, and 20–35%, when AC infusion rates are 0.8, 1.0, and 1.2 mL ACD-A/min/L TBV, respectively [11]. Inlet pump rate, AC flow rate, and/or the whole blood (WB)/AC ratio are three parameters that affect citrate concentrate in the circuit. An inlet pump delivers citrate blood to the centrifuge, which is then infused into the patient. The AC flow rate is the rate at which citrate is infused from the ACD-A bag to the inlet line containing the patient's blood. Increases in AC flow rate also increase citrate delivery to the circuit. In addition to these technical variables, the pump speed, the duration of the procedure, replacement fluids that contain citrate (e.g., FFP and RBC), and apheresis equipment are the other factors that control the amount of citrate [17, 18].

10.2.3 Adverse Effects of Citrate

Side effects/toxicity related to the use of citrate can be detected early and easily intervened by an experienced apheresis team. Since citrate binds to free calcium, the most frequent side effects are symptoms of hypocalcemia. Transient episodes of hypocalcemia associated with apheresis usually are well tolerated [19]. Symptoms of hypocalcemia occur when ionized calcium falls below the normal levels. Although complication rates are reported with different numbers in the literature (5–36%), they are generally below 5% [3, 6, 20]. The most common side effect is paranesthesia associated with hypocalcemia.

It may be in the form of headache, nervousness, irritability, drowsiness, nausea, vomiting, flushing, chest discomfort, and abdominal cramps [19–21]. Hypocalcemia can also trigger neuromuscular symptoms: loss of deep tendon reflexes, dysesthesia, muscle cramps, tremors, perioral and acral paraesthesias, involuntary muscle cramps, carpopedal spasm or tetany, laryngospasm, and even seizures may occur as the severity increases. At the same time, hypocalcemia can affect cardiac function. QT prolongation can be seen on EKG [22–24]. Although very rare, fatal arrhythmias have been reported in apheresis patients [25, 26].

10.2.4 Management of Citrate Toxicity

Citrate has a very specific antidote—calcium. Oral or intravenous calcium supplementation is recommended depending on ionized calcium levels and/or the presence of hypocalcemia symptoms [27]. Intravenous calcium infusion is preferred for patients who cannot tolerate oral calcium or have high citrate sensitivity such as patients with altered mental status and the pediatric group. Administration of 5–10 mL of 10% calcium gluconate intravenously over 10–15 min (IV push) is effective in reducing symptoms. In fact, prophylactic use of calcium will reduce the incidence of citrate-related hypocalcemia by less than 1% [20, 22, 23].

When blood products that have additive citrate are used as a replacement fluid, the risk of citrate-related complications may increase. Citrate toxicity may occur more frequently in patients who have impaired liver or renal function, or have low calcium levels, and the pediatric group [12]. Citrate does not cause systemic anticoagulation, so its use is not associated with a higher risk of hemorrhages [28].

10.3 Heparin Anticoagulation

Heparin prevents coagulation by binding to antithrombin III, which then inactivates coagulation enzymes thrombin and factor X. UH requires continuous infusions; activated partial prothrombin time (aPTT) monitoring is required when using UH. Heparin is metabolized mainly by the reticuloendothelial system. A low percentage of unchanged heparin is also excreted in the urine.

Heparin anticoagulation is preferred for pediatric apheresis, large-volume leukapheresis, membrane-based plasma exchange, LDL apheresis, and photopheresis [4, 29].

In contrast to citrate, heparin acts as a systemic anticoagulant due to its slow metabolization. Heparin overdose may cause prolongation of aPTT or bleeding. Hemorrhagic episodes are associated with the intensity of anticoagulation, concomitant use of antiplatelet therapy, gender (female > male), and comorbidities such as recent surgical or interventional procedures and coexisting hemostatic defects [30, 31].

The use of heparin is associated with more bleeding complications and the risk of developing heparin-related thrombocytopenia [22]. Moreover, heparin-induced thrombocytopenia should always be considered in case of unexplained thrombocytopenia and/or thrombosis [32].

Heparin can be used with ACD solution (5000 units to 500 mL ACD-A bag). Combining heparin with citrate anticoagulation does not eliminate citrate reactions; in one study, 39% of patients still experienced paresthesia due to citrate-related hypocalcemia [33].

Moreover, protamine sulfate is an antagonist of heparin.

While the apheresis procedure is planned, the patient should be evaluated in detail, especially before and during the procedure, to treat the patient effectively and to minimize the risk of complications. Calculations must be evaluated carefully, and each step of the process must be carefully applied.

References

1. Mokrzycki MH, Balogun RA. Therapeutic apheresis: a review of complications and recommendations for prevention and management. J Clin Apher. 2011;26(5):243–8.
2. Sutton DMC, Nair RC, Rock G, The Canadian Apheresis Study Group. Complications of plasma exchange. Transfusion. 1989;29:124–7.
3. Rodnitzky RL, Goeken JA. Complications of plasma exchange in neurological patients. Arch Neurol. 1982;39:350–4. [PubMed: 7092611].
4. Buchta C, Macher M, Bieglmayer C, Hocker P, Dettke M. Reduction of adverse citrate reactions during autologous large-volume PBPC apheresis by continuous infusion of calcium-gluconate. Transfusion. 2003;43:1615–21. [PubMed: 14617323].
5. Hirsh J, Bauer KA, Donati MB, Gould M, Samama MM, Weitz JI. Parenteral anticoagulants: American College of Chest Physicians Evidence-Based Clinical Practice Guidelines (8th edition). Chest. 2008;133:141S–59. [PubMed: 18574264].
6. Strauss RG. Mechanisms of adverse effects during hemapheresis. J Clin Apher. 1996;11:160–4. [PubMed: 8915821].

7. Flanigan MJ, Pillsbury L, Sadewasser G, Lim VS. Regional hemodialysis anticoagulation: hypertonic tri-sodium citrate or anticoagulant citrate dextrose-A. Am J Kidney Dis. 1996;27:519–24. [PubMed: 8678062].
8. Ludbrook J, Wynn V. Citrate intoxication; a clinical and experimental study. Br Med J. 1958;2:523–8. [PubMed: 13572825].
9. Farrokhi P, Farahmand H, Bismuth A, et al. How to stabilize the level of ionized calcium and citrate during plateletpheresis. Vox Sang. 1998;74:7–12. [PubMed: 9481853].
10. Kramer L, Bauer E, Joukhadar C, et al. Citrate pharmacokinetics and metabolism in cirrhotic and noncirrhotic critically ill patients. Crit Care Med. 2003;31:2450–5. [PubMed: 14530750].
11. Kishimoto M, Ohto H, Shikama Y, Kikuta A, Kimijima I, Takenoshita S. Treatment for the decline of ionized calcium levels during peripheral blood progenitor cell harvesting. Transfusion. 2002;42:1340.
12. Marques MB, Huang ST. Patients with thrombotic thrombocytopenic purpura commonly develop metabolic alkalosis during therapeutic plasma exchange. J Clin Apher. 2001;16:120–4. [PubMed: 11746537].
13. Hester JP, McCullough J, Mishler JM, Szymanski IO. Dosage regimens for citrate anticoagulants. J Clin Apher. 1983;1:149–57. [PubMed: 6546053].
14. Crookston KP, Novak DJ. Physiology of apheresis. In: McLeod BC, Szczepiorkowski ZM, Weinstein R, Winters JL, editors. Apheresis: principles and practice. Bethesda: AABB Press; 2010. p. 45–69.
15. Lee G, Arepally GM. J Clin Apher. 2012;27(3):117–25.
16. Weinstein R. Prevention of citrate reactions during therapeutic plasma exchange by constant infusion of calcium gluconate with the return fluid. J Clin Apher. 1996;11:204–10. [PubMed: 8986866].
17. Hester JP, Ayyar R. Anticoagulation and electrolytes. J Clin Apher. 1984;2:41–51. [PubMed: 6536658].
18. Penny A. Plasmapheresis procedure design operation: a consideration of citrate anticoagulant usage. Transfus Sci. 1989;10:51–6.
19. Puig LI, Mazzara R, Torras A, Castillo R. Adverse effects secondary to the treatment with plasma exchange. Int J Artif Org. 1985;8:155–8.
20. Strewler GJ, Rosenblatt M. Mineral metabolism. In: Felig P, Baxter JD, Frohman LA, editors. Endocrinology and metabolism. New York: McGraw-Hill; 1995. p. 1407–89.
21. Ziselman EM, Bongiovanni MB, Wurzel HA. The complications of therapeutic plasma exchange. Vox Sang. 1984;46:270–6.
22. Szymanski IO. Ionized calcium during plateletpheresis. Transfusion. 1978;18:701–8.
23. Olson PR, Cox C, McCullough J. Laboratory and clinical effects of the infusion of ACD solution during plateletpheresis. Vox Sang. 1977;33(2):79–87.
24. Mishler JM, Janes AW, Lowes B, Farfan C, Emerson PM. The utilization of a new strength citrate anticoagulant during centrifugal plateletpheresis. I. Assessment of donors effects. Br J Haematol. 1976;34:387–94.
25. Bunker JP, Bendixen HH, Murphy AJ. Hemodynamic effects of intravenously administered sodium citrate. N Engl J Med. 1962;266:372–7.
26. Klein HG. Therapeutic hemapheresis. In: Petz LD, Swisher SN, Kleinman S, Spence RK, Strauss RG, editors. Clinical practice of transfusion medicine. 3rd ed. New York: Churchill Livingstone; 1996. p. 1011–22.
27. Huestis DW. Risks and safety practices in hemapheresis procedures. Arch Pathol Lab Med. 1989;113:273–8.
28. McLeod BC. Apheresis: principles and practice. Bethesda: AAABB Press; 2003.
29. Bolan CD, Cecco SA, Wesley RA, et al. Controlled study of citrate effects and response to i.v. calcium administration during allogeneic peripheral blood progenitor cell donation. Transfusion. 2002;42:935–46. [PubMed: 12375668].
30. Schulman S, Beyth RJ, Kearon C, Levine MN. Hemorrhagic complications of anticoagulant and thrombolytic treatment: American College of Chest Physicians Evidence-Based Clinical Practice Guidelines (8th edition). Chest. 2008;133:257S–98S. [PubMed: 18574268].
31. Arepally GM, Ortel TL. Heparin-induced thrombocytopenia. Annu Rev Med. 2010;61:77–90.
32. Van de Wetering J, Westendorp RG, van der Hoeven JG, Stolk B, Feuth JD, Chang PC. Heparin use in continuous renal replacement procedures: the struggle between filter coagulation and patient hemorrhage. J Am Soc Nephrol. 1996;7:145–50. [PubMed: 8808122].
33. Reik RA, Noto TA, Fernandez HF. Safety of large-volume leukapheresis for collection of peripheral blood progenitor cells. J Clin Apher. 1997;12:10–3. [PubMed: 9097229].

Complications and How to Avoid Them During Apheresis

11

Ilknur Kozanoğlu

11.1 Background

Apheresis is used to obtain blood products such as plasma, platelets, and granulocytes from healthy people (voluntary blood donors). However, today, in addition to obtaining blood products, it has also found use in the treatment of various hematological and non-hematological diseases [1–3].

Severe complications rarely develop during apheresis (Table 11.1). In fact, in multicenter studies, the frequency of complications during apheresis was generally determined to be 3.9–4.75% [1–3]. In these studies, more than half of the complications recover with minor interventions, while the rate of complications serious enough to require the apheresis procedure to be stopped was noted to be 1% [1–3]. It has been observed that some complications occur less frequently when platelet apheresis is performed from volunteer blood donors who have previously received whole blood. For example, the rate of vasovagal syncope observed in volunteer blood donors who donated whole blood as their first blood product donation was lower when they subsequently donated platelet suspensions by apheresis. Similarly, hypotension is less common during apheresis. This is explained by the longer duration of apheresis compared to blood donation, which then facilitates the body's adaptation to hypovolemia [4]. The severe complications associated with apheresis occur in patients undergoing therapeutic apheresis rather than in voluntary blood donors. For example, numbness and tingling around the mouth and lips is a common complication during thrombopheresis from volunteer blood donors. However, the incidence rate of serious complications is higher than that during whole blood donation. Adverse events (AEs) were categorized into four grades: mild (if the AE was tolerated without medication), moderate (if the AE required medication), severe (if the AE required discontinuation of TA), or death (if the AE was responsible for the patient's death). A good knowledge of these complications can help to prevent them or to minimize their severity [4].

This chapter describes the complications that may occur in apheresis procedures, the management of these complications, and the recommendations to be made to reduce the side effects to a minimum.

I. Kozanoğlu (✉)
Adana Adult BMT Center, Baskent University, Adana, Türkiye

Acibadem Labmed Medical Laboratories, Hematology Laboratories, Istanbul, Türkiye
e-mail: ilknur.kozanoglu@acibademlabmed.com.tr

I. Kozanoglu (ed.), *Problem Solving in Apheresis Medicine*,
https://doi.org/10.1007/978-3-031-74081-7_11

Table 11.1 The most common complications associated with apheresis procedure

Apheresis-related complications	
• Associated with the vascular access	• Traumatic hemolysis
• Associated with circulatory system	• Infections
• Associated with citrate toxicity	• Lymphocytes, coagulation factors, plasma
• Technical side effects	• Decrease in proteins
• Allergic reactions	• Apheresis-related death
• Respiratory impairment, shortness of breath	• Disturbance in drug pharmacodynamics

11.2 Complications Related to Vascular Access

A good vascular access is one of the most important factors in the success of apheresis. In voluntary whole blood donors, venous access is established by means of 16-gauge "angiocut" or arteriovenous cannulas into superficial veins on the inner side of the forearm [3, 5]. During the insertion of these cannulas, skin hemorrhages, ecchymosis, and sometimes hematoma may occur, particularly in people with a tendency to bleed. This rare complication can be controlled using a hirudin pomade and an alcohol swab. Large-diameter cannulas remaining in the vein for more than 1 h of apheresis procedure increase the risk of venous spasm and collapse [3, 5].

If the venous veins on the inner side of the forearm are suitable for apheresis, they can be used as a vascular access for people who will undergo therapeutic apheresis. For this purpose, 20-gauge "angiocut" or arteriovenous cannulas can be used [6]. However, peripheral veins may not be suitable for long or multiple apheresis procedures. In this case, central venous catheters (CVC) placed in the vena jugularis, vena cava superior, or vena femoralis are preferred. In apheresis complications, most of the complications related to the vascular access are related to these CVCs [6].

A complication rate of 0.4% has been reported during catheter placement. Large vessel and even cardiac perforations, arteriovenous fistula development, and deep dissecting hematomas are reported in case reports. Pneumothorax, hemothorax, and hemorrhage may develop during catheter insertion. Thrombus may form after insertion or during withdrawal. Embolism may occur when this thrombus ruptures. Bacterial colonization may occur inside the catheter, which then may lead to septicemia. Cellulitis or tunnel infection may develop in the tissue where the catheter is inserted [7–11].

Reduced blood flow: Inability to maintain adequate pressure for apheresis has been determined to be the most common problem. It is usually caused by kinking of the CVC inside or outside the body and/or collapse or spasm of the vessel.

In cases where sufficient pressure for apheresis cannot be achieved, the blood flow rate can be increased with some of the following maneuvers [7] (Table 11.2):

1. The patient's arm is raised above the head and made to cough.
2. The patient is turned from one side to the other.
3. As the tip of the catheter may be resting against the vessel wall, it can be removed.
    - Saline is given.
    - The catheter can be gently withdrawn. This procedure can only be performed by an experienced surgeon.
4. The ends of the catheter are changed to allow blood to be taken in and out.

Despite these maneuvers, the blood flow rate may not be increased. In this case, the CVC may have to be removed and reinserted.

Sudden pressure reduction: If blood can be drawn from the catheter, this may be caused by the collapse of the vessel or a spasm of the vessel. In this case, the pump speed of the device is reduced, and the initial flow rate is slowly increased [7].

Table 11.2 Possible causes of symptoms and signs encountered during apheresis procedures and treatment approach

Symptoms and signs	Possible causes	Recommended treatment
Bradycardia ($N < 60$/min), hypotension, diaphoresis, nausea, vomiting, feeling of weakness	Vasovagal reaction, anxiety, bladder fullness	Place the patient in Trendelenburg position (if the seat is suitable, the patient's feet can be lifted so that the patient's head is upside down), rapid physiological saline to the patient, stimulation and mobilization of the patient, ammonia can be sniffed
Tingling, flushing, sweating, hypo/hypertension, tachycardia	Hyperventilation, anxiety	The patient can breathe into the paper, advised to breathe slowly and deeply; if hypotensive, physiological saline is given and placed in Trendelenburg position
Tachycardia, sweating, hypotension	Antihypertensive (beta-blocker, Ca-channel blocker) use, hypovolemia	Until the next procedure, antihypertensives are discontinued, IV saline is given, Trendelenburg position is taken, fluid balance is corrected, the type and volume of replacement fluids are re-evaluated; if crystalloid weight, the intravascular oncotic pressure is increased by increasing the colloid percentage
Numbness around the mouth, spreading throughout the body, chest tightness, nausea, vomiting, diarrhea, hypotension, increased QT, tetany	Citrate toxicity, hypocalcemia	The process is to decrease the blood flow rate, increase the whole blood: ACD rate is increased, ACD and heparin are coagulated, FFP delivery rate is decreased, per oral or intravenous Ca is given to the patient (slow pulse), Ca is added to replacement fluids (only in continuous flow devices, FFP and cryo-poor plasma are not added!!!)
Itching, rash, plaques, wheezing, facial edema, hypotension, tachycardia	Allergic reaction	The patient is administered intravenous antihistamine, intravenous corticosteroid, and subcutaneous epinephrine, which can be used if necessary
Back pain, hematuria, tachycardia, hypotension, hemolysis	Acute hemolytic transfusion reaction	Blood product administration is stopped urgently; hydration is increased; diuresis is closely monitored, and blood bank and transfusion consultant are informed urgently
Burning in the eyes, periorbital oedema	Ethylene oxide allergic reaction	Interrupt processing, double-prime, in such cases it is preferable to use sets that are close to expiry
Hot flushes and hypotension	ACE inhibitor reaction	Albumin lot number is changed; fresh frozen plasma or HES is switched; ACE inhibitor use is interrupted; therapeutic apheresis is performed 24–48 h after ACE inhibitor intake

ACD acid citrate dextrose, *FFP* fresh frozen plasma, *HES* hydroxyethyl starch, *ACE* angiotensin converting enzyme

In cases where blood cannot be taken from the catheter: a clot in the catheter opening or anywhere in the lumen should be considered. If a catheter blockage is suspected, streptokinase or tissue plasminogen activator may be used. This should be performed by an experienced physician. It should not be forgotten that pressure should not be applied with saline in removing the catheter obstruction. Otherwise, the clot may cause pulmonary embolism [8, 9].

In case of catheter-related vein thrombosis, pain, discoloration, and swelling of the limb where the CVC is located may occur. In this case, the procedure must be stopped (Table 11.2). To establish the diagnosis of catheter vein thrombosis, urgent angiography should be performed, and thrombolytic therapy should thereafter be planned [7–11].

11.3 Air Embolism

Loose connections or unrecognized separation of the catheter tip or set can lead to bleeding and, more importantly, to air embolism, which can cause a clinical picture of sudden respiratory distress. Modern apheresis devices are equipped with air sensors. However, it can occur if auxiliary pumps without air sensors are used and/or if the operator fails to observe safety mechanisms [12, 13].

Acute respiratory failure can cause problems ranging from chest pain, diaphoresis (excessive sweating), confusion, shock, or syncope (Table 11.2).

In treatment, the patient is placed on the left side and head down (this position directs air away from the pulmonary valve and into the right atrium). The patient is given oxygen, and the vascular access is kept open. If possible, a chest X-ray is taken (this will help with the diagnosis) [12, 13] (Table 11.2).

11.4 Undesirable Effects Related to the Circulatory System

Undesirable effects related to the circulatory system are relatively common complications of fluid imbalance. In this case, close monitoring of the patient and necessary interventions are recommended.

11.4.1 Hypotension

If more than 15% of the total blood volume is drawn into the apheresis device at any time during the procedure, the likelihood of hypotension increases. The Swedish study group reported a 20.5% incidence of hypotension in their study, summarizing 14,000 apheresis procedures. This is more common in pediatric, elderly, and small-sized patients. Reducing the speed, reclining the apheresis chair, and elevating the patient's feet are usually sufficient [3]. However, isotonic NaCl solutions may sometimes be necessary. In apheresis devices operating with intermittent flow, a large amount of blood is drawn from the patient and then centrifuged, and the desired product is collected in a separate bag after centrifugation, while the unwanted products are returned to the patient. Hypotension is more common in small-sized people when apheresis is performed in such devices. Hypotension may not be prevented even if the processing speed is kept at the lowest level. Therefore, filling the apheresis device set with a small amount of human albumin under such conditions prevents the device from drawing too much blood to start centrifugation, which,in turn, prevents the development of hypotension (Table 11.2). However, it should be borne in mind that the resulting product will be diluted [14].

11.4.2 Hypertension

Hypertension may develop if the volume of blood returned to the patient after being processed by the device is higher than the volume of blood taken into the device during apheresis. This situation becomes even more important in patients with previous hypertension. Close monitoring of the blood volume separated from the patient and returned to the patient during the procedure and regular blood pressure monitoring can prevent the development of hypertension. In case of unpreventable hypertension, the procedure should be interrupted [14, 15] (Table 11.2).

11.4.3 Vasovagal Reactions

A slight feeling of chilliness due to the use of room-temperature solutions and vasovagal reactions such as "I feel like I am sighing" or "I have a feeling of lightness in my head" are frequently observed, especially during plasma changes. Such complaints may also occur because of citrate. Slowing down the blood flow rate is an adequate approach. In the treatment, intravenous saline may be given; the patient is placed in the Trendelenburg position; the fluid balance is corrected; and the type and volume of replacement fluids are re-evaluated. If crystalloid is predominant, the intravascular oncotic pressure should be increased by increasing the percentage of colloid [16] (Table 11.2).

11.4.4 Arrhythmias

The administration of cold replacement fluids or fresh frozen plasma (FFP), especially via the CVC, may rarely cause arrhythmias. Therefore, it is deemed more appropriate to use warmed replacement fluids during apheresis [5] (Table 11.2).

11.4.5 Increase in Vasoactive Amine

Patients taking angiotensin-converting enzyme (ACE) inhibitors, which are frequently prescribed for hypertension or congestive heart failure, may experience nausea, vomiting, hot flushes, and hypotension due to increased levels of vasoactive amines which are not catabolized during apheresis. Therefore, ACE inhibitors should be discontinued 48–72 h before apheresis [1, 3, 5, 6] (Table 11.2).

11.5 Complications Related to Citrate

Citrate-induced hypocalcemia is one of the most common apheresis complications. In various studies, it has been reported that citrate toxicity is seen around 3% of the procedures, and 0.2–0.3% of these are severe enough to cause tetany and convulsions. Paresthesia and tingling sensation occur in the fingertips and around the mouth (Table 11.2). If the patient is undergoing plasma exchange and FFP, is used for this purpose, the citrate effect is more pronounced if hyperventilation, hypothermia, and hypomagnesemia are present. In fact, it has been observed that calcium balance can be easily maintained even during plasma exchange in people with normal parathyroid and liver function. This is because the body rapidly eliminates citrate [17–21].

It is mainly observed in patients with hepatic and renal dysfunction, acidosis, and alkalosis, patients with daily plasma exchange and/or FFP as replacement fluid, patients with renal damage, and patients with hyperventilation, hyperthermia, hypomagnesemia, and hypoalbuminemia [17, 19].

Symptoms may include Chvostek's sign, Trousseau's sign, severe muscle cramps, severe abdominal cramps, tremor, incontinence, fear of death, loss of consciousness, blurred or double vision, long QT interval, and severe ST abnormalities on ECG [17–21] (Table 11.2).

In treatment, it is necessary to reduce the blood flow rate of the procedure and increase the whole blood/ACD ratio. If necessary, ACD/heparin anticoagulation can be switched to. If fresh frozen plasma is given, the rate of FFP administration should be decreased. PO or IV Ca++ is given to the patient according to the condition (slow injection or infusion). Ca++ can be added to replacement fluids [17–21] (Table 11.2).

The rate of reinfusion is slowed down to reduce the short-term citrate side effect. Calcium is given before the procedure or in case of symptoms. Symptoms do not occur if the citrate infusion rate is less than 1 mg/kg per minute, while symptoms develop at a rate of 1.8/mg/kg/min and above. The response of patients to citrate concentration is different. Therefore, it is more important to adjust the infusion rate in relation to the clinic rather than calculating the citrate concentration according to the body structure with some mathematical formulas [17–21] (Table 11.2).

If the rate of reinfusion is not slowed down before the symptoms of citrate effect are recognized, these symptoms may become severe such as muscle contraction, shivering, nausea, vomiting, feeling of pressure in the chest, loss of consciousness, and shock. In patients with citrate-induced toxic effects, the rate of reinfusion should be reduced; calcium drinks should be given; hypothermia should be prevented by covering; and replacement solutions should be heated. If these measures are not sufficient, parenteral calcium preparations should be given. Although there are several studies showing that oral calcium administration has no effect on ionized calcium levels, effervescent calcium preparations are used in many centers primarily in response to the findings of citrate effect. High citrate concentrations can lead to serious cardiac arrhythmias. In this case, apheresis should be stopped immediately, and 10% calcium gluconate infusion should be given with rhythm monitoring. Some textbooks have suggested that routine prophylactic calcium infusion is not necessary. However, there are studies showing the benefit of prophylactic calcium infusions, especially during large-volume apheresis procedures [17–21].

It should be remembered that calcium preparations should not be administered directly intravenously and should not be administered through the vascular route of transfusion of blood or blood products. Depending on the clinical situation, calcium can be given in 10 cc ampoules of 10% calcium gluconate, usually 1–2 ampoules, as a short 10-minute infusion in 100 cc saline. It should not be forgotten to wash the vascular access with saline after the infusion [22–25].

Apheresis unit staff should be alert to citrate toxicity and should question whether there are signs such as twitching and tingling in the muscles during apheresis and then adjust the infusion rate according to the situation. In patients who cannot communicate, caution should be exercised, and the infusion rate should be kept low. QT intervals should be closely monitored in patients, especially in procedures performed in intensive care units [22–25].

11.6 Allergic Reactions

Allergic reactions (bronchospasm and dyspnea) may develop during the use of fresh frozen plasma (FFP) as a replacement fluid. Fortunately, this complication responds quickly to antihistamines and corticosteroid treatment. Diffuse urticarial reactions due to ethylene oxide gas used in the sterilization of apheresis bags are rare complications.

Anaphylaxis is a rare complication after apheresis. Anaphylaxis, which is a hypersensitivity reaction leading to sudden skin rashes, loss of consciousness, shock, and death, does not cause fever and can develop with as little as 1–2 mL of plasma (Table 11.2). Therefore, the procedure should be stopped immediately and antihistamines, and, if necessary, prednisolone should be given. If the need for plasmapheresis persists in people with a history of allergic reactions during previous apheresis, antihistamines should be given half to 1 h before the procedure. In severe allergic reactions, corticosteroids, aminophylline, and adrenaline may be required [2, 26] (Table 11.2).

In case of allergic reactions, the procedure should be stopped. Subsequent treatment depends on the type and severity of the reaction. Relatively simple reactions such as urticaria can be treated with oral or parenteral antihistamines. In anaphylactic reactions, intravenous infusion of isotonic NaCl is started. If the reaction is relatively mild, 0.3–0.5 mg epinephrine should be given subcutaneously; this dose can be repeated three times every 20–30 min. In addition, in patients with bronchospasm, 6 mg/kg aminophylline is given, and the infusion is continued at a dose of 0.5–1 mg/kg after the loading dose. Isotonic or lactated Ringer's solution may be given for hypotension. Oxygen therapy is started in patients with respiratory distress. In severe reactions, 0.5 mg epinephrine is given intravenously; this dose can be repeated every 5–10 min. If hypotension does not improve with fluid infusion, dopamine infusion is started. Airway should be kept open; intubation may be necessary in some cases [2, 26] (Table 11.2).

The prevalence of IgA deficiency, which is an important factor in anaphylaxis, is estimated to be 1/700–800 in the general population. Some drugs, plasma products containing complement proteins, hydroxyethyl starch (HES), and dextran solutions are also involved in the development of anaphylaxis [2, 27]. Apheresis should be stopped immediately, and adrenaline should be given subcutaneously or intramuscularly (adult dose: 1:1000 adrenaline 0.3–0.5 mg/kg) or intravenously (1/10000 adrenaline) in severe cases. Corticosteroids and aminophylline may be administered. Intubation for mechanical ventilation may be necessary. In patients with known IgA deficiency, only FFP or human albumin prepared from IgA-deficient donors should be used as replacement fluid [2, 27].

11.7 Respiratory Complications

The main respiratory-related complications are acute pulmonary edema, anaphylactic reaction, massive pulmonary embolism, and transfusion-related acute lung injury (TRALI). These complications are serious and require physician-supervised treatment. Acute pulmonary edema is easily diagnosed by hypertension, diffuse wet rales, and full neck veins. The procedure is stopped. Furosemide (40–120 mg) and nasal oxygen (4 L/min) are given (Table 11.2). TRALI is associated with symptoms including fever, dyspnea, cyanosis, cough, and hypotension. Lung radiography shows patchy infiltration. Right heart pressures are normal. Therefore, there are no signs of fluid overload. It is also associated with hypotension and unresponsive to diuretics. Unlike adult respiratory distress syndrome, clinical signs and symptoms resolve spontaneously within 24–48 h with supportive treatment. In addition, non-cardiogenic acute lung edema with the effect of vasoactive substances in colloid solutions obtained from FFP or human plasma may lead to respiratory distress, which may be fatal; it is also called adult respiratory distress syndrome [21, 28].

11.8 Changes in the Pharmacodynamics of Drugs

In patients undergoing plasma exchange for therapeutic purposes, blood levels of albumin-dependent drugs may be reduced. Indeed, although blood levels of some antiepileptic drugs and antibiotics have been found to be decreased, since the efficacy of most of these drugs is directly related to their concentration in tissues, there has been no clinical observation of an adverse effect of decreased drug levels due to apheresis. Nevertheless, it would be appropriate to review the medications taken by the patients and to postpone the administration of any medication that may be removed during apheresis until after the apheresis procedure, even if it is time to give it to the patient [29].

11.9 Traumatic Hemolysis

Folded tubes, defective caps, or improper wrapping of tubes in the device may lead to hemolysis of the blood during processing in the apheresis device. Several studies have reported a similar incidence of mechanical hemolysis in volunteer apheresis and therapeutic apheresis (0.07% and 0.06%). The technicians performing the procedure should be aware of such a complication and check the sets intermittently [1–3]. Hemolysis can also occur with ABO-incompatible blood products or inappropriate dilution of replacement fluids. If it is observed that the plasma collection set starts to turn pink during the procedure, mechanical hemolysis should be suspected, and the procedure should be stopped, and the system need to be checked [1–3].

11.10 Infections

If sepsis is not observed, phlebitis of superficial veins related to the apheresis procedure may occur and can usually be controlled with oral penicillin or cephalosporin. Viral and bacterial infections may develop, especially in the therapeutic apheresis where plasma is used as replacement fluid. Catheter-associated bacterial infections may also occur in patients with central venous catheters during repeated apheresis, requiring the removal of the catheter as well as broad-spectrum antibiotics [30, 31] (Table 11.1).

11.11 Lymphocyte, Coagulation Factors, and Plasma Protein Depletion

Especially with platelet apheresis, the collection of large amounts of leukocytes with platelets and plasma has raised concerns that it may cause problems in immunological memory due to lymphocyte depletion in healthy volunteers. However, no adverse effects on platelet, hemoglobin, lymphocyte counts, and T and B lymphocyte functions were detected, even in those who underwent frequent platelet apheresis [32, 33].

There have been several studies showing the changes in the plasma levels of coagulant and anticoagulant factors and activation of proinflammatory cytokines and platelets both in healthy volunteers and after therapeutic apheresis. Thus, to increase the safety of apheresis procedures, studies on these effects, which are rarely reported to cause bleeding and thrombosis, are still ongoing [34].

11.12 Late Side Effects (>6 h After the Procedure)

Viral infection due to blood products used during apheresis is one of the leading late side effects (Table 11.1). Other late side effects are listed below.

- Hepatitis B and C (usually occurs 4 months after procedures, detailed procedure and user analysis and feedback to the blood bank are important for follow-up [30, 31].
- HIV infection [31].
- Infection and severe sepsis (due to use of contaminated set, catheter, or replacement fluid) [31].
- Hypogammaglobulinemia (especially develops after repeated FFP procedures without FFP, and intravenous immunoglobulin (IVIG) may be recommended for its treatment [35–39].
- Electrolyte imbalance (close electrolyte monitoring after repeated FFP procedures, according to the nature of the replacement fluid used) [35–39].
- Coagulopathy (develops and is reversible, especially after repeated FFP procedures using HES) [35–39].

11.13 Death During Apheresis

It is known that patients undergoing therapeutic apheresis and in poor general condition, for example, leukapheresis for severe leukocytosis, may die during apheresis. However, death directly due to apheresis is reported to be extremely rare. In some studies, death rates due to apheresis are reported to be between 3 in 10.000 and 1 in 500 [40]. Most of the deaths occur during or immediately after the procedure due to cardiac arrhythmias or acute lung edema or adult respiratory distress syndrome. Death due to serious apheresis complications such as anaphylaxis, vascular perforation, hepatitis, sepsis, thrombosis, or hemorrhage is extremely rare [41–43].

11.14 Technical Problems

Some of the technical errors are determined in the disposable set to be inserted (outdated, torn packaging, sets without lot numbers), error messages given by the device during operation, and mechanical and electronic problems (it is recommended that the devices are connected to an uninterruptible power supply) [6, 31, 41] (Table 11.1).

Problems due to user-induced faults:

- Incorrect installation of the set
- Incorrect entry of the transaction
- Failure to respond to error messages in a timely and correct manner
- Problems such as poor monitoring of the procedure and the patient

Some correlations were found between reactions in apheresis donors and gender, device type, and citrate-related side effects. Being female was a risk factor for complications related to the site of entry. There was also an interesting correlation between donor weight and citrate-related reactions, depending on whether the device used was COBE Spectra or Fenwal CS3000: In low-weight donors, the rate of citrate reactions was lower with the Fenwal CS3000, whereas this rate was significantly higher with the COBE Spectra in heavier donors. This difference was attributed to the use of different variables to calculate the amount of anticoagulant required [44].

In summary, therapeutic apheresis procedures were reported to be acceptably safe even with older equipment; today, these procedures can be performed even more safely. In general, the most common complications are citrate-induced hypocalcemia and urticarial reactions due to the protein-containing replacement fluid. If the complications that may occur during the procedure are known, they can be monitored and sometimes prevented before they develop; thus, safer apheresis procedures can be performed.

References

1. Kiprov DD, Golden P, Rohe R, Smith S, Hofmann J, Hunnicutt J. Adverse reactions associated with mobile therapeutic apheresis: analysis of 17,940 procedures. J Clin Apher. 2001;16:130–3.
2. McLeod BC, Sniecinski I, Ciavarella D, et al. Frequency of immediate adverse effects associated with therapeutic apheresis. Transfusion. 1999;39:282–8.
3. Norda R, Stegmayr BG, Swedish Apheresis Group. Therapeutic apheresis in Sweden: update of epidemiology and adverse events. Transfus Apher Sci. 2003;29:159–66.
4. Gilcher RO. Apheresis: principles and practices. In: Rossi EC, Simon TL, Moss GS, Gould SA, editors. Principles of transfusion medicine. 2nd ed. Baltimore: Williams and Wilkins; 1995. p. 537–46.
5. Winters JL. Complications of donor apheresis. J Clin Apher. 2006;21:132–41.
6. McCarthy LJ. Evidence-based medicine for apheresis: an ongoing challenge. Ther Apher Dial. 2004;8(2):112.
7. Stegmayr B, Wikdahl AM. Access in therapeutic apheresis. Ther Apher Dial. 2003;7:209–14.
8. Haire WD, Edney JA, Landmark JD, Kessinger A. Thrombotic complications of subclavian apheresis catheters in cancer patients: prevention with heparin infusion. J Clin Apher. 1990;5:188–91.
9. Bozzetti F, Scarpa D, Terno G, et al. Subclavian venous thrombosis due to indwelling catheters: a prospective study on 52 patients. J Parenter Enter Nutr. 1983;7:560–2.
10. Lazarus HM, Lowder JN, Herzig RH. Occlusion and infection in Broviac catheters during intensive cancer therapy. Cancer. 1983;52:2342–8.
11. Oliver MJ, Callery SM, Thorpe KE, et al. Risk of bacteremia from temporary hemodialysis catheters by site of insertion and duration of use: a prospective study. Kidney Int. 2000;58:2543–5.
12. Grífols JR, Ferrà C, Sancho JM, Pujol M, Ribera JM. A case of non-lethal pulmonary air embolism after leukapheresis catheter removal. J Clin Apher. 2005;20(2):93–4. https://doi.org/10.1002/jca.20055. PMID: 15892083.
13. Boer WH, Hené RJ. Lethal air embolism following removal of a double lumen jugular vein catheter. Nephrol Dial Transplant. 1999;14(8):1850–2. https://doi.org/10.1093/ndt/14.8.1850. PMID: 10462261.
14. Kayashima M, Sakai K, Harada K, Kanetake J, Kubo M, Hamada E, Hayakawa M, Hatakeyama K, Matsumoto M. Strong association between insufficient plasma exchange and fatal outcomes in Japanese patients with immune-mediated thrombotic thrombocytopenic purpura. Int J Hematol. 2021;114(4):415–23.
15. Alhasan KA. Therapeutic plasma exchange for children with kidney disorders: definitions, prescription, indications, and complications. Saudi J Kidney Dis Transpl. 2019;30(2):291–8.
16. Tomita T, Takayanagi M, Kiwada K, Mieda A, Takahashi C, Hata T. Vasovagal reactions in apheresis donors. Transfusion. 2002;42:1561–6.
17. Weinstein R. Hypocalcemic toxicity and atypical reactions in therapeutic plasma exchange. J Clin Apher. 2001;16:210–1.
18. Makar YF, Butler MO, Cockersole GM, Gabra G, Serevitch JM. National audit of citrate toxicity in plateletpheresis donors. Transfus Med. 2002;12:187–91.
19. Bell AM, Nolen JF, Knudson CM. Severe citrate toxicity complicating volunteer apheresis platelet donation. J Clin Apher. 2007;22:15–6.
20. Altobelli C, Anastasio P, Cerrone A, Signoriello E, Lus G, Pluvio C, Perna AF, Capasso G, Simeoni M, Capolongo G. Therapeutic plasmapheresis: a revision of literature. Kidney Blood Press Res. 2022;48(1):66–78.
21. Mortzell Henriksson M, Newman E, Witt V, Derfler K, Leitner G, Eloot S, et al. Adverse events in apheresis an update of the WAA registry data. Transfus Apher Sci. 2016;54(1):2–15.
22. Bolan CD, Leitman SF. Management of anticoagulation associated toxicity during large-volume leukapheresis of peripheral blood stem cell donors. Blood. 2002;99:1878.
23. Weinstein R. Prevention of citrate reactions during therapeutic plasma exchange by constant infusion of calcium-gluconate with the return fluid. J Clin Apher. 1996;11:204–10.
24. Bolan CD, Cecco SA, Wesley RA, et al. Controlled study of citrate effects and response to i.v. calcium administration during allogeneic peripheral blood progenitor cell donation. Transfusion. 2002;42:935–46.
25. Kishimoto M, Ohto H, Shikama Y, et al. Treatment for the decline of ionized calcium levels during peripheral blood progenitor cell harvesting. Transfusion. 2002;42:1340–7.
26. Leitman SF, Boltansky H, Alter HJ, et al. Allergic reactions in healthy plateletpheresis donors caused by sensitization to ethylene oxide gas. N Engl J Med. 1986;315:1192–6.
27. McLeod BC, Price TH, Owen H, et al. Frequency of immediate adverse effects associated with apheresis donation. Transfusion. 1998;38:938–43.
28. Kracalik I, Mowla S, Basavaraju SV, Sapiano MRP. Transfusion-related adverse reactions: data from the National Healthcare Safety Network Hemovigilance Module—United States, 2013-2018. Transfusion. 2021;61(5):1424–34. https://doi.org/10.1111/trf.16362. Epub 2021 Apr 20. PMID: 33880771.

29. Binns TC, Sostin N, Tormey CA. State of the evidence: drug removal via apheresis. Transfus Med Rev. 2023;37(1):16–20.
30. Depcik-Smith ND, Hay SN, Brecher ME. Bacterial contamination of blood products: factors, options, and insights. J Clin Apher. 2001;16:192–201.
31. Kaplan A. Complications of apheresis. Semin Dial. 2012;25(2):152–8.
32. Strauss RG. Effects on donors of repeated leukocyte losses during plateletpheresis. J Clin Apher. 1994;9:130–4.
33. Lewis SL, Kutvirt SG, Bonner PN, Simon TL. Effect of long-term platelet donation on lymphocyte subsets and plasma protein concentrations. Transfus Sci. 1997;18:205–13.
34. Karadogan I, Ozdogan M, Undar L. Single automated donor plateletpheresis increases the plasma level of proinflammatory cytokine tumor necrosis factor-alpha which does not associate with endothelial release markers von Willebrand factor and fibronectin. Transfus Sci. 2000;23:171–5.
35. Heal JM, Horan PK, Schmitt TC, Bailey G, Nusbacher J. Long- term follow-up of donors cytapheresed more than 50 times. Vox Sang. 1983;45:14–24.
36. Stohlawetz P, Kapiotis S, Seidl D, Hergovich N, Zellner M, Eichler HG, Stiegler G, Leitner G, Hocker P, Jilma B. Safety issues of plateletpheresis: comparison of the effects of two cell separators on the activation of coagulation, fibrinolysis, and neutrophils and on the formation of neutrophil-platelet aggregates. Transfusion. 1999;39:420–7.
37. Kobayashi I, Hamaoka S, Ozawa H, Ihno M, Tamura K, Tanaka Y, Sakamoto Y, Nakamura A, Ueno A. Hypercoagulable state induced by thrombocytapheresis. J Clin Apher. 1993;8:147–52.
38. Tek I, Arslan O, Arat M, Ozcan M, Akdag B, Ilhan O. Effects of replacement fluids on coagulation system used for therapeutic plasma exchange. Transfus Apher Sci. 2003;28:3–7.
39. Flaum MA, Cuneo RA, Appelbaum FR, Disseroth AB, Engel WK, Gralnick HR. The hemostatic imbalance of plasma exchange transfusion. Blood. 1979;54:694–702.
40. Huestis DW. Mortality in therapeutic haemapheresis (letter). Lancet. 1983;1:1043.
41. Rock G, Clark B, Sutton D, CAG, CAAN. The Canadian Apheresis Registry. Transfus Apher Sci. 2003;29:167–77.
42. Aufeuvre JP, Morin-Hertel F, Cohen-Solal M, Lefloch A, Baudelot J. Hazards of plasma exchange. In: Sieberth HG, editor. Plasma exchange. Stuttgart: FK Schattauer Verlag; 1980. p. 149–57.
43. Aufeuvre JP, Mortin-Hertel F, Cohen-Solal M, Lefloch A, Baudelot J. Clinical tolerance and hazards of plasma exchanges: a study of 6200 plasma exchanges in 1033 patients. In: Beyer JH, Burgerg H, Fuchs C, Nagel GA, editors. Plasmapheresis in immunology and oncology. Basel: Karger; 1982. p. 65–77.
44. Despotis GJ, Goodnough L, Dynis M, et al. Adverse events in platelet apheresis donors: a multivariate analysis in a hospital based program. Vox Sang. 1999;77:24–32.

12 Complications During Adsorptive Cytapheresis Treatment

Piero Vernia and Filippo Vernia

12.1 Background

Adsorptive cytapheresis (AC) is a non-pharmacological procedure performed to remove selected cell populations from peripheral blood using specific filters and reduce inflammation. Different approaches have been used, resulting in differences in the amount and type of leukocytes removed. The two most used and most widely studied ones are selective granulocyte-monocyte apheresis (GMA) [1] and leukocytapheresis (LCAP) [2]. More recently, a novel device, Immunopure, has become clinically available [3].

GMA (Adacolumn™, JIMRO, Takasaki, Japan) uses 335 mL columns containing 2-mm cellulose diacetate beads in isotonic saline, selectively adsorbing the activated granulocytes and monocytes expressing Fcγ, C3a, and C5a immune complexes [4]. Nonetheless, the overall number of granulocytes remains to be stable, due to the relative increase of CD10-, naïve, non-activated cells [5, 6]. This is paralleled by the downregulation of pro-inflammatory cytokines and IFγ by direct adsorption in the column; upregulation of CD4+, CD25+, Foxp3+ T-reg cells; and reduced myeloid and plasmacytoid dendritic cell populations. A reduction of IL8, acting as a chemotactic factor for granulocytes, is also observed. This eventually results in lessened acute and chronic inflammatory processes [7, 8].

LCAP (Cellsorba, Asahi Kasei Kuraray Medical, Tokyo, Japan), using nonwoven polyester fiber filters in isotonic saline, removes granulocytes, monocytes, and lymphocytes, as well as platelets [9, 10].

Immunopure (NIKKISO Co., Ltd. Tokyo, Japan) utilizes polyarylate resin beads to adsorb granulocytes, monocytes, activated lymphocytes, and platelets [2].

All devices were proven effective in removing considerable amounts of selected leucocytes from the blood flow. GMA, following a standard 1 h, 30 mL/min session filtering 1800 mL blood, adsorbs 25% activated granulocytes, 20% monocytes, 2–7% lymphocytes, and virtually no erythrocytes [11].

LCAP sessions use higher blood flow rates (50 mL/min) as compared to GMA and filter more blood, thus removing 90% granulocytes, 79% monocytes, over 55% platelets, as well as an average of 50% lymphocytes [9]. The level of proinflammatory cytokines is also reduced. Immunopure (30 mL/min, 1-h sessions) demonstrates intermediate values, adsorbing 35% granulocytes, 45% monocytes, 45% platelets and 3% lymphocytes [2]. The removal of platelets and

P. Vernia (✉)
Department of Translational and Precision Medicine, Sapienza University of Rome, Rome, Italy

F. Vernia
Division of Gastroenterology, Department of Life, Health and Environmental Sciences, University of L'Aquila, L'Aquila, Italy

I. Kozanoglu (ed.), *Problem Solving in Apheresis Medicine*,
https://doi.org/10.1007/978-3-031-74081-7_12

platelet aggregates seems to be particularly effective [10].

12.2 Treatment Goals and Efficacy

By far, the main clinical application of AC is represented by inflammatory bowel disease (IBD), ulcerative colitis (UC), and Crohn's disease (CD). Favorable effects have also been documented in rheumatoid arthritis, other forms of inflammatory and reactive arthritis [11–13] and various skin diseases, associated or not to IBD. They include pustular psoriasis [14], pyoderma gangrenosum [15], Behçet's disease, systemic lupus erythematosus, allergic vasculitis and hidradenitis suppurativa [16].

Studies in UC and the meta-analysis from Habermalz [17], reporting response rates from 60 to 80%, have confirmed the efficacy in improving clinical scores and endoscopic findings. Due to difficulties in performing randomized, sham-controlled, double-blind studies, only two studies were carried out. A significantly favorable outcome (80% vs 33%) was reported with LCAP [18], but not with GMA (remission 17% vs 11%, response rate 44% vs 39%) [19]. The reason of the latter finding remains unclear, but methodologic biases are likely involved, including high drop-out rate and the inclusion of patients with minimal active inflammation.

AC is effective in steroid-dependent and steroid-refractory patients for achieving clinical response and remission [20–22]. The addition of apheresis to standard steroid therapy improves efficacy [23]. Significant differences between GMA, LCAP, and Immunopure have not been documented, and similar results can be expected using these three devices [24, 25].

Mucosal healing attained by intensive, twice-a-week regimen without the concomitant use of steroids results in long-term maintenance of remission [26, 27], and AC works again in case of relapse.

AC is effective in pediatric UC patients unresponsive to conventional therapy [28–30] as well as in elderly patients [31, 32], with response rates comparable to that in adults. In older patients, however, a delay in the onset of efficacy is not rare [33]. The few data available in pregnancy suggest that this condition does not represent a contraindication to apheresis [34–36], and the response rate is good.

Long-term benefit is documented in patients with steroid-dependent chronically active UC, resistant or intolerant to immunosuppressants and/or TNF inhibitors [37]. A recent paper [38] summarized the efficacy of AC in relation to the use of immunomodulators (IM) or biologics. Previous exposure to IM does not reduce response to cytapheresis, while lower efficacy has been associated with previous exposure to biologics (from 44.2 to 29.4%). In patients showing loss of response or inadequate response to biologics, the association of AC induces clinical remission/response and steroid-free remission in about 40% of cases. These results could be anticipated, considering the lowering effect on proinflammatory cytokines as well as the reduced migration of leucocytes in the inflamed areas. Increased trough levels of biologics and reduced levels of anti-infliximab antibodies have also been reported [39].

Acceptable, but less clear, is the efficacy of AC in Crohn's disease [40–42]. Recent CD diagnosis and intensive, twice-a-week regimen have been associated with favorable response rates.

With few exceptions [14, 15, 43], data on AC in dermatology are derived from case reports and small series. A recent review indicates that a favorable response may be expected in about two-thirds of patients [16].

Treatment of inflammatory arthritis with GMA proved effective in old series [11, 12], but efficacy and cost/effectiveness of biologic drugs limited its use in recent years [44]. A role may still be present in selected patients, alone or in combination with biologics [45].

12.3 Adverse Events

Adverse event (AE) is defined as any undesirable experience associated with the use of a drug or a medical product, in this case procedure, in humans, whether or not considered drug- or procedure-related [46] (CFR312.32). An adverse reaction that results in death, is life-threatening, requires hospitalization, results in persistent or significant disability or incapacity, or a birth defect is considered serious (sAE). AEs due to technical problems related to the procedure, including difficulties in blood access, system operation, venous pressure abnormalities, and coagulation in the apheresis system lines, are separately classified as feasibility problems (FP) in some papers, or considered as AE in others. Similarly, unwanted side effects directly resulting from the use of anticoagulants used represent a separate problem, but have often been included in AE. Their occurrence accounts for a significant proportion of AE observed in AC. A large study has focused on this issue including 832 patients, wherein 2.7% incidence of decreased platelet count and 1.8% for both nasal congestion and pain in the vascular access site were reported when using heparin [47]. Nafamostat mesylate, which is not available in several countries, was associated with mild headache in 2.2%, nausea in 1.3%, and fever in 0.9%. No serious AE was observed in this series [47]. All these considerations explain the wide variability in the prevalence of AE reported in the literature.

12.3.1 General Considerations

Only few serious AEs have been reported, and their occurrence, or definition, is in some instances debatable. For example, 24 patients out of 894 in Yamamoto series experienced worsening of the disease, as well as few more in other trials [19, 23, 48, 49]. This may well be considered as treatment failure, more than procedure-related sAE. One case of severe pneumonia and one of spontaneous abortion were also reported [23, 50]. Thus, the number and type of sAE confirm the excellent security profile of AC.

The reported occurrence of mild and moderate AE is widely variable in the literature. Pooling or comparing different series is not always feasible, as the exact definition of AE is often omitted, and data have been expressed, in turn, as AE per patient or AE per procedure. Moreover, the number of procedures in each individual patient changed in different protocols and in real-world experience, and the number of AE in the same patient was not invariably reported.

Most data concerning AE refer to GMA and inflammatory bowel disease, mainly UC, and will be considered first.

12.3.2 Ulcerative Colitis

Mild-moderate AE in GMA ranged from 2 to 95% of the cases [19, 51] and from 2.3 to 36% per procedure [49, 52]. The wide range of reported AE reflects the fact that AE were mild and did not affect the feasibility of the procedure. Minor symptoms were likely considered irrelevant by some authors and thus not reported. The opposite occurred in those series in which minor AEs were reported in almost all patients and controls [19].

Feasibility problems, related to blood access or system operation problems, were observed in 5–20% of the patients [50] and 0.3–2.3% of the procedures [52]. In some cases, a central line was required.

The need for stopping apheresis sessions did not exceed 2% of procedures and was mainly due to headache or fever. In most instances, it did not prevent further treatment as mild to moderate AE subsided reducing the blood flow rate or following brief suspension of the procedure. Patient adhesion to apheresis was not affected by AE, and apheresis was a well-accepted therapeutic option, often preferred to conventional pharmacological treatment [53]. The presence or absence of minor AE during the procedure did not affect the response rate (48% vs 47%) [48].

The most common AEs occurring in UC patients are reported in Table 12.1. The safety profile was invariably better than that of conventional treatment, including steroids, immunosuppressants and biologics [21, 28, 38, 55–57, 60]. The addition of apheresis to conventional pharmacological or biological therapy, while increasing efficacy, did not result in significant increase of reported AEs [53, 61–63].

Table 12.1 Occurrence of adverse events in adult patients who suffer from ulcerative colitis

	Per patient	Per procedure	Main references
Overall AE	2–95%	2.3–36%	[3, 19, 21, 23, 31, 37, 41, 48–52, 54–59]
Severe AE	0–2.6%[a]	n.a.	[48]
Feasibility problems	5–20%	1–2.3%	[50, 52]
Procedure stop	0–4%	0–0.3%	[55, 59]
Headache	10–33%	3.9–14%	[41]
Lightheadedness	0–14%	0–4.7%	[23, 54]
Fatigue	0–18%	0–0.4%	[6, 19, 48, 49]
Hypotension	0.29–26%	0–4.7%	[19, 23, 52]
Nausea	6–21.8%	n.a.	[19, 48]
Nasopharyngitis	0–9%	n.a.	[49]
Itching	0–9%	n.a.	[57]
Anemia, elevated ALT AST	0–1%		[52]

The table reports on the most observed AE in adult patients treated with GMA. The occurrence of AE is expressed as percent of patients or procedure. Main references are reported in the right column

Data referring to LCAP, or particular situations, including pediatric and elderly patients or pregnant women, have not been included

[a] Mainly consisting of worsening of the underlying disease

Data available for LCAP indicate a safety profile comparable to that of GMA, with few reported sAEs (0–0.6%). Mild to moderate AEs were observed in 4.5–10.3% of patients in clinical studies and post-marketing surveillance [58, 64–67] and approximately 2% of apheresis sessions. Mild transient lymphopenia was occasionally reported, as expected considering the mechanism of action of LCAP [68].

The safety profile of Immunopure is based on the data from a limited number of treated patients [3, 69] presenting with mild AE in 10% of cases.

12.3.3 UC: Particular Situations

AEs in special situations have recently been evaluated in a large multicenter cohort study [31]. Data confirm and expand observation in smaller studies, data extracted from subgroup of patients in other series, or case reports. The occurrence of serious AE in elderly patients using GMA or LCAP is higher than that of younger patients (about 5%). However, a proportion of them is related to underlying severe diseases or concomitant medication (thiopurine, calcineurin inhibitors, and biologics). Conversely, the prevalence of mild to moderate AE in elderly patients is comparable to that in the younger age groups, with the overall odd ratio for AE being 1.3 (CI 0.61–2.79) [31, 32, 58, 65, 70, 71].

The safety profile is good in pediatric patients. This holds true both for GMA (32–61% of patients) [29–31] and LCAP (61% [67]), despite a moderately increased odd ratio (OR 2.6, CI 1.03–6.54). In over 50% of the reported cases, they derived from blood access and feasibility problems or pain at the infusion site. Mild transient headache and nausea were also common. Slightly reduced red blood cell count was occasionally reported.

The use of AC in a small number of pregnant or lactating women proved safe and was not associated with severe AE. Mild AEs were observed in 6% of GMA procedures, consisting of mild fever or chest discomfort, which did not prompt suspension of therapy [71]. In other case reports, AE did not occur [34–36].

12.3.4 Crohn's Disease

The safety profile in CD does not differ from that in UC, and data are often included in IBD series, without separate analysis of the two diseases. Like UC, the incidence of AE in CD is variable, ranging from 0 [72] to 93.5% [73]. Noticeably, in the double-blind sham-controlled study by Sands, reporting the highest figures, the occurrence of AE was identical in the two treatment arms. They were usually related to the procedure, consisting of mild reduction of blood pressure and hypotension. In most other series, the overall occurrence of mild-moderate AE was 5–10% [74–76], with transient headache and fatigue being the most frequently reported.

No increase in AE is observed when apheresis was used in combination with biologics [64, 77, 78] and, when present, resulted from the use of immunomodulators and biologics.

12.3.5 Arthritis and Dermatological Disease

Limited evidence supports the use of AC in dermatological and rheumatological diseases. Three cases of sAE were reported in 27 patients with rheumatoid arthritis [44]. Only one of them could be attributed to the procedure, consisting in severe sepsis due to vein catheter manipulation, which led to the suspension of apheresis after four cycles. No AE was reported in 23 patients with joint lesions associated with dermatological diseases [79]. Few mild AEs were reported in small series or case reports in patients with arthritis.

The largest series of dermatological diseases reported no AE in 44 patients [79] as well as in 22 patients with generalized pustular psoriasis [14]. In the 15 patients of Ikeda's series [43], one severe case of allergy to nafamostat mesylate was observed. Dizziness, lightheadedness, and headache occurred in three more patients. Five out of 19 patients with pyoderma gangrenosum presented with transient hypertension, and a decrease in blood flow was needed in 5 more patients [15]. Other dermatological conditions listed in a recent review paper [16] including case reports and small series suggest that the safety profile of AC is good and does not differ from that in IBD.

12.4 Illustration of Clinical Case

A 16-year-old adolescent presenting with cortisone-dependent left-sided ulcerative colitis, following an ineffective course of the anti-TNFα infliximab was considered eligible for AC. His body weight was 47 kg, and his body mass index was 18.2. Laboratory data were normal, except for mild iron-deficiency anemia (Hb 12.3 g/dL, MCV 82 fL) and elevated white blood cell (WBC), erythrocyte sedimentation rate (ESR), and C-reactive protein (CRP). Shortly after beginning the first AC session, using the standard 30 mL/min blood flow rate, he experienced mild headache, nausea, and reduced blood pressure (from 120/72 to 102/60 mmHg). The procedure was stopped for a few minutes and then uneventfully reinstituted at 20 mL/min filtration rate.

Young age, bodyweight below normal, and the coincident presence of anemia identify patients at increased risk for AE. Beginning the procedure with a lower-than-normal blood filtration rate would likely have prevented the occurrence of this mild AE. In the absence of AEs, the filtration rate could have been safely increased to normal values.

12.5 Considerations, Pearls, and Pitfalls

Severe anemia, hypercoagulability state, and systemic infections contraindicate the procedure. Oral coagulants should be switched to heparin before and during AC [80, 81]. The flow rate of 30 mL/min should be maintained to avoid hypotension, although some evidence suggests that higher flow rates up to 50 mL/min may be used in selected cases, under strict clinical monitoring. The processed blood volume is 1800 mL of the blood during the standard 90′ GMA procedure and should not exceed 13% of the patient's blood volume. Total volume and flow rates may be adjusted in pediatric patients, but the standard procedure was used without problems in children-adolescents weighing over 30 kg [29]. Conversely, preliminary evidence suggests that adjusting the overall treated volume in relation to body weight, particularly in overweight adult subjects, may ensure better results [82]. LCAP uses flow rates of 30–50 mL/min, thus processing 2–3 L of blood in each session [83], and general considerations do not differ from those in GMA.

As a reduction in blood volume may result in dizziness and hypotension, the optimal circulating blood volume should be preserved, priming the column with 300–500 mL of saline. Monitoring blood pressure and other vital signs before, during, and at the end of the procedure is mandatory to minimize flow and volume-related problems [80]. Low-molecular-weight heparin seems to be the anticoagulant associated with less AE, compared to nafamostat mesylate [47], while citrate anticoagulants, potentially lowering efficacy of adsorptive mechanisms, are better avoided.

References

1. Shimoyama T, Sawada K, Tanaka T. Granulocyte and monocyte apheresis with the G-1 column in the treatment of patients with active ulcerative colitis. Jpn J Apher. 1999;18:117–31.
2. Kanai T, Hibi T, Watanabe M. The logics of leukocytapheresis as a natural biological therapy for inflammatory bowel disease. Expert Opin Biol Ther. 2006;6:453–66. https://doi.org/10.1517/14712598.6.5.453.
3. Ramlow W, Waitz G, Sparmann G, Prophet H, Bodammer P, Emmrich J. First human application of a novel adsorptive type cytapheresis module in patients with active ulcerative colitis: a pilot study. Ther Apher Dial. 2013;17(3):339–47. https://doi.org/10.1111/1744-9987.12007.
4. Saniabadi AR, Hanai H, Fukunaga K, Sawada K, Shima C, Bjarnason I, Lofberg R. Therapeutic leukocytapheresis for inflammatory bowel disease. Transfus Apher Sci. 2007;37:191–200. https://doi.org/10.1016/j.transci.2007.08.003.
5. Kashiwagi N, Sugimura K, Koiwai H, Yamamoto H, Yoshikawa T, Saniabadi AR, Adachi M, Shimoyama T. Immunomodulatory effects of granulocyte and monocyte adsorption apheresis as a treatment for patients with ulcerative colitis. Dig Dis Sci. 2002;47:1334–41. https://doi.org/10.1023/a:1015330816364.
6. Saniabadi AR, Hanai H, Takeuchi K, Umemura K, Nakashima M, Adachi T, Shima C, Bjarnason I, Lofberg R. Adacolumn, an adsorptive carrier-based granulocyte and monocyte apheresis device for the treatment of inflammatory and refractory diseases associated with leukocytes. Ther Apher Dial. 2003;7(1):48–59. https://doi.org/10.1046/j.1526-0968.2003.00012.x.
7. Pai RK, Hartman DJ, Rivers CR, et al. Complete resolution of mucosal neutrophils associates with improved long-term clinical outcomes of patients with ulcerative colitis. Clin Gastroenterol Hepatol. 2020;18:2510–7.
8. Eberhardson M, Marits P, Jones M, et al. Treatment of inflammatory bowel disease by chemokine receptor-targeted leukapheresis. Clin Immunol. 2013;149(1):73–82. https://doi.org/10.1016/j.clim.2013.05.021.
9. Sawada K, Ohnishi K, Kosaka T, Chikano S, Yokota Y, Egashira A, et al. Leukocytapheresis with leukocyte removal filter as new therapy for ulcerative colitis. Ther Apher. 1997;1(3):207–11.
10. Schneider M, Waitz G, Prophet H, Schober HC, Ramlow W. Adsorptive cytapheresis for ulcerative colitis with focus on removing platelets and platelet-aggregates. Ther Apher Dial. 2023;27:452. https://doi.org/10.1111/1744-9987.13942.
11. Fujimori J, Yoshino S, Koiwa M, Hirai H, Shiga H, Hayama N, Iino Y. Improvement in rheumatoid arthritis following application of an extracorporeal granulotrap column, G-1. Rheumatol Int. 1996;15:175–80. https://doi.org/10.1007/BF00290518.
12. Kashiwagi N, Hirata I, Kasukawa R. A role for granulocyte and monocyte apheresis in the treatment of rheumatoid arthritis. Ther Apher. 1998;2(2):134–41. https://doi.org/10.1111/j.1744-9987.1998.tb00091.x.
13. Kitagaichi M, Kusaoi M, Tsukahara T, Murayama G, Nemoto T, Sekiya F, Kon T, Ogasawara M, et al. Safety and efficacy of the leukocytapheresis procedure in eighty-five patients with rheumatoid arthritis. Transfus Apher Sci. 2016;55:225–32. https://doi.org/10.1016/j.transci.2016.07.019.
14. Ohnishi H, Kadowaki T, Mizutani Y, Nishida E, Tobita R, Abe N, et al. Genetic background and therapeutic response in generalized pustular psoriasis patients treated with granulocyte and monocyte adsorption apheresis. Eur J Dermatol. 2018;28:108–11. https://doi.org/10.1684/ejd.2017.3174.
15. Higashi Y, Ibusuki A, Baba N, Hatanaka M, Tada KI, Kanekura T. Granulocyte and monocyte adsorptive apheresis for pyoderma gangrenosum. Ther Apher Dial. 2021;26:450–5. https://doi.org/10.1111/1744-9987.13720.
16. Gnesotto L, Mioso G, Alaibac M. Use of granulocyte and monocyte adsorption apheresis in dermatology (review). Exp Ther Med. 2022;24:536–47. https://doi.org/10.3892/etm.2022.11463.
17. Habermalz B, Sauerland S. Clinical effectiveness of selective granulocyte, monocyte adsorptive apheresis with the Adacolumn device in ulcerative colitis. Dig Dis Sci. 2010;55:1421–8. https://doi.org/10.1007/s10620-009-0845-x.
18. Sawada K, Kusugami K, Suzuki Y, Bamba T, Munakata A, Hibi T, et al. Leukocytapheresis in ulcerative coli-

tis: results of a multicenter double-blind prospective case-control study with sham apheresis as placebo treatment. Am J Gastroenterol. 2005;100:1362–9. https://doi.org/10.1111/j.1572-0241.2005.41089.x.
19. Sands B, Sandborn WJ, Feagan B, Lofberg R, Hibi T, Wang T, et al. A randomized, double-blind, sham-controlled study of granulocyte/monocyte apheresis for active ulcerative colitis. Gastroenterology. 2008;135:400–9. https://doi.org/10.1053/j.gastro.2008.04.023.
20. Yoshino T, Nakase H, Minami N, Yamada S, Matsuura M, Yazumi S, et al. Efficacy and safety of granulocyte and monocyte adsorption apheresis for ulcerative colitis: a meta-analysis. Dig Liver Dis. 2014;46(3):219–26. https://doi.org/10.1016/j.dld.2013.10.011.
21. Dignass A, Akbar A, Hart A, Subramanian S, Bommelaer G, Baumgart DC, Grimaud JC, Cadiot G, et al. Safety and efficacy of granulocyte/monocyte apheresis in steroid-dependent active ulcerative colitis with insufficient response or intolerance to immunosuppressants and/or biologics [the ART trial]: 12-week interim results. J Crohns Colitis. 2016;10:812–20. https://doi.org/10.1093/ecco-jcc/jjw032.
22. Sacco R, Romano A, Mazzoni A, Bertini M, Federici G, Metrangolo S, et al. Granulocytapheresis in steroid-dependent and steroid-resistant patients with inflammatory bowel disease: a prospective observational study. J Crohns Colitis. 2013;7:e692–7. https://doi.org/10.1016/j.crohns.2013.06.012.
23. Domènech E, Panés J, Hinojosa J, Annese V, Magro F, Sturniolo GC, the ATTICA Study Group. Addition of granulocyte/monocyte apheresis to oral prednisone for steroid-dependent ulcerative colitis: a randomized multicentre clinical trial. J Crohns Colitis. 2018;12:687–94. https://doi.org/10.1093/ecco-jcc/jjy023.
24. Sakata Y, Iwakiri R, Amemori S, Yamaguch K, Fujise T, Otani H, Shimoda R, Tsunada S, et al. Comparison of the efficacy of granulocyte and monocyte/macrophage adsorptive apheresis and leukocytapheresis in active ulcerative colitis patients: a prospective randomized study. Eur J Gastroenterol Hepatol. 2008;20(7):629–33. https://doi.org/10.1097/MEG.0b013e3282f5e9a4.
25. Endo Y, Yonekawa M, Kukita K, Katagiri M, Matsumoto T, Kawasaki K, Yanai S, Kato S, et al. Novel adsorptive type apheresis device Immunopure for ulcerative colitis from clinical perspectives based on clinical trials: Japan and Europe. Ther Apher Dial. 2021;25:432–6. https://doi.org/10.1111/1744-9987.13661.
26. Fukuchi T, Kawashima K, Koga H, Utsonomiya R, Sugiyama K, Shimatsu K, Eguchi T, Ishihara S. Induction of mucosal healing by intensive granulocyte/monocyte adsorptive apheresis without the use of corticosteroids in patients with ulcerative colitis: long-term remission maintenance after induction by GMA and efficacy of GMA re-treatment upon relapse. J Clin Biochem Nutr. 2022;70(2):197–204. https://doi.org/10.3164/jcbn.21-112.
27. Iitzuka M, Etou T, Shimodaira Y, Hatakeyama T, Sagara S. Cytapheresis re-induces high-rate steroid-free remission in patients with steroid-dependent and steroid-refractory ulcerative colitis. World J Gastroenterol. 2021;27(12):1194–212. https://doi.org/10.3748/wjg.v27.i12.1194.
28. de Carpi JM, Vilar P, Prieto G, Garcia Novo MD, Ribes C, Varea V. Safety and efficacy of granulocyte and monocyte adsorption apheresis in paediatric inflammatory bowel disease: a prospective pilot study. J Pediatr Gastroenterol Nutr. 2008;46(4):386–91. https://doi.org/10.1097/MPG.0b013e31815604e5.
29. Ruuska T, Küster P, Grahnquist L, Lindgren F, Wewew AV. Efficacy and safety of granulocyte, monocyte/macrophage adsorptive in pediatric ulcerative colitis. World J Gastroenterol. 2016;22(17):4389–96. https://doi.org/10.3748/wjg.v22.i17.4389.
30. Rolandsdotter H, Eberhardson M, Fagerberg UL, Finkel Y. Granulocyte and monocyte apheresis for induction of remission in children with new-onset inflammatory bowel colitis. J Pediatr Gastroenterol Nutr. 2018;66:84–9. https://doi.org/10.1097/MPG.0000000000001641.
31. Motoya S, Tanaka H, Shibuya T, Osada T, Yamamoto T, Hongo H, et al. Safety and effectiveness of granulocyte and monocyte adsorptive apheresis in patients with inflammatory bowel disease in special situations: a multicentre cohort study. BMC Gastroenterol. 2019;19:196. https://doi.org/10.1186/s12876-019-1110-1.
32. Komoto S, Matsuoka K, Kobayashi T, Yokoyama Y, Suzuki Y, Hibi T, et al. Safety and efficacy of leukocytapheresis in elderly patients with ulcerative colitis: the impact in steroid-free elderly patients. J Gastroenterol Hepatol. 2018;33:1485–91. https://doi.org/10.1111/jgh.14116.
33. Shibuya T, Nomura O, Nomura K, Okahara K, Haga K, Ishikawa D, Sakamoto N, Ogihara T, Osada T, Nagahara A. Effectiveness of cytapheresis for ulcerative colitis in special situations: delayed onset of optimum efficacy in elderly patients. Digestion. 2020;101:46–52. https://doi.org/10.1159/000504091.
34. D'Ovidio V, Meo D, Gozer M, Bazuro ME, Vernia P. Ulcerative colitis and granulocyte-monocyte-apheresis: safety and efficacy of maintenance therapy during pregnancy. J Clin Apher. 2015;30:55–7. https://doi.org/10.1002/jca.21349.
35. Takahashi H, Sugawara K, Sugimura M, Iwabuchi M, Mano Y, Ukai K, et al. Flare up of ulcerative colitis during pregnancy treated by adsorptive granulocyte and monocyte apheresis: therapeutic outcomes in three pregnant patients. Arch Gynecol Obstet. 2013;288:341–7. https://doi.org/10.1007/s00404-013-2748-5.
36. Shibuya T, Haga K, Kamei M, Okahara K, Ito S, Takahashi M, et al. Successful remission of ulcerative colitis flare-up during pregnancy with adsorp-

tive granulomonocytapheresis plus tacrolimus. Intest Res. 2018;16:484–8. https://doi.org/10.5217/ir.2018.16.3.484.
37. Dignass A, Akbar A, Baumgart DC, Bommelaer G, Bouguen G, Cadiot G, Gillessen A, Grimaud JC, et al. Granulocyte/monocyte adsorptive apheresis for the treatment of therapy-refractory chronic active ulcerative colitis. Scand J Gastroenterol. 2018;53(4):442–8. https://doi.org/10.1080/00365521.2018.1447598.
38. Iizuka M, Etou K, Sagara S. Efficacy of cytapheresis in patients with ulcerative colitis showing insufficient or lost response to biologic therapy. World J Gastroenterol. 2022;28(34):4959–72. https://doi.org/10.3748/wjg.v28.i34.4959.
39. Yokoyama Y, Sawada K, Aoyama N, Yoshimura N, Sako M, Hirai F, et al. Efficacy of granulocyte and monocyte adsorptive apheresis in patients with inflammatory bowel disease showing lost response to infliximab. J Crohns Colitis. 2020;14:1264–73. https://doi.org/10.1093/ecco-jcc/jjaa051.
40. Fukuda Y, Matsui T, Suzuki Y. Adsorptive granulocyte and monocyte apheresis for refractory Crohn's disease: an open multicenter prospective study. J Gastroenterol. 2004;39:1158–64. https://doi.org/10.1007/s00535-004-1465-z.
41. Bresci G, Parisi G, Bertoni M, Mazzoni A, Scatena F, Capria A. Treatment of active steroid-refractory inflammatory bowel diseases with granulocytapheresis: our experience with a prospective study. World J Gastroenterol. 2006;14:2201–4. https://doi.org/10.3748/wjg.v12.i14.2201.
42. Fukuchi T, Nakase H, Ubukata S, Matsuura M, Yoshino T, Toyonaga T, et al. Therapeutic effect of intensive granulocyte and monocyte adsorption apheresis combined with thiopurines for steroid- and biologics-naïve Japanese patients with early-diagnosed Crohn's disease. BMC Gastroenterol. 2014;14:124–8. https://doi.org/10.1186/1471-230X-14-124.
43. Ikeda S, Takahashi H, Suga Y, Eto H, Etoh T, Okuma K, Takahashi K, Kanbara T, et al. Therapeutic depletion of myeloid lineage leukocytes in patients with generalized pustular psoriasis indicates a major role for neutrophils in the immunopathogenesis of psoriasis. J Am Acad Dermatol. 2013;68:609–17. https://doi.org/10.1016/j.jaad.2012.09.037.
44. Sanmartí R, Marsal S, Valverde J, Casado E, Lafuente R, Kashiwagi N, et al. Adsorptive granulocyte/monocyte apheresis for the treatment of refractory rheumatoid arthritis: an open pilot multicentre trial. Rheumatology. 2005;44(9):1140–4. https://doi.org/10.1093/rheumatology/keh701.
45. Martínez AVC, Chiva LM, Villarino MR. Granulocyte and monocyte/macrophage apheresis for the treatment of immune-mediated inflammatory arthropathies: case reports. Drugs Context. 2021;10:2021-8-5. https://doi.org/10.7573/dic.2021-8-5.
46. Code of Federal Regulations. Title 21, Volume 5. 21CFR312.32.
47. Sawada K, Ohdo M, Ino T, Nakamura T, Numata T, Shibata H, Sakou J, Kusada M, Hibi T. Safety and tolerability of nafamostat mesylate and heparin as anticoagulants in leukocytapheresis for ulcerative colitis: post hoc analysis of a large-scale, prospective, observational study. Ther Apher Dial. 2016;20:197–204. https://doi.org/10.1111/1744-9987.12357.
48. Yamamoto T, Iida T, Ikeya K, Kato M, Matsuura A, Tamura S, Takano R, Tani S, Osawa S, Sugimoto K, Shimoyama T, Hanai H. A multicenter retrospective study aiming to identify patients who respond well to adsorptive granulomonocytapheresis in moderately to severely active ulcerative colitis. Clin Transl Gastroenterol. 2018;9:170. https://doi.org/10.1038/s41424-018-0037-0.
49. Dignass AU, Eriksson A, Kilander A, Pukitis A, Rhodes JM, Vavricka S. Clinical trial: five or ten cycles of granulocyte-monocyte apheresis show equivalent efficacy and safety in ulcerative colitis. Aliment Pharmacol Ther. 2010;31:1286–95. https://doi.org/10.1111/j.1365-2036.2010.04295.x.
50. Cabriada J, Domenech L, Ibargoyen N, Hernandez V, Clofent J, Ginard G, Gutierrez-Ibarluzea I, Hinojosa J. Leukocytapheresis for steroid-dependent ulcerative colitis in clinical practice: results of a nationwide Spanish registry. J Gastroenterol. 2012;47(4):359–65. https://doi.org/10.1007/s00535-011-0499-2.
51. Ishiguro Y, Ohomori T, Umemura K, Iizuka M. Factors associated with the outcomes in ulcerative colitis patients undergoing granulocyte and monocyte adsorptive apheresis as remission induction therapy: a multicenter cohort study. Ther Apher Dial. 2021;25:502–12. https://doi.org/10.1111/1744-9987.13594.
52. Hibi T, Sameshima Y, Sekiguchi Y, Hisatome Y, Maruyama F, Moriwaki K, Shima C, Saniabadi AR, Matsumoto T. Treating ulcerative colitis by Adacolumn therapeutic leucocytapheresis: clinical efficacy and safety based on surveillance of 656 patients in 53 centres in Japan. Dig Liver Dis. 2009;41:570–7. https://doi.org/10.1016/j.dld.2008.11.020.
53. Rodríguez-Lago I, Benítez JM, Sempere L, Sáez-González E, Barreiro-de Acosta M, de Zárate JO, Cabriada JL. The combination of granulocyte-monocyte apheresis and vedolizumab: a new treatment option for ulcerative colitis? J Clin Apher. 2019;34:680–5. https://doi.org/10.1002/jca.21746.
54. Hanai H, Watanabe F, Yamada M, Sato Y, Takeushi K, Iida T, Tozawa K, Tanka T, et al. Adsorptive granulocyte and monocyte apheresis versus prednisolone in patients with corticosteroid-dependent moderately severe ulcerative colitis. Digestion. 2004;70:36–44. https://doi.org/10.1159/000080079.
55. Passalacqua S, Ferraro PM, Bresci G, D'Ovidio V, Astegiano M, Principi MB, Testa R, D'Incà R, et al. The Italian registry of therapeutic apheresis: granulocyte-monocyte apheresis in the treatment of inflammatory bowel disease. A multicentric study. J Clin Apher. 2011;26:332–7. https://doi.org/10.1002/jca.20315.

56. Tominaga K, Nakano M, Hoshino M, Kanke K, Hiraiashi H. Efficacy, safety and cost analyses in ulcerative colitis patients undergoing granulocyte and monocyte adsorption or receiving prednisolone. BMC Gastroenterol. 2013;13:41–7. https://doi.org/10.1186/1471-230X-13-41.
57. Fukunaga K, Yokoyama Y, Kamokozuru K, Nagase K, Nakamura S, Miwa H, Matsumoto T. Adsorptive granulocyte/monocyte apheresis for the maintenance of remission in patients with ulcerative colitis: a prospective randomized, double blind, sham-controlled clinical trial. Gut Liver. 2012;6(4):427–33. https://doi.org/10.5009/gnl.2012.6.4.427.
58. Yokoyama Y, Matsuoka K, Kobayashi T, Sawada K, Fujiyoshi T, Ando T, Ohnishi I, Ishida T, et al. A large-scale, prospective, observational study of leukocytapheresis for ulcerative colitis: treatment outcomes of 847 patients in clinical practice. J Crohns Colitis. 2014;8(9):981–91. https://doi.org/10.1016/j.crohns.2014.01.027.
59. Li N, Mao J, Tang H, Zhu L, Tan X, Bi J, Wu H, Chen X, et al. Efficacy and safety of adsorptive granulomonocytapheresis in Chinese patients with ulcerative colitis: a retrospective analysis of 50 cases with focus on factors impacting clinical efficacy. J Clin Apher. 2020;35:271–80. https://doi.org/10.1002/jca.21787.
60. Bresci G. Granulocytapheresis in the treatment of patients with active ulcerative colitis. Expert Rev Gastroenterol Hepatol. 2008;2(5):639–43. https://doi.org/10.1586/17474124.2.5.639.
61. Scrivo B, Vitello A, Cappello M. Response to the combination therapy with cytapheresis plus vedolizumab in a corticosteroid-dependent patient with ulcerative colitis and previous anti-TNF alfa failure. Dig Liver Dis. 2018;50:1103–4. https://doi.org/10.1016/j.dld.2018.05.001.
62. Rodríguez-Lago I, Sempere L, Gutiérrez A, Núñez A, Leo Carnerero E, Hinojosa E, Mora M, Cañete F, et al. Granulocyte-monocyte apheresis: an alternative combination therapy after loss of response to anti-TNF agents in ulcerative colitis. Scand J Gastroenterol. 2019;54:459–64. https://doi.org/10.1080/00365521.2019.1600715.
63. Tanida S, Mizoshita T, Ozeki K, Katano T, Tanaka M, Nishie H, Shimura T, Okamoto Y, et al. Combination therapy with intensive granulocyte and monocyte adsorptive apheresis plus ustekinumab in patients with refractory Crohn's disease. Ther Apher Dial. 2018;22:295–300. https://doi.org/10.1111/1744-9987.12697.
64. Sawada K, Muto T, Shimoyama T, Satomi M, Sawada T, Nagawa H, Hiwatashi N, Asakura H, et al. Multicenter randomized controlled trial for the treatment of ulcerative colitis with a leukocytapheresis column. Curr Pharm Des. 2003;9(4):307–21. https://doi.org/10.2174/1381612033391928.
65. Naganuma M, Yokoyama Y, Motoya S, Watanabe K, Sawada K, Hirai F, Yamamoto T, Hanai H, CAPTAIN Study Group. Efficacy of apheresis as maintenance therapy for patients with ulcerative colitis in an open-label prospective multicenter randomized controlled trial. J Gastroenterol. 2020;55:390–400. https://doi.org/10.1007/s00535-019-01651-0.
66. Nishioka C, Aoyama N, Maekawa S, Shirasaka D, Nakahara T, Tamura T, Fukagawa M, Umezu M, et al. Leukocytapheresis therapy for steroid naïve patients with active ulcerative colitis: its clinical efficacy and adverse effects compared with those of conventional steroid therapy. J Gastroenterol Hepatol. 2005;20:1567–71. https://doi.org/10.1111/j.1440-1746.2005.03907.x.
67. Fukunaga K, Kamikozuru K, Yokoyama Y, Hida N, Ohda Y, Takeda N, Yoshida K, Iimuro M, et al. Optimal apheresis treatment volume for the efficacy and safety of leukocytapheresis with Cellsorba in patients with active ulcerative colitis. J Clin Apher. 2011;26:326–31. https://doi.org/10.1002/jca.20314.
68. Sáez-González E, Moret I, Alvarez-Sotomayor D, Díaz-Jaime FC, Cerrillo E, Iborra M, Nos P, Beltrán B. Immunological mechanisms of adsorptive cytapheresis in inflammatory bowel disease. Dig Dis Sci. 2017;62:1417–25. https://doi.org/10.1007/s10620-017-4577-z.
69. Kruis W, Nguyen P, Morgenstern J, Ramlow W, Dignass A, Stallmach A, Drebber U. Novel leucocyte/thrombocyte apheresis for induction of steroid-free remission in ulcerative colitis: a controlled randomized pilot study. J Crohns Colitis. 2019;13(7):949–53.
70. Ito A, Omori T, Hanafusa N, Tsuchiya K, Nakamura S, Tokushige K. Efficacy and safety of granulocyte adsorption apheresis in elderly patients with ulcerative colitis. J Clin Apher. 2018;33:514–20.
71. Yanagisawa K, Murakami M, Kondo Y, Oguma S, Kobayashi S, Miyasaka H, Shinohara T, Tomori A, et al. Efficacy and safety of adsorptive granulocyte and monocyte apheresis in elderly and pregnant patients with ulcerative colitis. Ther Apher Dial. 2019;23(3):217–23. https://doi.org/10.1111/1744-9987.12818.
72. Nagase K, Fukuanga K, Yokoyama Y, Kamikozuru K, Miwa H, Nakamura S. Questionnaire based assessment of patients' acceptability of leukocytapheresis for the treatment of inflammatory bowel disease. Ther Apher Dial. 2013;17:490–7. https://doi.org/10.1111/1744-9987.12115.
73. Sands BE, Katz S, Wolf DC, Feagan BG, Wang T, Gustofson LM, Wong C, Vandervoort MK, et al. A randomized, double-blind, sham-controlled study of granulocyte/monocyte apheresis for moderate to severe Crohn's disease. Gut. 2013;62:1288–94. https://doi.org/10.1136/gutjnl-2011-300995.
74. Domènech E, Hinojosa J, Esteve-Comas M, Gomollón F, Herrera JM, Bastida G, et al. Granulocytaphaeresis in steroid-dependent inflammatory bowel disease: a prospective, open, pilot study. Aliment Pharmacol Ther. 2004;20:1347–52. https://doi.org/10.1111/j.1365-2036.2004.02288.x.
75. Sacco R, Romano A, Mazzoni A, Bertini M, Federici G, Metrangolo S, Parisi G, Nencini C, et al. Granulocytapheresis in steroid-dependent and

steroid-resistant patients with IBD: a prospective study. J Crohns Colitis. 2013;7(12):e692–7. https://doi.org/10.1016/j.crohns.2013.06.012.
76. Bresci G, Romano A, Mazzoni A, Scatena F, Altomare E, Capria A, Sacco R. Feasibility and safety of granulocytapheresis in Crohn's disease: a prospective cohort study. Gastroenterol Clin Biol. 2010;34(12):682–6. https://doi.org/10.1016/j.gcb.2010.09.009.
77. Ozeki K, Tanida S, Mizoshita T, Tsukamoto H, Ebi M, Mori Y, Kataoka H, Kamiya T, et al. Combination therapy with intensive granulocyte and monocyte adsorptive apheresis plus adalimumab: therapeutic outcomes in 5 cases with refractory Crohn's disease. Case Rep Gastroenterol. 2012;6:765–71. https://doi.org/10.1159/000346312.
78. Fukunaga K, Matsumoto T. Current status and future perspectives of leukocytapheresis for inflammatory bowel disease. J Gastroenterol Hepatol. 2012;27:997–1003. https://doi.org/10.1111/j.1440-1746.2012.07119.x.
79. Sakanoue M, Takeda K, Kawai K, Kanekura T. Granulocyte and monocyte adsorption apheresis for refractory skin diseases due to activated neutrophils, psoriasis, and associated arthropathy. Ther Apher Dial. 2013;17:477–83. https://doi.org/10.1111/1744-9987.12113.
80. Domènech E, Grífols JR, Akbar A, Dignass A. Use of granulocyte/monocytapheresis in ulcerative colitis: a practical review from a European perspective. World J Gastroenterol. 2021;27(10):908–18. https://doi.org/10.3748/wjg.v27.i10.908.
81. Adacolumn. CE0123. Instructions for use. 2021. https://www.adacyte.com/wp-content/uploads/2021/02/63-17-English.pdf.
82. Eberhardson M, Karlén P, Linton L, Jones P, Lindberg A, Kostalla MJ, Lindh E, Odén A, et al. Randomised, double-blind, placebo-controlled trial of CCR9-targeted leukapheresis treatment of ulcerative colitis patients. J Crohns Colitis. 2017;11:534–42. https://doi.org/10.1093/ecco-jcc/jjw196.
83. Pineda AA. Developments in the apheresis procedure for the treatment of inflammatory bowel disease. Inflamm Bowel Dis. 2006;12(Suppl 1):S10–4. https://doi.org/10.1097/01.MIB.0000195386.19268.B3.

Basic Principles and Problems in Donor Lymphocyte Collection

13

Meltem Kurt Yüksel

13.1 Background

Allogeneic hematopoietic stem cell transplantation (AHSCT) is the pioneering adoptive immunotherapy. The immune system plays a crucial role in both engraftment or graft rejection, involving all its components, such as cells and cytokines. T cells are of utmost importance, as they mediate the graft-versus-malignancy (GVM) and graft-versus-host disease (GVHD) effects, immune reconstitution, and tolerance following AHSCT. Relapse after AHSCT remains a major challenge, with limited therapeutic options. Donor lymphocyte infusion (DLI) is a procedure that can address relapse by infusing donor lymphocytes to stimulate an immune response.

DLI, a form of cellular therapy, can induce graft-versus-leukemia effect following AHSCT, especially in cases of chimerism loss, minimal residual disease (MRD), or overt relapse, sometimes in combination with chemotherapy or epigenetic therapy.

In January 1987, Slavin et al. provided the first evidence of DLI's efficacy in chronic myeloid leukemia (CML) [1]. Weiden et al. also studied DLI in long-term canine radiation chimeras [2], while Kolb et al. subsequently treated not only CML relapses but also other diseases relapsing after AHSCT using DLI [3, 4].

The collection of lymphocytes via apheresis and their infusion into patients has led to the elimination of tumor cells, even in patients with hematologic malignancies resistant to ablative conditioning regimens.

Alloreactive lymphocytes, which mediate antitumor effects following the induction of host-versus-graft tolerance by donor stem cell transplantation, can trigger GVM effects, often accompanied by GVHD. To reduce the risk of GVHD and improve outcomes, the Sloan Kettering Transplantation group developed a dose-escalation schedule for DLI [5].

13.2 Pathophysiological Background and Treatment Goals and Principles

13.2.1 Pathophysiological Background

The GVM effect occurs when donor cells exert alloreactivity against a recipient's leukemic cells, primarily through the recognition of minor histocompatibility antigens (mHAgs) and tumor antigens by donor cells. This effect is largely driven by the T-cell compartment, including cytotoxic T cells (CD8+) or T helper cells (CD4+), although

M. K. Yüksel (✉)
Division of Internal Medicine, Department of Hematology and Stem Cell Transplantation Unit, Ankara University School of Medicine, Ankara, Turkey
e-mail: mkyuksel@ankara.edu.tr

I. Kozanoglu (ed.), *Problem Solving in Apheresis Medicine*,
https://doi.org/10.1007/978-3-031-74081-7_13

dendritic cells, natural killer (NK), and B cells may also play key roles [6, 7].

T-cell receptor (TCR) signaling is a critical step in this process; however, T-cell activation and differentiation are not solely dependent on TCR signaling. Instead, they reflect the cumulative effect of graded signals from various receptors in response to ligands from antigen-presenting cells (APCs) and other accessory cells. The outcome depends on the strength, duration, timing, and frequency of these signals. In the context of AHSCT, both major and minor human leukocyte antigen (HLA) disparities generate a broad range of T-cell responses. Naive T-cell activation involves (1) TCRs, (2) receptors engaging co-stimulatory molecules on APCs, and (3) cytokine receptors [6].

After cytokine signaling, naive CD4 and CD8 cells differentiate into multiple subsets. For naive CD4 cells, these subsets include T helper (Th1, Th2, Th17), T follicular helper (Tfh), Tr1, TH9, and induced FoxP3^{+} regulatory T (Treg) cells. Naive CD8 cells can differentiate into analogous subsets. The regulation of CD8 responses influences the differentiation into effector and memory T cells. Following initial antigen activation, CD8 cells proliferate extensively and subsequently contract, with a subset persisting as long-term memory cells. Persistent inflammation favors short-term effector differentiation, whereas reduced inflammation increases the likelihood of CD8 cells differentiating into memory cells [6, 7].

13.2.1.1 Donor Lymphocyte Type

Tumor-specific T cells are present in patients, and through simple cloning techniques, various donor-derived T-cell clones can be isolated from patients with GVHD. These include cytotoxic T lymphocytes (CTLs) that recognize and kill tumor cells without affecting normal cells, CTLs that target normal host cells but not tumor cells, CTLs reactive against both host and tumor cells, and CTLs that are non-reactive to both, which reflect different correlations of GVL and GVHD—such as GVL without GVHD, GVL associated with GVHD, and progressive tumors in patients with persistent GVHD [7, 8].

The efficacy of DLI may be enhanced by nonspecific or specific activation of donor lymphocytes with cytokines. Future research should aim to develop methods for maximizing tumor-specific responses while protecting normal host cells from nonspecific and harmful anti-host responses, which can lead to acute and chronic GVHD and present major barriers to successful DLI immunotherapy. Using specifically immune, rather than naive, donor lymphocytes appears to be the most promising strategy to optimize outcomes in adoptive allogeneic cell therapy for cancer. Interestingly, donor lymphocyte immunotherapy may also be applied to treat nonmalignant diseases, as alloreactive donor lymphocytes can effectively eliminate all host-origin hematopoietic cells [7–9].

An alternative approach may involve non-alloreactive, tumor-reactive donor lymphocytes, similar to tumor-infiltrating lymphocytes (TIL), as previously described [8]. Tumor-specific GVL effects, without associated GVHD, could be mediated by T cells or CTLs induced in vitro to respond exclusively, or predominantly, against tumor-specific or tissue-specific antigens [8, 9].

In cases of suboptimal or absent GVL responses following allogeneic blood and marrow transplantation (BMT) in patients without GVHD, donor T cells may fail to respond to tumor cells due to clonal deletion, anergy, TCR blockade, or active suppression from immunosuppressive agents used for GVHD prophylaxis or factors secreted by tumor cells. Additionally, the absence of GVHD and GVL might stem from a low frequency of cytotoxic T-lymphocyte precursors (CTLp) or a complete match between donor and host at all mHAgs, which are significant factors in both GVHD and GVL [8, 9].

13.2.1.2 DLI Content

In addition to dose adjustment, a better understanding of DLI composition could improve outcomes, particularly by reducing toxicity.

Studies related to DLI content include naive T cell (T_N)-depleted DLI, which targets naive T cells as significant drivers of GVHD, and CD45RA+ depleted DLI, developed in TCR alpha-/beta-depleted transplantation settings to reduce infection rates. Modifying DLI composition in other ways may also improve outcomes. Tregs (CD3 + CD4 + CD25^{high} + Foxp3 + CD127−), which help maintain immune homeostasis and prevent autoimmune events, have been shown to offer protection from GVHD. Moreover, studies indicate that a lower proportion of Tregs in DLI is associated with a higher response rate [10]. In another study, Treg-depleted DLI [7, 11] was found to be safe and capable of inducing alloreactivity after transplantation. Another approach to reduce GVHD involves removing donor CD8+ T cells from DLI [7, 12–14].

Depending on the donor HLA matching status—whether haploidentical, matched, or mismatched unrelated donors—the DLI approach may vary. Combining immunosuppressive prophylaxis (ISP) with DLI is one option for controlling GVHD. A group of Chinese researchers published a retrospective comparative study on the use of DLI with and without ISP in haploidentical transplantation with in vivo T-cell depletion (TCD) [15]. They found no difference in relapse risk, with grade 2–4 acute GVHD being lower in the ISP plus DLI cohort. This group also suggested a preference for methotrexate over cyclosporine as the ISP for DLI [16]. Another study reported achieving complete donor chimerism in patients receiving DLI while maintaining ISP [17].

GVHD is the primary complication after DLI, but it can be modulated by various methods. One approach involves using suicide gene-transduced donor T lymphocytes. Transduced killer (TK) alloreactive lymphocytes are genetically engineered to express a suicide gene, which supports early immune reconstitution, prevents leukemic relapse, and controls GVHD. The effect of TK cells is regulated by antiviral therapy targeting the suicide gene-carrying cells. The San Raffaele Group [18] pioneered the use of the herpes simplex virus thymidine kinase (HSV-TK) gene, the most extensively studied suicide gene. In a phase I–II clinical trial, 30 adult patients with TCD haploidentical AHSCT received one or two infusions of TK-engineered T cells. GVHD occurred in 11 patients, and in all cases, the TK/GCV (ganciclovir) mechanism was effective, leading to complete resolution of GVHD [19].

13.2.2 Treatment Goals and Principles

The goal of AHSCT is the development of immune tolerance. Tolerance after HCT is functionally defined as the presence of immune reactivity without rejection or overt GVHD, in the absence of immunosuppressive medications. At any given time, immune reactivity potentially involves three main populations of T cells in the recipient: residual recipient T cells, the progeny of mature T cells contained in the allograft, and donor-derived T cells that mature from donor progenitor cells in the thymus [6].

In case of disease recurrence, donor-derived lymphocytes become diminished both functionally and quantitatively. To rebalance the process in favor of GVM and treat relapse, DLI is one of the options. DLI aims to promote the GVM effect without inducing GVHD. DLI can be categorized into two main groups. First, if there is manipulation of the donor or apheresis product before or after donor T-cell apheresis, the terminology is mobilized/modified DLI. Second, if the DLI is administered based on the status of the disease, the terminology is prophylactic/preemptive or therapeutic DLI (tDLI). Relapse after AHSCT can be categorized as overt relapses with varying percentages of blasts in the peripheral blood or bone marrow, MRD positivity, and loss of chimerism. In patients with mixed chimerism (MC) and molecular relapse, preemptive DLI (pDLI) or prophylactic DLI (prDLI) may be used as maintenance therapy for malignancies in patients with high-risk hematological malignancies (Fig. 13.1) [7].

The European Society for Blood and Marrow Transplantation (EBMT) registry study, which included 48,111 patients after the first allogeneic transplants, hypothesized that comparing the correlation between GVHD and relapse might provide a surrogate marker for the susceptibility

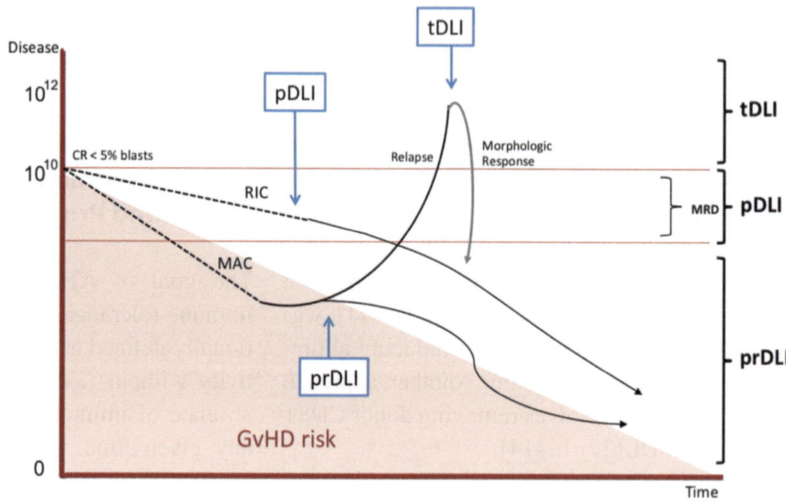

Fig. 13.1 Diagram displaying the use of tDLI, pDLI, and prDLI. (Taken from Guillermo Orti et al., *Experimental Hematology* 2017;48:1–11)

of diseases to alloimmune effects, such as DLI. These results confirm previous observations of potent graft-versus-tumor (GvT) effects associated with GVHD. The strength of the GVHD/GvT correlation differs significantly between hematological malignancies. In chronic myeloid leukemia (CML), the relapse risk declined clearly and proportionally with the severity of acute and chronic GVHD. Acute lymphoblastic leukemia and BCR-ABL-negative myeloproliferative neoplasms were comparably sensitive to GVHD as CML, whereas myelodysplastic syndromes and lymphoproliferative disorders showed intermediate sensitivity. GVHD was only associated with modest reductions in relapse risk in acute myeloid leukemia (AML) and plasma cell disorders (PCDs). The parallel drop in relapse rates across different diseases, despite differences in GVHD/GvT ratios, suggests that GvT effects might operate in the absence of GVHD, particularly in AML [20].

DLI response and efficacy depend on the patient, disease, and DLI factors [21]. Although not as significant as in CML, there is evidence of the GVL effect in AML and myelodysplastic syndrome (MDS). Maintained responses can be achieved with DLI in these malignancies (15–20%), but global outcomes remain poor and unpredictable. The reasons DLI is less effective in AML than in CML may include the high proliferative kinetics of AML cells or immune evasion mechanisms, such as loss of HLA [4, 6, 7, 21].

The optimal DLI dose, timing, and frequency are significant concerns. DLI can be administered on an outpatient basis while the patient is off any posttransplant immunosuppression. The starting dose for patients is 10^5 T cells/kg, which is considered the dose level at BMT, beyond which patients are at risk of developing GVHD. Subsequent doses of DLI can consist of 10^6, 10^7, and 10^8 T cells/kg, as needed, until measurable tumor cell markers or residual host cells are eliminated or until GVHD becomes apparent. Additional nonspecific activation of donor effector cells with cytokines such as rIL-2, interferon-a (IFN-a), possibly IL-12, or combinations thereof, or tumor- or tissue-specific activation of donor lymphocytes should be considered for patients with residual or resistant disease and no GVHD who are not responding to DLI [7, 22]. Interestingly, responses have also been observed in the absence of GVHD [5].

The duration of DLI and the interval between DLIs is another concern. Studies have demonstrated that the dose escalation protocols may not depend on the total dose of infused lymphocytes but rather how they are infused, which is relevant to the development of GVHD. Given the limited data, there is no clear recommendation on when to stop DLI if the patient has not developed GVHD and GVL has not been observed [7, 22, 23].

The time interval between DLI infusions varies among institutional protocols and has not been adequately assessed. An 8-week time interval is generally accepted, but this may depend on when the first dose is administered (i.e., the time interval from AHSCT to DLI). In addition, DLIs are typically not given within the first 3 months after AHSCT, except in cases of relapse [23]. A time interval of 2 years between AHSCT and DLI has been reported as relevant for GVHD development [24], but other cutoff time points have also been suggested [25, 26]. In pDLI, protocols exist where DLI is scheduled within the first 6 months after AHSCT, which has been reported as feasible [7, 25]. What seems clear from these studies is that the earlier DLIs are given, the higher the chance of developing GVHD.

The unsatisfactory results of tDLI prompted some groups to introduce DLI to harness the GVL effect before relapse. Two strategies can be identified: pDLI, a T-cell infusion administered for MC or any state of MRD, and prDLI, where T cells are given prophylactically before any signs of relapse or progression (Fig. 13.1 schematically describes the use of DLI, pDLI, and prDLI). In myeloablative transplantations for AML, whole blood and T-cell MC have been associated with relapse [27, 28]. However, the presence of MC in TCD AHSCT is not uncommon, and in this setting, full donor chimerism has been linked to lower overall survival (OS) [29]. Notably, the interpretation of chimerism differs depending on the conditioning regimen, transplant platform, or type of TCD. Apart from certain nonmalignant diseases in which stable MC can be "allowed," T-cell MC (the loss of donor T-cell MC) should be reverted. This can be done through ISP withdrawal or by DLI; outcomes have been reported in Hodgkin's lymphoma [30] and in AML and MDS [31].

A recent study reported on the use of pDLI in 113 patients diagnosed with myeloid malignancies who received TCD (mostly alemtuzumab)-reduced intensity conditioning (RIC) AHSCT [32]. Patients received either pDLI or tDLI. Patients receiving pDLI had a 5-year OS of 80%, whereas patients who received tDLI had a 5-year OS of 40%. Notably, patients receiving early pDLI (<6 months) did not develop more GVHD compared to those receiving late DLI (>6 months). Interestingly, the relapse rates at 5 years were similar for both tDLI and pDLI (69% and 65%, respectively). Schmid et al. [33], on behalf of the EBMT ALWP (Acute Leukemia Working Party), reported data on preemptive lymphocyte infusions at the 2015 American Society of Hematology meeting. The investigators presented a cohort of 343 patients diagnosed with acute leukemia (mainly AML) treated with pDLI for MRD or MC. In this study, about half of the patients with MRD and 70% of the patients with MC who received pDLI did not relapse during a follow-up of 5 years, suggesting a clinically meaningful effect of pDLI in AML patients. The investigators also found that the development of GVHD depends on the time interval between AHSCT and DLI (the cutoff time point was 6 months). Other groups have also recently reported on prDLI [34] in a retrospective study, and the cohort of 46 patients who received prDLI had a remarkable 7-year OS of 67% [31, 33].

The use of either pDLI or prDLI is gaining importance in myeloid malignancies. The best timing, dosing, and product manipulation require further investigation. Studies so far have shown that early DLI in AML or MDS is feasible, although variably effective. The limited efficacy achieved with tDLI suggests that pDLI and prDLI may play a role in AML and MDS relapses, particularly in TCD and nonmyeloablative transplantation platforms [7, 22, 31, 33].

13.2.3 Patient and Donor Education

Patient and donor education regarding donor lymphocyte infusion begins before the initiation of the AHSCT procedure. Transplantation complications should be thoroughly explained in detail during the family meeting. The rationale for stem cell transplantation, follow-up care, and solutions to related complications should be discussed. Patients should understand that the aim of an AHSCT is to replace diseased bone marrow with healthy, functioning marrow. When all new blood cells are derived from donor stem cells, this is called full chimerism; sometimes, a mixture of donor and host (patient) stem cells will occur, known as MC. When a stem cell transplant is performed for a hematological malignancy (blood cancer), the goal is to replace all of the patient's marrow with donor cells, i.e., achieving full chimerism. T lymphocytes, a type of leukocyte, are responsible for full chimerism. They are collected by apheresis and form the content of DLI. There are two main reasons why DLI may be given: (1) to destroy any residual disease and (2) to treat MC [35].

13.2.3.1 Collecting the Donor Lymphocytes

Sometimes the transplant center will have collected donor lymphocytes at the time of the original stem cell harvest and frozen and stored them. If this is the case, there will be no need to collect additional cells. There is no difference between fresh or cryopreserved DLI in terms of count or clinical effect [35–37]. Donor lymphocytes are easy to collect from the blood of a donor, as they are present in considerable numbers. Generally, no medications are required to increase the number of lymphocytes. The donor will undergo a full physical examination and blood tests, including screening for viruses such as HIV and hepatitis. Blood tests will also be done to ensure there is no risk of clotting or bleeding problems before the donor undergoes the cell apheresis process [36]. The donor will have two intravenous lines placed, one in each arm. Blood is drawn through one line and passed through the machine, where it is mixed with an anticoagulant to prevent blood clotting and assist in separating the cells [37]. The blood is spun in the machine and separated into red, white, and plasma cells. Special pumps collect lymphocytes into a sterile bag attached to the machine, while the remaining red, white, and plasma cells are returned to the donor through the other line. The collection process typically takes 2–3 h, with a total lymphocyte volume of about 200 mL. The collection bag is then separated from the machine, labeled, and sent to the laboratory for checking and cell counting. Usually, only one collection is required, and the lymphocytes are frozen in several small bags containing different doses of cells. However, it is possible that the donor may need to undergo this process again [35]. The collection facility minimizes donation-related discomforts and ensures adequate mononuclear cell (MNC) collection, which will be further processed before clinical use. The most common complaints associated with the lengthy procedure include activity restriction on the donation bed or chair, limited arm movement when peripheral access is used, and symptoms caused by citrate toxicity, including numbness, tingling, muscle cramping, hypotension, and arrhythmia. The establishment of a predictive model could help avoid underestimating MNC yield, increasing the chances of obtaining adequate MNCs and preventing unnecessary prolongation of the procedure [36, 37].

13.2.3.2 Patient Receiving DLI

Before receiving DLI, the patient will undergo a complete physical examination. Blood tests will also be conducted to check the function of other organs, such as the kidneys and liver, and to screen for viruses [35, 36].

The infusion can be administered through a central line if one is already in place. Otherwise, a small temporary line will be inserted into a vein in the arm and removed before the patient goes home. The cells are given slowly over 10–30 min through the line or in a syringe, depending on the number of infused cells. If the cells have been frozen, there is a small chance of reacting to the preservative dimethyl sulfoxide (DMSO). Once the infusion is complete, the lines are removed, or the central line is flushed [35, 36].

A nurse will supervise the procedure and monitor for any reactions to the infusion. An injection of antihistamine is given before the infusion to minimize the risk of reaction. This may cause drowsiness, so it is advisable not to drive to and from the appointment. Reactions to the transfusion are very uncommon, but nurses will always be present. Patients should not hesitate to inform them if they experience any discomfort or have concerns [35, 36].

Patients should be aware of the early signs of GVHD, which include the following: rashes or redness of the skin, upset stomach or loss of appetite, nausea or diarrhea, soreness in the mouth and tongue, and infections in the mouth. Blood tests may show alterations in liver function.

DLI can suppress the bone marrow (myelosuppression), leading to a reduced number of blood cells and resulting in symptoms such as anemia, increased bruising and bleeding, and greater susceptibility to infection [37].

Progress must be carefully monitored by the transplant team, who are experienced in assessing and recognizing potential problems. Approximately 8 weeks after the first dose of donor lymphocytes is given, the response is assessed in terms of disease status or chimerism. If there is still evidence of disease or MC, and no significant GVHD has developed, a slightly higher dose of donor lymphocytes may be given. Further doses are typically administered at 3-month intervals. In some cases, multiple doses of donor lymphocytes are given until the desired effect is achieved or until significant GVHD develops [23, 35].

13.2.4 Considerations

13.2.4.1 Considerations for the Apheresis Team

Cellular collections are a rapidly expanding area of apheresis. As soon as DLI is indicated, the first step should be to check whether cryopreserved lymphocytes are available and if the patient has venous access. If cryopreserved DLI is not available, the next step is to contact the donor, who may be a relative or an unrelated donor from a donor registry. Donors should be invited to the apheresis unit for the collection. To facilitate these procedures, the choice of vascular access is critical. Several factors, including the adequacy of peripheral veins, the patient's medication administration needs, the duration and frequency of procedures, and the skills of the apheresis team, should be carefully considered before making vascular access decisions. As protocols refine and cellular therapies expand for new indications, these decisions will play a significant role in ensuring safe and effective leukocyte apheresis [7, 38, 39].

Cellular collections require steady blood flow to process two to four or more blood volumes to collect the desired target cell components. In allogeneic donors, the leukocyte apheresis procedure is performed solely for the recipient's benefit, and every effort should be made to minimize risks to the donor [36, 38].

13.2.4.2 Venous Access

Patient and donor evaluation should begin with a detailed assessment of peripheral vein location and size. In patients with adequate peripheral venous access, large bore needles (typically 16–18 gauge [G]) are used to draw and return blood to the donor. Challenges with peripheral access are often encountered in small and overweight/obese individuals. Many programs reserve central vascular access for such patients/donors. Essential considerations for peripheral vascular access include (1) the use of warmers to dilate peripheral vessels, (2) ensuring patients/donors are well-hydrated, (3) the patient being able to remain in a supine position with an outstretched arm (if antecubital access) for prolonged periods, and (4) well-trained staff with experience in venous cannulation using large bore needles [38, 39].

13.2.4.3 DLI Procurement

There are several alternatives for obtaining DLI from either related or unrelated donors. In the case of related donors, when low-dose DLIs are requested (10^4–10^5 T-cells/kg), a small aliquot of freshly collected blood from a familiar donor may be used for immediate release. For small aliquots of whole blood (1–2 mL), donor-recipient major ABO incompatibility is generally not life-threatening and does not represent an absolute contraindication. In contrast, when DLIs are obtained from a registry donor, longer times are needed for authorization and collection; thus, only DLIs from lymphocytapheresis should be considered.

MNC collection is similar to peripheral hematopoietic progenitor cell (HPC) collection because HPCs are also MNCs. However, there are some important differences between these two procedures. First, MNC collection is performed without mobilization, unlike HPC collection. As a result, the number of circulating cells is much lower in MNC collection, leading to a thinner buffy coat (also known as the interface). Second, circulating MNCs decrease faster during collection compared to HPC collection because of the lack of active MNC replenishment from bone marrow mobilization.

Moreover, the collection time of MNCs is normally shorter than that of HPC collections because fewer MNCs are required. There is no consensus regarding processing volume or collection time among apheresis facilities, sponsors, or processing laboratories. In many institutions, a fixed "standard" volume is used unless a specific target number is mandated by experimental study protocols [39, 40].

DLI may be harvested through normal or large-volume leukapheresis, especially when further immunomagnetic selection procedures are needed to obtain the selected T-cell population [41]. In other clinical settings, such as haploidentical transplantation, where G-CSF-stimulated peripheral blood stem cells are harvested, DLI may be collected from the negative fraction of the CD34+-hematopoietic stem cell selection [42]. From a technical standpoint, recently released cell separators provide very satisfactory lymphocyte-enriched yields. According to published reports [43–45], differences among the latest-generation devices are minimal. Most of the investigated cell separators (COBE Spectra, Amicus, Fresenius COM.TEC, and Spectra Optia) produce a highly lymphocyte-enriched yield, with very low erythrocyte contamination and, in some cases [43, 45], reduced platelet content. Furthermore, when performing lymphocyte collection in a low-weight donor, devices with a low extracorporeal blood volume should be chosen. The lymphocyte-enriched harvest is then subdivided into aliquots containing increasing doses of DLI, according to the different clinical protocols. These aliquots are kept frozen until thawing and infusion [38–40, 45].

13.2.4.4 Apheresis Devices/Collection Efficiency (CE) and MNC Collection

The apheresis devices used to collect MNCs vary in their hardware specifications and separation technologies, but they all require good flow rates to process adequate volumes of blood and achieve the target cell dose. Commonly used devices in the United States include the Spectra Optia (Terumo BCT) and the Amicus (Fresenius Kabi). Due to the proximity of the platelet layer to MNCs, platelet depletion can be a significant clinical concern. The Spectra Optia collects MNCs continually or through cyclical harvest, depending on the protocol used. The Amicus operates through intermittent collection of MNCs [39, 40].

13.3 MNC CE and Factors Affecting MNC Yield

Modern apheresis instruments can effectively differentiate MNC from whole blood using an automated MNC program based on gravity and/or cell size. Routine clinical procedures using manufacturer-suggested instrument settings demonstrate the feasibility and safety of MNC apheresis with two successive technological generations of apheresis systems. Performance differences between the technologies are relatively minor and likely clinically irrelevant.

CE is a tool used to assess the capacity of apheresis to extract circulating cells and has been widely used in peripheral blood progenitor cell (PBPC) collection studies. CE1 is the most critical parameter for apheresis outcomes. Variations in CE1 are, in part, donor-dependent. The calculation of CE1% is below.

"Total collected cells" were calculated based on product volume and the concentration of the respective cell type in the apheresis product. CE1 for MNCs was calculated using the following formula, as previously reported [40, 45–47]:

$$\text{CE1}(\%) = (\text{MNC } \mu L \text{ product} \times \text{PV}) / (((\text{MNCpre} + \text{MNCpost})2) \times \text{TPV}),$$

where PV is product volume, MNCpre is MNC/μL peripheral blood before apheresis, MNCpost is MNC/μL peripheral blood after apheresis, and TPV is total processed blood volume. CE1 for lymphocytes or monocytes was calculated accordingly.

Lymphocytes are the primary cells of interest in most MNC collection procedures. Different formulas exist to assess the predictive capability of pre-MNC values for the collection yield of MNCs, lymphocytes, and monocytes. Predicting the number of CD3+ T cells to be collected is a key objective. Shaz et al. have shown that the TBV processed during collections for DLIs can be predicted using a linear correlation function between TBV and CD3+ T-cell yield from previous collections. They used this linear correlation to determine the TBV to be processed to collect the requested number of CD3+ T cells. Their study demonstrated that this approach can be safely and effectively implemented using a linear function that incorporates TBV processed and cellular yield data from the least efficient collection in the reference group. The application of this function resulted in significantly reduced leukapheresis procedure time and product discard compared to the previous collection protocol, where three times the donor's TBV was processed as standard [46].

Schulz et al. 1 compared unstimulated MNC apheresis (DLIs; healthy donors) and extracorporeal photopheresis (ECP; patients), specifically lymphocyte collections randomly performed with either the Spectra Optia MNC or COBE Spectra MNC. The comparison focused on target cell yield and CE, product volume, nontarget cell contamination, platelet (PLT) attrition, and various process variables such as process volume and time [45]. The results showed that for most relevant apheresis outcomes, differences between the devices were, at best, marginal. Spectra Optia MNC collections in patients, but not in donors, took 10% longer to achieve the target process volume. PLT attrition with Spectra Optia MNC was markedly lower in donors. ECP apheresis outcome variability was significantly donor-dependent, regardless of the device used. In conclusion, both apheresis systems were safe, robust, and equally suitable for unstimulated MNC collections, and both could be successfully run with manufacturer-recommended settings and algorithms [45].

Adaptive cellular immunotherapy may be the fastest-growing field in cancer therapy. It includes not only DLI but also chimeric antigen receptor (CAR) T cells, NK cells, and cancer vaccines using dendritic cells (DC) [48]. Peripheral blood MNC collection by apheresis is the first step for all these treatments.

13.3.1 Considerations for Clinicians

Favorable prognostic factors influencing outcomes after DLI include the use of related donor, chronic GVHD (cGVHD), favorable karyotype, female gender, young patient age, low disease burden, acute and chronic GVHD, low-risk disease, and the time between AHSCT and DLI. However, the optimal time between AHSCT and DLI varies across studies.

The effectiveness of DLI varies widely depending on the malignancy. Chronic myeloid leukemia is sensitive to the graft-versus-malignancy effect, and the use of DLI in combination with chemotherapy has shown success. Responses have been reported in patients with follicular lymphoma and myeloma, though there is less success with aggressive lymphomas. Acute lymphoblastic leukemia has less sensitivity to the graft-versus-malignancy effect, and DLI is not often beneficial in this setting. Studies have clearly demonstrated that DLI, whether used alone or in combination with conventional chemotherapy or hypomethylating drugs, is effective in late relapse after AHSCT when leukemia burden is low or relapse is detected at the molecular level and when a complete response (CR) can be achieved [38].

Transplantation from bone marrow and peripheral blood donors allows the subsequent use of donor T cells. However, this situation differs for umbilical cord blood (UCB) transplantation, as the entire product is infused on day 0. Strategies such as UCB third-party donor-expanded Tregs or using Tregs from multiple pooled UCBs have been adopted to address this issue [7, 38].

Haploidentical transplantation (haplo-SCT) using T-replete platforms has renewed interest in these alternative donors, and DLI has been used in this clinical setting. Most of the clinical data has been reported from the Chinese experience [7, 22, 38]. The central aspect of the Chinese experience was the use of modified DLI (mDLI) harvested after stimulation of a haploidentical donor with G-CSF. G-CSF-stimulated lymphocytes exhibited distinct functional characteristics: Th2 polarization, induction of Tregs, and tolerogenic DCs. Likely due to the high incidence of GVHD, the Beijing group tested the use of a short course of immunosuppression after mDLI with cyclosporine A or methotrexate.

DLI was also tested using the Baltimore platform with posttransplant cyclophosphamide (PT-Cy) [7, 22, 38]. In this setting, Zeidan et al. reported on 40 patients receiving unmodified tDLI after relapsing following haplo-SCT with PT-Cy. The starting dose was 1×10^5 CD3 cells/kg of the recipient, and all patients were off immunosuppression. Most patients had received chemotherapy or radiotherapy before tDLI, and the CR rate was 30%. The incidence of grade 2–4 acute GVHD (aGVHD) was 25%. The authors suggested that a safe starting dose for tDLI could be 1×10^6 CD3 cells/kg. As with tDLI from other donors, a response was observed when DLIs were combined with chemotherapy and when patients were treated for MRD. Ghiso et al. analyzed 42 patients who relapsed after haplo-SCT. Three groups were identified: AML patients in MRD relapse, AML patients in hematological relapse, and Hodgkin lymphoma patients. Only MRD relapses were treated with tDLI alone without chemotherapy ($n = 20$). The response rates were 45%, 33%, and 70%; the incidence of grade 2–3 aGVHD was 15%, 17%, and 10%, and the 2-year OS rates were 43%, 19%, and 80%, respectively. In this study, patients initially received a low dose of CD3 (1×10^3/kg), which was gradually increased to 1×10^5/kg–1×10^6/kg. Again, in AML, the burden of disease had a significant impact on response and survival [7, 22, 38].

DLI from an unrelated donor appears to be as safe as its use in sibling AHSCT [7, 22, 38]. Although concerns arise about potentially higher rates of GVHD in DLI from mismatched donors compared to matched donors, some data suggest that its use might be equally safe.

13.3.2 Fresh and Cryopreserved DLI

Viability is becoming a standard in progenitor cell laboratories and cell therapy in general. However, for DLI, parameters such as post-thawing CD3+ viability have not been adequately evaluated. DLI viability may be affected after cryopreservation, which could alter its effectiveness or toxicity. A group from Philadelphia performed a retrospective analysis of 63 patients who received fresh or cryopreserved DLI. They found similar outcomes when comparing both cohorts, although the small sample size suggest that further evidence is needed [49].

13.3.3 Stimulated and Modified DLI

G-CSF exerts an intense immunoregulatory effect on T cells, shifting from the Th1 to the Th2 phenotype with a higher production of anti-inflammatory cytokines. The T-cell compartment of donors exposed to G-CSF may experience Th2 polarization, resulting in different outcomes. For instance, aGVHD is mainly caused by Th1 T cells, whereas Th2 T cells seem more involved in cGVHD. Interestingly, the immunomodulation caused by G-CSF appears to differ between bone marrow and peripheral blood donation. Considering these data, Abbi et al. compared patients who received either granulocyte colony-stimulated factor primed DLI (G-DLI) or conventionally collected DLI (C-DLI) and found no difference between the cohorts [50].

Modified tDLIs have been altered to optimize the therapeutic window, enhancing the GvT effect and reducing the GVHD effect. Several methods have been tested, mainly in the context of haploidentical transplantation, such as growth factor-stimulated DLI, the insertion of suicide genes into T lymphocytes (HSV-TK or inducible caspase-9), the depletion of alloreactive T-cell subsets, the use of DLI against specific tumor antigens (mHAgs, leukemia-associated antigens, or tissue-associated antigens), and the infusion of T cells engineered with high-affinity TCRs against specific antigens or engineered with CAR [38, 48, 50].

13.3.4 Pearls and Pitfalls of Complications

Allogeneic cell therapy with DLI for treatment of early relapse and possibly for relapse prevention in patients at risk is recommended, especially following the transplantation of T cell-depleted allografts (either by negative or positive selection of stem cells), purified stem cells, or nonalloreactive donor-derived bone marrow or blood stem cells. At the time of DLI administration, no concomitant anti-GVHD prophylaxis should be used to avoid interfering with developing GVL or GvT effects. Graded increments of donor peripheral blood lymphocytes (PBL) are recommended to prevent uncontrolled GVHD, starting with 10^5 or no more than 10^7 T cells/kg in patients with stable or slowly progressing tumors. One order of magnitude increment of donor PBL should be made every month, depending on clinical urgency, the time interval between BMT and DLI, and the desired risk–benefit ratio. Administration of higher doses of DLI should be considered ahead of time when treating aggressive relapse or rapidly proliferating tumors. The longer the time interval between BMT and DLI, the less risk of GVHD is anticipated [22, 25, 33, 38]. The onset of GVHD is a relative contraindication for the continuation of DLI. Patients with high-risk disease or rapidly progressing tumors who show no signs of GVHD may benefit from a short course of cytoreductive agents before administering donor cells activated nonspecifically in vivo or in vitro using lymphokine-activated killer (LAK) cells, or both, with rIL-2. Ultimately, as discussed subsequently, the optimal use of DLI may involve the use of specifically immune donor lymphocytes rather than naive cells with low CTLp to maximize reactivity against undesirable host cells while minimizing or avoiding GVHD [7, 33, 38].

GVHD may or may not be present along with GVL. In the post-DLI setting, GVHD rates have been reported to be as high as 50–60% in several studies, depending on the transplantation characteristics, cell dose, DLI, and timing [5, 21–27]. The absolute effect of DLI on GVL vs. GVHD is difficult to predict [7]. DLI affects the exhausted resident T cells, stimulating them to proliferate [51, 52].

In addition, severe GVHD is associated with increased mortality, with DLI-related (GVHD) mortality rates of approximately 10% reported [33, 38, 53]. However, GVHD is not the only complication that patients receiving DLI may experience. The development of pancytopenia, a relatively infrequent complication, has been reported with an incidence of about 20% [33, 38], though its physiopathology remains largely unknown. Patients receiving DLI for hematological relapse are more likely to develop pancytopenia [33, 38] than those receiving DLI for early relapses.

13.4 Management of Complications After DLI Involves Addressing GVHD and Pancytopenia

DLI is frequently, but not consistently, associated with depression of bone marrow function [33, 38]. Mild marrow aplasia often reverses spontaneously, but in some cases, bone marrow aplasia can be severe and occasionally fatal. Marrow dysfunction can be treated with hematopoietic growth factors and, if indicated, stem cells from the original donor without additional conditioning [33, 38].

Based on earlier animal data suggesting that the incidence of GVHD decreases as the time interval from BMT to DLI increases [33, 38], a simple, cost-effective way to control the incidence, intensity, and severity of GVHD is to administer graded increments of donor PBL. Thus, lower doses of donor T cells can be initiated early on, preferably when the risk of acute GVHD is higher, while increasing the T-cell dose as the time interval from BMT increases. Furthermore, different doses of T cells may be required for each patient, depending on the differential sensitivity of tumor cells and normal host somatic cells to immunocompetent donor T cells. In addition, donor NK or NKT cells, which may also play a role in inducing less effective GVL and GvT effects independently of GVHD, may also be involved.

As a result, optimal treatment of relapse should be started prophylactically or as soon as molecular evidence of disease or reappearance of host markers is confirmed [33]. In patients with low tumor burden or slowly progressive disease, DLI could be initiated with a low, potentially suboptimal but safer T-cell dose, such as 10^5 T cells/kg, which should be escalated by a factor of 10 at 2- to 4-week intervals for patients receiving no anti-GVHD prophylaxis, as long as they have no signs of GVHD [54].

GVHD is the most frequent expected complication. The incidence of aGVHD is higher than that of cGVHD. In particular, the median incidence of aGVHD was 31% (range 4–61%) when tDLI was used and 42% (range 6–45%) when pDLI was used. cGVHD was reported less frequently, with a median incidence of 40% (range 20–59%). The median time from the first DLI to GVHD onset was 30 days (range 17–138). A detailed analysis of GVHD occurrence was published. Sixty-eight patients with various hematological diseases received DLI in an escalated schedule, starting from 0.5 to 1 × 10^6/kg CD3. The overall incidence of aGVHD was 32%, with grades 2–4 at 26%. The most frequently affected organ was the skin (82%), followed by the liver and gut (41%). All patients received steroids as first-line therapy, with an overall response rate (ORR) of 55%. The DLI-related death rate was 22%. The incidence of de novo cGVHD was 38%, with the skin and oral mucosa being the most commonly affected organs. Steroids were used as first-line therapy in most cases, and the CR rate was 62%. Only one patient died from cGVHD [33, 38]. As reported in some studies, DLIs were infused after donor stimulation with G-CSF (mDLI). This approach was developed by Chinese groups, mainly in the haplo-SCT setting. In the initial reports, the incidence of aGVHD and cGVHD after mDLI was relatively high (42% and 45%, respectively) [7]. This high incidence has been reduced by using short-course immunosuppression with cyclosporin A or methotrexate, both in relapsed [7, 21, 22, 33, 38] and prophylactic settings [46]. Notably, methotrexate prophylaxis reduced the relapse rate and improved disease-free survival [7, 33, 38]. DLI from another donor has also been shown to be effective in patients with MC and secondary graft failure [55].

Not all T cells appear to produce the same level of alloreactivity. Specific T-cell phenotypes have been reported in in vitro experiments to cause GVHD but not (or only very limited) GVL [56]. Regarding the different states of T-cell differentiation, murine studies suggest that the T_N compartment is more capable of producing alloreactivity compared with memory T cells [57]. Given these findings, investigating the T_N or memory T-cell compartments within DLI might provide valuable insights into its effectiveness or the development of GVHD. Further cell adjustments are under study; modifying Tregs, NK cells, and γδ (gd) T cells with DLI content might also influence outcomes. γδ T cells, a small subset of T cells with allogeneic cytolytic effect and less specific recognition mechanisms, along with NK+ cells, do not seem to be the primary initiators of GVHD [58]. Since DLIs are unfractionated T-cell infusions (mainly consisting of αβ T cells, which make up the majority of circulating lymphocytes), selecting a γδ DLI could help retain the GVL effect while reducing GVHD. Fine-tuning DLI is still an area of ongoing research, and insights gained from these studies could also be applied to other immunotherapies. Further investigation is needed into the role of DLI in malignancies such as t(15; 17), inversions in chromosome 3, FLT3 mutations (ITD [internal tandem duplication] and TKI [tyrosine kinase inhibitor] domains), and core-binding factor AML [38, 56–58].

13.4.1 DLI in Extramedullary Relapses

Extramedullary relapses (ERs) in AML or myeloid sarcomas are rare but challenging for physicians. Relapses in sanctuary sites such as the testis, ovary, or central nervous system are generally associated with a poor prognosis. Although not fully understood, the presence of AML cells in these sites may reflect immune system evasion through inefficient lymphocyte homing [7, 59] or the expression of the CD56+ adhesion molecule, which is associated with extramedullary leukemia and seen in t(8; 21) AML. Consistent with the potential lack of GVL in sanctuary sites, it has been reported that patients with ER had a higher rate of chronic GVHD compared to patients with systemic relapse (79% vs. 49%, respectively) [7, 59]. In acute lymphoblastic leukemia, ER after AHSCT and buffy coat infusions were reported back in 1996. In AML patients, sustained responses have been observed with DLI plus chemotherapy for ER [7]. However, responses are somewhat erratic, and treatment for this scenario remains unclear; in clinical practice, the approach combines chemotherapy, radiotherapy, and DLI. Given that ER is associated with diminished GVL, durable responses are limited. A group from Korea reported a concerning pattern of relapse in their cohort of AML patients receiving DLI for relapsed AML, observing 5 relapses out of 16 patients; all 5 had an ER (3 in the central nervous system and 2 in the skin). Notably, three of these five patients also had extramedullary leukemia at the time of relapse after initial AHSCT. Interestingly, all five relapsed patients developed GVHD after DLI [7].

13.5 Clinical Results

The early cumulative international experience with DLI in Europe (Fig. 13.2) was presented in 2001 and demonstrated the effectiveness of DLI not only in CML but also in various types of hematologic malignancies. Nowadays, CML is a rare indication for AHSCT. The response and OS after tDLI are shown in Table 13.1.

In the last 10 years, alternative donor transplantation has increased dramatically. DLI after haploidentical transplantation has been a topic of debate. Ultimately, the effect of DLI on transplantation outcomes has been demonstrated by the EBMT registry, as shown in Fig. 13.3 [60]. This study compared reasons for DLI—prophylactic, preemptive, and therapeutic (Table 13.2). Better response rates were obtained in patients treated at the stage of MRD. Therefore, it is highly recommended to monitor patients at risk frequently during the first year or two after transplantation, with molecular assessments of host, disease, and donor-specific markers [60]. Survival rates remain relatively low in patients with active disease. While the cumulative incidence of aGVHD appears acceptable, a high incidence of cGVHD was observed in the prophylactic group compared to the pDLI and tDLI groups [60]. OS after the first DLI was 61% (46–75%) for prophylactic, 40% (19–61%) for preemptive, and 22% (13–31%) for therapeutic. The cumulative incidence of 2–4 aGVHD and cGVHD was 17% (7–27%) and 53% (40–67%) for the prophylactic, 20% (2–38%) and 21% (3–39%) for the preemptive, and 17% (9–24%) and 24% (15–33%) for the therapeutic group, respectively [60].

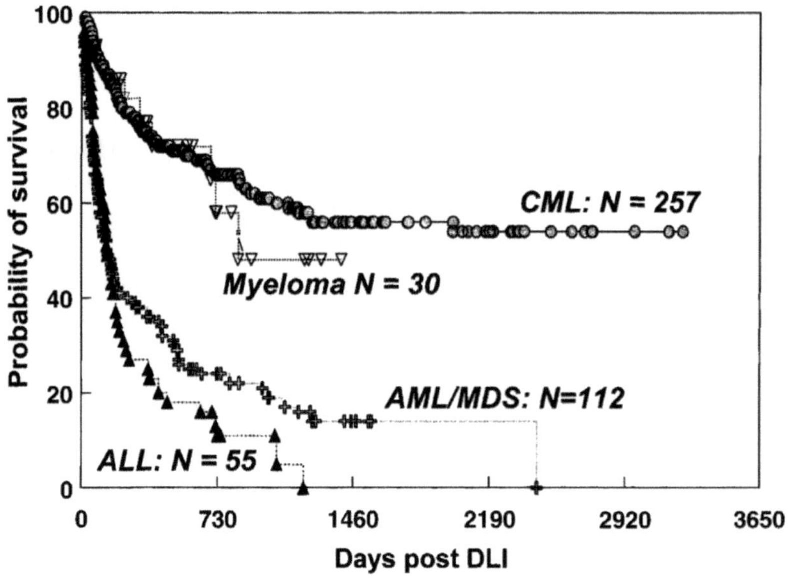

Fig. 13.2 The first report on the long-term effects of DLI in leukemia and myeloma, EBMT registry data results from 2001

Table 13.1 tDLI in patients with AML/MDS and ALL

Diagnosis	*N*	Therapy pre-DLI	Response rate	OS
AML/MDS	16/0	CT in 16 pts	63%	2y, 31%
AML/MDS	399/0	CT in 124 pts	43%	2y, 21%
AML/MDS	263/0	CT in 40	27%	2y 12%
AML/MDS	58/65	CT in 35/51	66%	5y 40%
AML/MDS	124/28	Aza in 154 pts	33%	2y 29%
AML/MDS	62/10	Aza in 72 pts	54%	108 days
AML/MDS	19/12	Aza in 31 pts	35%	153 days
AML/MDS	44/0	CT in 32 pts	NR	2y 36%
AML/MDS	1788/0	CT in 660 pts	NR	1, 23%
ALL	44	28 pts	NR	3y 13%
ALL	23	NR	25%	2y 5%

AML acute myeloid leukemia; *MDS* myelodysplastic syndrome; *ALL* acute lymphoblastic leukemia; *Pts* patients; *CT* chemotherapy; *Aza* azacytidine; *NR* not reported
Table is adapted from L Castagna et al. *Transfusion and Apheresis Science* 54 (2016)345–355

DLI can produce GvT effects to treat relapse after allogeneic hematopoietic cell transplantation; however, durable responses remain uncommon. A systematic review and meta-analysis are needed to clarify whether DLI collected after stimulation with G-CSF (G-DLI) can improve clinical outcomes. Moreover, 16 studies (4 controlled) involving 585 patients were identified in a systematic search up to 17 September 2020. A meta-analysis demonstrated no significant difference in the risk of all-cause mortality (RR, 0.94; 95% CI 0.52–1.68; $p = 0.82$; $n = 3$ studies) or relapse-related mortality (RR, 0.72; 95% CI 0.44–1.18; $p = 0.19$; $n = 3$ studies) between G-DLI and C-DLI groups. G-DLI products had similar mean CD3+ cells compared to C-DLI products, but the median CD34+ cells/kg was increased. No improvement in disease progression, CR rates, or risk of developing GVHD was observed with G-DLI; however, higher significant non-relapse mortality was noted compared to C-DLI. Alternative approaches to enhancing GvT effects are needed.

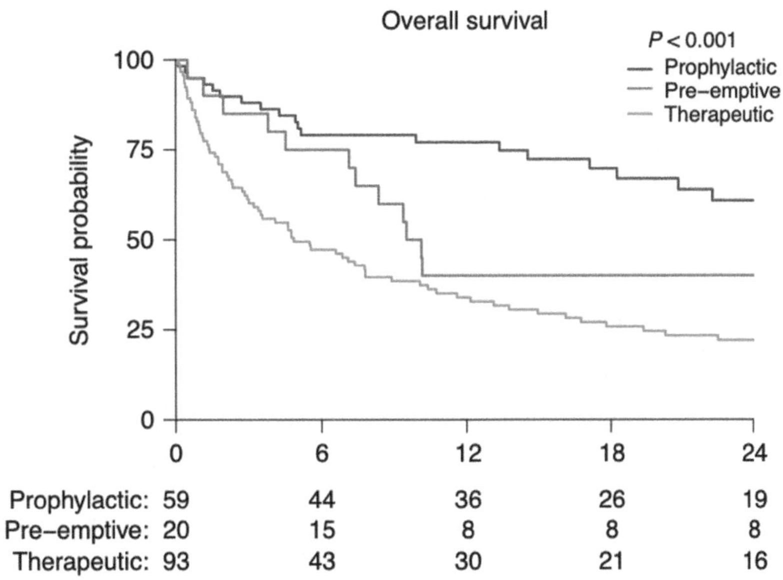

Fig. 13.3 OS after haploidentical AHSCT according to DLI type. (Figure taken from Santoro N et al., *Bone Marrow Transplant.* 2023 Jan;58(1):54–60)

Table 13.2 Comparison of the three different DLI features after AHSCT

	Prophylactic *n* = 59	Preemptive *n* = 20	Therapeutic *n* = 93
Median number of doses (IQR)	1 (1–2.5)	2 (1–3)	1 (1–3)
Median first CD3+ T cell dose/kg (IQR)	0.1 × 106 (0.1–0.5)	0.5 × 106 (0.1–1)	1 × 106 (0.2–51)
Median first CD3+ T cell dose/kg (IQR)	0.5 × 106 (0.5–1)	1 × 106 (07–1)	1.1 × 106 (0.5–5)
Interval between HCT and DLI (months)	3.1 (2.6–4.4)	6.1 (2.8–9.8)	7.2 (4.9–12.5)
Median time between the first and second dose IQR	2.1 (1.8–2.5)	1.5 (1.2–1.6)	1.2 (1.0–1.8)
Median time between the second and third dose IQR	2.6 (15–3)	1.9 (1.5–2.7)	1.5 (0.8–2.3)
Diagnosis			
AML	31 (52.5)	7 (35)	42 (45.2)
ALL	5 (8.5)	5 (25)	18 (19.4)
MDS	12 (20.3)	1 (5)	7 (7.5)
HL	5 (8.5)	2 (10)	13 (14)
NHL	5 (8.5)	3 (15)	9 (9.6)
CLL	0	2 (10)	0
MM	0	0	3 (3.2)
CML	1 (1.7)	0	1 (1.1)
Chemotherapy preDLI	7 (11.9)	6 (30	58 (63.0)
Stop immunosuppression before DLI	13 (22)	12 (60)	62 (69.7)

AML acute myeloid leukemia; *MDS* myelodysplastic syndrome; *ALL* acute lymphoblastic leukemia; *HL* Hodgkin lymphoma; *NHL* non-Hodgkin lymphoma; *CLL* chronic lymphocytic leukemia; *MM* multiple myeloma; *CML* chronic myeloid leukemia; *IQR* interquartile range

Adapted from *Bone Marrow Transplantation* (2023) 58:54–60

13.6 Illustrative Clinical Case

A 46-year-old man with secondary AML in the first complete remission (CR1) underwent allogeneic peripheral AHSCT from his haploidentical, blood group-compatible 30-year-old brother. On the 28th day posttransplantation, bone marrow evaluation revealed MRD by flow cytometry. The patient is on immunosuppressive treatment with tacrolimus and mycophenolate mofetil. Should DLI be planned for this patient?

The first step is to discontinue all immunosuppressive drugs and monitor for the development of GVHD. In the meantime, check whether cryopreserved donor lymphocytes are available in the apheresis unit. If not, the collection of lymphocytes from the donor should be arranged. Close cooperation between the attending physician and the apheresis staff is crucial, as each lymphocytapheresis procedure must be tailored to the patient's needs to avoid unnecessary, lengthy, and stressful procedures for the donor [38].

If GVHD does not develop, tDLI is planned for MRD+ relapsed disease. Before DLI, treatment to reduce tumor burden is recommended. However, there is no consensus on the type of chemotherapy or the number of courses before DLI. One or two courses of conventional chemotherapy or newer active drugs could be used, followed by DLI in subsequent courses. The timing of DLI could be 1–2 weeks after chemotherapy to optimize the synergistic effect. However, the schedule may vary with drugs that are administered continuously, such as thalidomide or lenalidomide, allowing DLI to be infused at any time [38].

Cryopreserved and freshly infused DLI have similar efficacy. Escalating the schedule is the preferred approach for infusion. The initial dose should be 1×10^6 CD3/kg, followed by logarithmic escalation. If the patient was not in CR1 at the time of transplantation, pDLI should be administered. The goal of tDLI, prDLI, and pDLI remains the same: to monitor patients closely. Those receiving DLI should be carefully followed for GVHD and pancytopenia. Second or third courses of DLI can be given in an escalated manner according to disease status. G-DLIs might be preferred, as they can trigger better immunomodulation. DLI can be activated in patients with impending relapse after AHSCT. These patients include those with positive MRD in leukemia (or some forms of lymphoma) or positive PET scans in lymphoma patients. In this scenario, DLI can be effective because the tumor burden is low. Furthermore, in some diseases (Ph + ALL [Philadelphia-positive acute lymphoblastic leukemia], B-cell lymphoma, multiple myeloma, chronic lymphocytic leukemia), DLI can be combined with active and well-tolerated drugs [38].

References

1. Slavin S, Morecki S, Weiss L, OR R. Donor lymphocyte infusion: the use of alloreactive and tumor-reactive lymphocytes for immunotherapy of malignant and nonmalignant diseases in conjunction with allogeneic stem cell transplantation. J Hemotherapy Stem Cell Res. 2022;11:265–76.
2. Weiden PL, Storb R, Tsoi MS, Graham TC, Lerner KG, Thomas ED. Infusion of donor lymphocytes into stable canine radiation chimeras: implications for mechanism of transplantation tolerance. J Immunol. 1976;116:1212–9.
3. Kolb HJ, Mittermüller J, Clemm C, Holler E, Ledderose G, Brehm G, Heim M, Wilmanns W. Donor leukocyte transfusions for treatment of recurrent chronic myelogenous leukemia in marrow transplant patients. Blood. 1990;76(12):2462–5.
4. Kolb HJ, Schattenberg A, Goldman JM, et al. Graft-versus-leukemia effect of donor lymphocyte transfusions in marrow grafted patients. Blood. 1995;86:2041–50.
5. Mackinnon S, Papadopoulos EB, Carabasi MH, et al. Adoptive immunotherapy evaluating escalating doses of donor leukocytes for relapse of chronic myeloid leukemia after bone marrow transplantation: separation of graft-versus-leukemia responses from graft-versus-host disease. Blood. 1995;86:1261–8.
6. Formani SJ, Negrin RS. Overview of hematopoietic cell transplantation immunology. Thomas' hematopoietic cell transplantation, 5th ed. p. 102.
7. Orti G, Barba P, Fox L, Salamero O, Bosch F, Valcarcel D. Donor lymphocyte infusions in AML and MDS: enhancing the graft-versus-leukemia effect. Exp Hematol. 2017;48:1–11.
8. Huang XJ, Liu DH, Liu KY, Xu LP, Chen H, Han W. Donor lymphocyte infusion for the treatment of leukemia relapse after HLA-mismatched/haploidentical T-cell-replete hematopoietic stem cell transplantation. Haematologica. 2007;92:414–7.
9. Yan CH, Wang JZ, Liu DH, et al. Chemotherapy followed by modified donor lymphocyte infusion as a treatment for relapsed acute leukemia after haploidentical hematopoietic stem cell transplantation without in vitro T-cell depletion: superior outcomes compared with chemotherapy alone and an analysis of prognostic factors. Eur J Haematol. 2013;91:304–14.
10. Hicheri Y, Bouchekioua A, Hamel Y, et al. Donor regulatory T cells identified by FoxP3 expression but also by the membranous CD4þCD127low/neg pheno-

type influence graft-versus-tumor effect after donor lymphocyte infusion. J Immunother. 2008;31:806–11.
11. Maury S, Lemoine FM, Hicheri Y, Rosenzwajg M, Badoual C, Cheraï M, Beaumont JL, Azar N, Dhedin N, Sirvent A, Buzyn A, Rubio MT, Vigouroux S, Montagne O, Bories D, Roudot-Thoraval F, Vernant JP, Cordonnier C, Klatzmann D, Cohen JL. CD4+CD25+ regulatory T cell depletion improves the graft-versus-tumor effect of donor lymphocytes after allogeneic hematopoietic stem cell transplantation. Sci Transl Med. 2010;2(41):41ra52.
12. Soiffer RJ, Alyea EP, Hochberg E, et al. Randomized trial of CD8+ T-cell depletion in the prevention of graft-versus-host disease associated with donor lymphocyte infusion. Biol Blood Marrow Transplant. 2002;8:625–32.
13. Meyer RG, Britten CM, Wehler D, et al. Prophylactic transfer of CD8-depleted donor lymphocytes after T-cell-depleted reduced-intensity transplantation. Blood. 2007;109:374–82.
14. Orti G, Lowdell M, Fielding A, et al. Phase I study of high-stringency CD8 depletion of donor leukocyte infusions after allogeneic hematopoietic stem cell transplantation. Transplantation. 2009;88:1312–8.
15. Huang XJ, Wang Y, Liu DH, et al. Administration of short-term immunosuppressive agents after DLI reduces the incidence of DLI-associated acute GVHD without influencing the GVL effect. Bone Marrow Transplant. 2009;44:309–16.
16. Yan CH, Xu LP, Liu DH, et al. Low-dose methotrexate may preserve a stronger antileukemic effect than that of cyclosporine after modified donor lymphocyte infusion in unmanipulated haploidentical HSCT. Clin Transpl. 2015;29:594–605.
17. Solomon R, Sizemore C, Zhang X, et al. Preemptive DLI without withdrawal of immunosuppression to promote complete donor T-cell chimerism results in favorable outcomes for high-risk older recipients of alemtuzumab-containing reduced-intensity unrelated donor allogeneic transplant: a prospective phase II trial. Bone Marrow Transplant. 2014;49:616–62.
18. Bonini C, Ferrari G, Verzeletti S, et al. HSV-TK gene transfer into donor lymphocytes for control of allogeneic graft-versus-leukemia. Science. 1997;276:1719–24.
19. Ciceri F, Bonini C, Stanghellini MT, et al. Infusion of suicide-gene-engineered donor lymphocytes after family haploidentical haemopoietic stem cell transplantation for leukaemia (the TK007 trial): a non-randomised phase I-II study. Lancet Oncol. 2009;10:489–500.
20. Stern M, de Wreede LC, Brand R, van Biezen A, Dreger P, Mohty M, de Witte TM, Kröger N, Ruutu T. Sensitivity of hematological malignancies to graft-versus-host effects: an EBMT megafile analysis. Leukemia. 2014;28(11):2235–40. https://doi.org/10.1038/leu.2014.145. Epub 2014 Apr 30.
21. Harada K. Pre-emptive and prophylactic donor lymphocyte infusion following allogeneic stem cell transplantation. Int J Hematol. 2023;118:158–68.
22. Dholaria B, Savani BN, Labopin M, Luznik L, Ruggeri A, Mielke S, Al MM, Malki PK, Fuchs E, Huang X-J, Locatelli F, et al. Clinical applications of donor lymphocyte infusion from an HLA-haploidentical donor: consensus recommendations from the Acute Leukemia Working Party of the EBMT. Haematologica. 2020;105(1):47–58.
23. Marks DI, Lush R, Cavenagh J, et al. The toxicity and efficacy of donor lymphocyte infusions given after reduced-intensity conditioning allogeneic stem cell transplantation. Blood. 2002;100:3108–14.
24. Chalandon Y, Passweg JR, Schmid C, et al. Outcome of patients developing GVHD after DLI given to treat CML relapse: a study by the Chronic Leukemia Working Party of the EBMT. Bone Marrow Transplant. 2010;45:558–64.
25. Porter DL, Antin JH. Donor leukocyte infusions in myeloid malignancies: new strategies. Best Pract Res Clin Haematol. 2006;19:737–55.
26. Bar M, Sandmaier BM, Inamoto Y, et al. Donor lymphocyte infusion for relapsed hematological malignancies after allogeneic hematopoietic cell transplantation: prognostic relevance of the initial CD3+T cell dose. Biol Blood Marrow Transplant. 2013;19:949–57.
27. Lee HC, Saliba RM, Rondon G, et al. Mixed T lymphocyte chimerism after allogeneic hematopoietic transplantation is predictive for relapse of acute myeloid leukemia and myelodysplastic syndromes. Biol Blood Marrow Transplant. 2015;21:1948–54.
28. Huisman C, de Weger RA, de Vries L, Tilanus MG, Verdonck LF. Chimerism analysis within 6 months of allogeneic stem cell transplantation predicts relapse in acute myeloid leukemia. Bone Marrow Transplant. 2007;39:285–91.
29. Roux E, Dumont-Girard F, Starobinski M, et al. Recovery of immune reactivity after T-cell-depleted bone marrow transplantation depends on thymicactivity. Blood. 2000;96:2299–303.
30. Peggs KS, Kayani I, Edwards N, et al. Donor lymphocyte infusions modulate relapse risk in mixed chimeras and induce durable salvage in relapsed patients after T-cell-depleted allogeneic transplantation for Hodgkin's lymphoma. J Clin Oncol. 2011;29:971–8.
31. de Lima M, Bonamino M, Vasconcelos Z, et al. Prophylactic donor lymphocyte infusions after moderately ablative chemotherapy and stem cell transplantation for hematological malignancies: high remission rate among poor prognosis patients at the expense of graft-versus-host disease. Bone Marrow Transplant. 2001;27:73–8.
32. Krishnamurthy P, Potter VT, Barber LD, et al. Outcome of donor lymphocyte infusion after T cell-depleted allogeneic hematopoietic stem cell transplantation for acute myelogenous leukemia and myelodysplastic syndromes. Biol Blood Marrow Transplant. 2013;19:562–8.
33. Schmid C, Labopin M, Nagler A, et al. Donor lymphocyte infusion in the treatment of first hematological relapse after allogeneic stem-cell transplantation

in adults with acute myeloid leukemia: a retrospective risk factors analysis and comparison with other strategies by the EBMT Acute Leukemia Working Party. J Clin Oncol. 2007;25:4938–45.
34. Jedlickova Z, Schmid C, Koenecke C, et al. Long-term results of adjuvant donor lymphocyte transfusion in AML after allogeneic stem cell transplantation. Bone Marrow Transplant. 2016;51:663–7.
35. https://nssg.oxford-haematology.org.uk/bmt/donor/B-2-28-dli.pdf.
36. Aljurf M, Snowden JA, Hayden P, Orchard KH, McGrath E. Quality management and accreditation in hematopoietic stem cell transplantation and cellular therapy: the JACIE guide. Cham, CH: JACIE; 2021.
37. Stenzinger M, Bonig H. Risks of leukapheresis and how to manage them—a non-systematic review. Transfus Apher Sci. 2018;57:628–34. https://doi.org/10.1016/j.transci.2018.09.008.
38. Castagna L, Sarina B, Bramanti S, Perseghin P, Mariotti J, Morabito L. Donor lymphocyte infusion after allogeneic stem cell transplantation. Transfus Apher Sci. 2016;54:345–55.
39. Padmanabhan A. Cellular collection by apheresis. Transfusion. 2018;58:598–604. https://doi.org/10.1111/trf.14502.
40. Chen J, Cheryl Goss MD, Avecilla ST, Hong H, Walsh E, Wuest D, Maslak P, Pessin MS. Evaluation of peripheral blood mononuclear cell collection by leukapheresis. Transfusion. 2019;59(5):1765–72. https://doi.org/10.1111/trf.15186.
41. Kumar AJ, Hexner EO, Frey NV, Luger SM, Loren AW, Reshef R, et al. Pilot study of prophylactic ex vivo costimulated donor leukocyte infusion after reduced-intensity conditioned allogeneic stem cell transplantation. Biol Blood Marrow Transplant. 2013;19:1094.
42. Lewalle P, Triffet A, Delforge A, Crombez P, Selleslag D, De Muyinck H, et al. Donor lymphocyte infusion in adult haploidentical transplant: a dose finding study. Bone Marrow Transplant. 2003;31:39–44.
43. Perseghin P, Incontri A. Mononuclear cell collection in patients treated with extracorporeal photochemotherapy by using the off-line method: a comparison between COBE spectra AutoPbsc version 6.1 and amicus cell separators. J Clin Apher. 2010;25:310–4.
44. Steininger PA, Strasse EF, Weiss D, Achenbach S, Zimmermann R, Eckstein R. First comparative evaluation of a new leukapheresis technology in non-cytokine stimulated donors. Vox Sang. 2013;106:248–55.
45. Schultz M, Biallck H, Thorausch K, Bug G, Dünziger U, Seifred E, et al. Unstimulated leukapheresis in patients and donors: comparison of two apheresis systems. Transfusion. 2014;54:1622–9.
46. Shaz B, Goodarzi K, Malynn E, Uhl L. Improved strategy for mononuclear cell collection for donor lymphocyte infusions. TRANSFUSION. 2006;46:1044–8. https://doi.org/10.1111/j.1537-2995.2006.00840.x.
47. Putensen D, Smith R, Pilcher L, Trandafir G. Comparison of the CMNC and MNC apheresis protocol for the collection of T-cells showed comparable outcome: an observational study in a single centre. J Clin Apher. 2018;33:349–56.
48. Worel N, Holbro A, Vrielink H, Ootjers C, Le Poole K, Beer-Wekking I, Rintala T, Lozano M, Bonig H. A guide to the collection of T-cells by apheresis for ATMP manufacturing—recommendations of the GoCART coalition apheresis working group. Bone Marrow Transplant. 2023;58(7):742–8. https://doi.org/10.1038/s41409-023-01957-x.
49. Schäfer AK, Waterhouse M, Follo M, Duque-Afonso J, Duyster J, Bertz H, Finke J. Phenotypical and functional analysis of donor lymphocyte infusion products after long-term cryopreservation. Transfus Apher Sci. 2020;59(1):102594. https://doi.org/10.1016/j.transci.2019.06.022. Epub 2019 Jul 10
50. Kirkham AM, Bailey AJM, Masurekar A, Shorr R, Bredeson C, Sabloff M, Allan DS. Can GCSF-stimulated donor lymphocyte infusions improve outcomes for relapsed disease following allogeneic hematopoietic cell transplantation? A systematic review and meta-analysis. Leuk Lymphoma. 2022;63(14):3276–87.
51. Wherry EJ. T cell exhaustion. Nat Immunol. 2011;12:492.
52. Bachireddy P, Hainz U, Rooney M, et al. Reversal of in situ T-cell exhaustion during effective human antileukemia responses to donor lymphocyte infusion. Blood. 2014;123:1412.
53. Keil F, Haas OA, Fritsch G, Kalhs P, Lechner K, Mannhalter C, et al. Donor leukocyte infusion for leukemic relapse after allogeneic marrow transplantation: lack of residual donor hematopoiesis predicts aplasia. Blood. 1997;89(9):3113.
54. Ros-Soto J, Snowden JA, Szydlo R, Nicholson E, Madrigal A, Easdale S, Potter M, Ethell M, Anthias C. Infusion in patients with hematological malignancies: donor characteristics matter. Transplant Cell Therapy. 2022;28:183.
55. Ren RR, Ma LM, Xie YX, Tian WW, Wang T. Effect of donor lymphocyte infusion from two types of donors on mixed Chimerism with secondary graft failure after allogeneic hematopoietic stem cell transplantation. Transplant Cell Ther. 2022;28(3):152.e1–7. https://doi.org/10.1016/j.jtct.2021.12.017. Epub 2021 Dec 29.
56. Ortí G, Palacio-Garcia C, García-Cadenas I, Sanchez-Ortega I, Jimenez MJ, Azqueta C, Villacampa G, Ferra C, Parody R, Martino R, Bosch F, Querol S, Valcarcel D. Analysis of cell subsets in donor lymphocyte infusions from HLA identical sibling donors after allogeneic hematopoietic cell transplant. Transplant Cell Therapy. 2021;27:53.e153.e8.
57. Dutt S, Tseng D, Ermann J, et al. Naive and memory T cells induce different types of graft-versus-host disease. J Immunol. 2007;179:6547–54.
58. Lamb LS Jr, Lopez RD. Gamma delta T cells: a new frontier for immunotherapy? Biol Blood Marrow Transplant. 2005;11:161–8.

59. Shimoni A, Rand A, Shem-Tov N, Yerushalmi R, Hardan I, Nagler A. Isolated extra-medullary relapse of acute leukemia after allogeneic stem-cell transplantation; different kinetics and better prognosis than systemic relapse. Biol Blood Marrow Transplant. 2009;15(2 Suppl):59.
60. Santoro N, Mooyaart JE, Devillier R, Koc Y, Vydra J, Castagna L, Gülbas Z, Martin JD, Araujo MC, Kulagin A, Arat M, Arroyo CH, Martelli MP, Di Ianni M, Hoogenboom JD, de Wreede LC, Ruggeri A, Chabannon C. Donor lymphocyte infusions after haploidentical stem cell transplantation with PTCY: a study on behalf of the EBMT cellular therapy & immunobiology working party. Bone Marrow Transplant. 2023;58(1):54–60. https://doi.org/10.1038/s41409--022-01839-8. Epub 2022 Oct 10. Erratum in: Bone Marrow Transplant. 2022 Dec 14.

Part IV

Complications During Plasma Exchange and Plasmapheresis Therapy

Complications During Apheresis in Patients with Hematologic Diseases

14

Nihan Alkış and H. Atilla Özkan

14.1 Complications During Plasma Exchange and Plasmapheresis Therapy

14.1.1 Introduction

Therapeutic plasmapheresis (TP) is an extracorporeal treatment method that enables the removal of pathogenic substances with high molecular weight (>150 kDa), such as immunoglobulins, immune complexes, or inflammatory mediators, from plasma. TP is used to treat various conditions, from autoimmune diseases to intoxications [1]. The first step in plasmapheresis is separating the plasma portion of the blood from its cellular components, which is achieved by centrifugation or filtration through semipermeable membranes [2].

After the plasma has been separated, three types of plasmapheresis can be applied: "nonselective plasmapheresis," where plasma is removed and replaced with an equal volume of replacement solutions using a nonselective technique called therapeutic plasma exchange (TPE); "selective plasmapheresis," where pathogens are removed using specific binders (e.g., immunoadsorption, lipoprotein apheresis, plasma adsorption perfusion); and "semi-selective plasmapheresis" (double-filtration plasmapheresis), in which both pathogenic substances and some beneficial molecules are removed using nonselective techniques [1].

Complications and adverse events (AEs) can occur during or after therapeutic apheresis (TA). The frequency and types of complications depend on the patient's general condition, the number of procedures performed, the replacement fluid used, the type of anticoagulant, and the vascular access route. According to the World Apheresis Association (WAA) registry, AEs occurred in 7142 out of 50,846 TA procedures. These AEs were categorized into four grades: mild (if tolerated without medication), moderate (if requiring medication), severe (if requiring discontinuation of TA), and death (if resulting in the patient's death). AEs were mild in 2.4%, moderate in 3%, and severe in 0.4%, with an overall incidence of 5.8%. The most common AEs were paresthesias (from citrate-related hypocalcemia) and vascular access-related complications [3]. In a study evaluating over 15,000 AEs in TPE treatment, replacement fluids were compared, showing that AEs occurred more frequently with plasma replacement than with albumin replacement (20% vs. 1.4%) [4]. The overall mortality rate reported for TPE is 0.03–0.05% [5].

TPE-related complications are classified as those related to vascular access, anticoagulants, replacement fluids, blood products (e.g., fresh

N. Alkış
Bursa Şehir Hastanesi, Erişkin Hematoloji Kliniği, Bursa, Turkey

H. A. Özkan (✉)
Bahçeşehir Üniversitesi Tıp Fakültesi, Medicalpark Göztepe Hastanesi, İstanbul, Turkey

I. Kozanoglu (ed.), *Problem Solving in Apheresis Medicine*,
https://doi.org/10.1007/978-3-031-74081-7_14

frozen plasma [FFP] or therapeutic donor plasma [TDP]), blood volume, post-TPE changes in blood components, and anaphylactoid reactions associated with angiotensin-converting enzyme inhibitor (ACEi) use.

14.1.2 Complications During Plasma Exchange and Plasmapheresis Therapy

14.1.2.1 Vascular Access Route-Related Complications

The vascular access must provide adequate blood flow to the plasmapheresis device. Without this, apheresis may have disadvantages, such as longer procedure times and reduced efficiency, or may not be feasible. Apheresis applications require low blood flows (60–120 mL/min). The vasculature should not collapse from high negative pressure or sustain injury from high positive pressure. In a peripheral vein, single-needle access is possible with TPE using centrifugation, though it may extend treatment time [6]. Central catheters placed in peripheral veins are unsuitable because their narrow diameter may close under the negative pressure applied during TPE [7]. Membrane filtration TPE devices generally require a higher exchange rate, necessitating larger diameter catheters, such as temporary hemodialysis catheters or large double-lumen catheters (e.g., 13.5 French) [8]. The choice of catheter depends on technical requirements (urgency, number and frequency of procedures, plasma volume exchanged) and clinical factors (vascular anatomy, underlying disease, consciousness level, hygiene, inpatient/outpatient status, or critical illness) [2]. Potential complications of central venous catheters include infection, pain, nerve damage, thrombosis, perforation, hematomas, air embolism, or arteriovenous fistulas. Some of these complications can also occur when peripheral veins are used. Peripheral vein access may avoid central-catheter related complications but typically prolongs procedure time due to slower blood flow. For this reason, peripheral veins are sometimes not suitable. Verifying correct placement of central catheters helps reduce these complications and is recommended by the Association for the Advancement of Blood and Biotherapies (AABB) and Foundation for Cellular Therapy (FACT) [9].

14.1.2.2 Complications Related to the Anticoagulant Used

Anticoagulation is used to prevent clotting in the extracorporeal circuit. The choice of anticoagulant depends on the apheresis method, comorbid conditions (e.g., cirrhosis, renal failure, thrombocytopenia) and any need for systemic anticoagulation for other indications (e.g., extracorporeal membrane oxygenation [ECMO]). Citrate and heparin are standard anticoagulants [10]. Epoprostenol may be used when citrate is unavailable and heparin is contraindicated.

Citrate

Citrate is the preferred agent due to its localized effect, short half-life (30–60 min), and favorable safety profile. It prevents coagulation by binding to ionized calcium, thereby inhibiting the coagulation cascade. During the procedure, it is infused into the circuit before the pump. In centrifugation-based TPE, the risk of citrate toxicity is low, as 80% of citrate is discarded with the waste plasma. In membrane filtration TPE, however, citrate use is higher due to the rapid speed, making side effects more common. In addition, less plasma removal allows more citrate to enter the patient's systemic circulation [11], increasing the risk of citrate toxicity, especially in patients with liver or kidney disease. In such cases, heparin is preferable. The most commonly used commercial citrate solutions are Anticoagulant Citrate Dextrose Solution A (ACD-A) and ACD-B, with whole blood-to-anticoagulant ratios of 10:1–14:1. The ratio can be adjusted to add more anticoagulant if clotting occurs, though this increases the likelihood of citrate toxicity [10].

Citrate-Induced Hypocalcemia: Citrate binds ionized calcium to form soluble calcium citrate, reducing ionized and total serum calcium levels. In patients with normal liver function, citrate is usually metabolized within approximately 1.5 h. However, due to the extended duration of most TPE procedures, symptoms of citrate toxicity often arise unless the exchange rate is reduced. Symptoms typically begin with perioral and acral paresthesias. Hyperventilation may cause respiratory alkalosis, worsening the paresthesias. Tetany presents with both sensory and muscular dysfunction. Motor symptoms of tetany include stiffness, jerkiness, myalgia, and muscle cramps or spasms. In the hands, carpal spasm manifests with forced adduction of the thumb, flexion of the metacarpophalangeal joints and wrists, and finger extension. Spasms of the respiratory muscles and glottis (laryngismus stridulous) may cause cyanosis. Severe reactions include tetany, QT interval prolongation, arrhythmias, and hypotension [12]. Electrocardiographic monitoring and intra-procedural evaluation of ionized calcium levels may be appropriate in patients receiving intravenous calcium infusion, those who become symptomatic, those at risk of citrate toxicity, those with mental status changes, or pediatric patients [13]. To reduce the risk of citrate-induced hypocalcemia, the initial approach is to decrease the exchange rate during the procedure. Starting 15 min after the onset of TPE, a 10-mL ampoule of 10% calcium chloride can be administered slowly via intravenous infusion over 15–30 min. Calcium infusion may be repeated if the treatment duration exceeds 1 h [4, 14]. With this approach, the incidence of symptomatic hypocalcemia decreased from 9.1% to 1% [4]. In some cases, such as with stable outpatients, oral calcium supplements before and during the procedure may effectively manage mild hypocalcemia. Intravenous calcium infusion may be required for patients unable to take oral calcium, those who develop severe hypocalcemia, or those with symptoms unresponsive to oral calcium. Rapid administration of calcium chloride or calcium gluconate can lead to muscle contractions [13]. Continuous infusion of 10 mL of 10% calcium gluconate per liter of non-plasma fluid has been shown to prevent citrate toxicity [15]. Additionally, 1 g of calcium gluconate per liter of non-plasma infusion fluid can prevent citrate-related symptoms [16].

Citrate-Induced Metabolic Alkalosis: Metabolic alkalosis can develop in patients with concomitant renal failure as another citrate-related complication. Citrate is metabolized to bicarbonate, which cannot be sufficiently excreted in patients with renal failure, potentially leading to metabolic alkalosis. In these cases, TPE followed by hemodialysis may be required to restore the acid-base and fluid-electrolyte balance. This condition can be managed with hemodialysis [17].

Heparin

Heparin has a short half-life (23–168 min) and is nearly completely cleared during TPE. A bolus of 3000–5000 U is administered at the start of treatment, followed by a bolus of 1000 U/h if necessary. Heparin is the preferred anticoagulant in membrane filtration TPE. Due to its systemic administration, bleeding is more common than with citrate. Heparin-related thrombocytopenia may develop, but this is not specific to the procedure [10].

14.1.2.3 Replacement Fluid-Related Complications

The volume of fluid removed from the patient during apheresis should be replaced to prevent significant volume depletion. Albumin (5%), normal saline, or a combination of albumin and normal saline are the preferred replacement fluids in most cases. The optimal choice usually depends on the clinical situation, with albumin being the most commonly used. Normal saline is preferred in cases of hyperviscosity. If cost is a consideration, a combination of albumin and normal saline may be used. TDP is generally recommended as a replacement fluid when plasma components are required, such as in thrombotic thrombocytopenic purpura (TTP). Albumin is frequently preferred because it is associated with fewer allergic or immune reactions compared to TDP, and there is no risk of transfusion-transmitted diseases [18, 19]. However, dilutional coagulopathy may occur after apheresis due to decreased clotting factors, and immunoglobulin loss may be observed. Normal saline alone provides insufficient oncotic pressure and can lead to severe edema and/or hypotension. Therefore, 5% albumin or a combination of albumin and normal saline is preferred.

Hypokalemia: Replacement fluids other than fresh frozen plasma may cause a 25% decrease in plasma potassium concentration due to dilution in the post-apheresis period [20]. In individuals at risk of hypokalemia (e.g., due to dilution or citrate-induced alkalosis), potassium levels should be checked immediately after the procedure and treated if hypokalemia develops.

Hypocalcemia: Infusion of large volumes of albumin has been implicated in the development of hypocalcemia. In a 32-patient randomized trial, 10% pentastarch given during the first half of apheresis was compared with 5% albumin. Hypocalcemic symptoms were less frequent with pentastarch than with albumin (8% vs. 33%, respectively). The cause of hypocalcemia is the binding of calcium to the infused albumin [21].

Metabolic Acidosis: When albumin is used as a replacement solution, metabolic acidosis may occur after a TPE session because albumin has an acidic profile [22].

Hypotension: Crystalloids are the replacement fluid of choice for cost-effectiveness and in patients with hyperviscosity syndrome. However, if the amount of crystalloid exceeds 30% of the total replacement fluid, replacing plasma with crystalloid carries a risk of hypotension. In this situation, water moves from the intravascular space to the extravascular space following a concentration gradient. If crystalloid is used as part of the replacement, it should be administered at the beginning of the apheresis procedure to avoid significant fluid shifts and hypotension [23].

14.1.2.4 Complications Related to the Blood Product Used (FFP or TDP)

Anaphylactic Reactions: Anaphylaxis can develop in IgA-deficient patients due to the presence of anti-IgA antibodies that react with IgA in donor plasma. In these patients, it is necessary to use plasma obtained from IgA-deficient donors. Anaphylactic reactions to plasma have been reported as a serious complication and a possible cause of death associated with TPE [24, 25]. These reactions have been observed in 21% of patients. Common symptoms include fever, chills, urticaria, wheezing, and hypotension. Cardiopulmonary collapse is rare [26, 27]. The possibility of anaphylaxis is high when one of the two criteria defined by the World Allergy Organization is met:

1. A disease of acute onset (minutes to several hours) with involvement of skin, mucosal tissue, or both (e.g., generalized urticaria, itching or flushing, swollen lips, tongue, or uvula) and at least one of the following:
   - Signs of airway obstruction (e.g., dyspnea, wheezing, bronchospasm, stridor, decreased peak expiratory flow, hypoxemia)
   - Circulatory dysfunction: Decreased blood pressure or associated symptoms of end-organ dysfunction (e.g., hypotonia, collapse, syncope, incontinence)
   - Severe gastrointestinal symptoms during allergen exposure (e.g., severe cramping abdominal pain, repeated vomiting)
2. Acute hypotension[1] or bronchospasm or laryngeal symptoms (e.g., stridor, voice changes, odynophagia) after re-exposure to the allergen (minutes to several hours), even in the absence of a typical skin reaction, in patients who developed an allergic-anaphylactic reaction upon previous exposure to the allergenic agent

The procedure is immediately stopped. Airway patency is ensured, and respiration and circulation are evaluated. The lips, tongue, and oropharynx are evaluated for angioedema. The skin is examined for urticaria or angioedema.

The first step in managing anaphylaxis involves a rapid assessment of the patient's airway:

- Initially, oxygen should be administered by mask at 15 L/min.
- If there is any airway obstruction or significant edema of the oropharyngeal tissues,

[1]Hypotension is defined as a decrease in systolic blood pressure (BP) by more than 30% compared to that individual's baseline value. For adults and children over 10 years old, hypotension can also be defined as systolic BP <90 mmHg [28].

including the tongue, or if voice changes have occurred, prepare for early intubation.
- Intubation should be performed urgently in the presence of stridor or respiratory distress due to upper airway obstruction.
- If severe upper airway edema prevents access to the glottic opening, even with the use of a video laryngoscope, emergency cricothyroidotomy may be required to secure the airway [29].

All anaphylaxis patients should receive fluid therapy via the intravenous (IV) route. Hypotension may develop as approximately 35% of the intravascular volume shifts into the extravascular space within minutes due to increased vascular permeability [30]. In the initial minutes of treatment, 1–2 L of normal saline should be administered rapidly intravenously. Large volumes of fluid (e.g., up to 7 L) may be required. Normal saline is preferred due to the disadvantages of other fluids. Lactated Ringer's (LR) solution may contribute to metabolic alkalosis. However, large volumes of normal saline can lead to hyperchloremic metabolic acidosis. Therefore, when very large volumes are required, normal saline can be switched to LR. Dextrose rapidly extravasates from the circulation into interstitial tissues. Colloid solutions (e.g., albumin or hydroxyethyl starch) do not provide a survival advantage in patients with hypotensive shock and are more costly. Patients should be carefully and continuously monitored for clinical response and volume overload [31]. Epinephrine is the first and most important treatment for anaphylaxis. In the emergency treatment of anaphylaxis in adults, it should be administered as soon as anaphylaxis is recognized to prevent the progression of life-threatening symptoms. Intramuscular (IM) injection is the preferred route in most cases and for patients of all ages [32]. The recommended dose of epinephrine is 0.01 mg/kg (maximum dose 0.5 mg) IM into the mid outer part of the thigh (vastus lateralis muscle). IM epinephrine can be repeated at 5–15-min intervals if there is no response or inadequate response [33]. Large volume fluid resuscitation should be given to every patient with hypotension who does not respond immediately or completely to IM epinephrine [29]. IV bolus epinephrine causes significant dosing errors and cardiovascular complications compared to IM epinephrine and should be avoided as much as possible [34]. If patients do not respond to IM injections, slow, continuous infusion is preferred [35]. IV epinephrine infusion is started with 0.1 mcg/kg/min (range, 0.05–0.2 mcg/kg/min) and increased by 0.05 mcg/kg/min every 2–3 min until blood pressure and perfusion improve. The maximum dose is unknown and varies by patient, but patients rarely require a dose exceeding 1 mcg/kg/min. The infusion rate is increased by half the initial rate every few minutes. The dose should be titrated based on continuous noninvasive blood pressure monitoring. When blood pressure increases by 10–15%, the infusion rate is maintained at this level for 3–5 min to observe if improvement continues. The infusion rate is then adjusted accordingly [29]. Glucocorticoids are often given to treat anaphylaxis, but there is little evidence of benefit. Glucocorticoids take several hours to take effect, so they do not relieve the initial signs and symptoms of anaphylaxis. One theoretical justification for giving them is to prevent prolonged reactions that occur in some cases of anaphylaxis, though a systematic review found no evidence for this effect [29]. Routine administration of glucocorticoids is not recommended in patients who respond well to epinephrine and other measures and are expected to be discharged. However, glucocorticoids may be useful in patients with severe symptoms requiring hospitalization or with known asthma and significant bronchospasm that persists after other symptoms of anaphylaxis have resolved. If given, a dose of 1–2 mg/kg/day of methylprednisolone is sufficient for 1–2 days. Thereafter, glucocorticoids can be discontinued without reduction.

Allergic Reactions, Urticaria: Allergic reactions characterized by urticaria and/or pruritus can usually be treated by temporarily interrupting the procedure and administering diphenhydramine and/or glucocorticoids. If symptoms resolve, the procedure can be resumed. Allergic reactions such as urticaria are thought to result from IgE-type antibodies previously developed in the recipient or donor, which react with an allergen in the donor or recipient, respectively [36, 37].

Transfusion-Related Acute Lung Injury (TRALI): TRALI is an acute, noncardiogenic pulmonary edema characterized by hypoxia that occurs during or after transfusion [38]. It is the leading cause of death related to blood transfusions, as documented by the US Food and Drug Administration (FDA). A TRALI event develops in 1 in 5000 units of erythrocyte suspension, 1 in 2000 of plasma-containing components, and 1 in 400 units of platelet concentrate derived from whole blood. TRALI is diagnosed clinically and usually confirmed by radiographic findings. The diagnostic criterion is the occurrence of symptoms during or within 6 h of transfusion, without any risk factors for acute lung injury, such as sepsis, aspiration, or shock [39]. Clinical features include acute dyspnea, hypoxemia, fever, hypotension, tachycardia, and laboratory leukopenia and thrombocytopenia. Bilateral exudative infiltrates are present on chest radiography. Normal pulmonary artery occlusion pressure is noted, indicating non-cardiogenic pulmonary edema. A ratio of partial oxygen pressure to fractional inspired oxygen concentration ($PaO2/FiO2 <300$ mmHg) and $SpO2 <90\%$ on room air supports hypoxemia. Low BNP (B-type natriuretic peptide) levels and transient leukopenia develop in approximately 30% of patients [40, 41]. TRALI is caused by antibodies in the donor blood against the recipient's human neutrophil antigen (HNA) or human leukocyte antigens (HLA). Pulmonary vascular space is damaged by neutrophils. The storage of blood products leads to the accumulation of proinflammatory mediators involved in the development of TRALI, and neutrophil sequestration occurs in the pulmonary vascular space. Neutrophils activate and damage the endothelial layer, causing leakage of protein and fluid into the alveolar space [42]. A higher incidence of TRALI has been reported with plasma from female donors, as multiple HLA antibodies, anti-HLA class II, and HNA-positive antibodies are present in the plasma of female donors who have given birth. Blood products with high plasma content have been associated with an increased rate of TRALI [43]. If TRALI is suspected, the procedure should be stopped immediately, and oxygen should be administered to correct hypoxemia. Noninvasive respiratory support with continuous positive airway pressure (CPAP) or bilevel positive airway pressure (BiPAP) may be sufficient in milder cases. However, invasive mechanical ventilation and endotracheal intubation are often necessary [44]. Hypovolemia and related hypotension frequently develop in patients with TRALI. The primary aim of hemodynamic support is to ensure end-organ perfusion, which can be achieved through fluid resuscitation and/or vasoactive support [45]. The efficacy of corticosteroids has not been demonstrated in prospective clinical studies. However, case reports suggest that high-dose corticosteroids may be beneficial. Therefore, routine administration of corticosteroids is not recommended when TRALI is suspected. Given evidence suggesting that initiating corticosteroids late during acute respiratory distress syndrome (ARDS) (>14 days after the onset of the syndrome) is harmful, corticosteroid therapy should not be used once lung damage is fully established and more than 2 weeks have elapsed [46, 47].

Transfusion-Transmitted Infections

Transmission of hepatitis B, hepatitis C, human immunodeficiency virus (HIV), and hepatitis D may occur in relation to TDP used during the procedure [48].

14.1.2.5 Complications Associated with Blood Volume

Hypotension: Reduced intravascular volume can occur with any procedure. Approximately 200 mL of patient blood remains in the apheresis kit tubing and centrifuge during and after the procedure. The extracorporeal volume of each kit type is listed in the manufacturer's information. With continuous flow technology, the extracorporeal volume is usually no more than 15% of the patient's intravascular volume. However, instruments using intermittent flow technology may have higher extracorporeal volumes. Additional intravascular fluid infusion, slowing the procedure, or increasing the rate of return may help restore blood pressure to baseline.

Transfusion-Associated Circulatory Overload (TACO): TACO is one of the causes of transfusion-related respiratory failure. Although it is most commonly reported in elderly individuals and young children, TACO can occur in all age groups. Risk factors for TACO include impaired cardiac function, positive fluid balance, renal dysfunction, emergency surgery, and rapid blood product administration [49]. TACO typically presents with respiratory distress (dyspnea, orthopnea), especially in patients with known or unknown underlying heart failure, undergoing apheresis in a positive fluid balance environment. The severity can range from mild dyspnea to acute respiratory decompensation. TACO should be suspected in any patient with new or worsening respiratory distress during apheresis or within 12 h after its completion [50]. Examination findings may include hypoxia, hypertension, tachycardia, wide pulse pressure, and/or jugular venous engorgement. An S3 heart sound may be heard on cardiac examination, and rales are often present on lung examination. A small study evaluating N-terminal pro-hormone BNP (NT-pro BNP) found that 94% of patients who developed TACO had elevated NT-pro BNP levels even before transfusion [51]. Treatment is similar to cardiogenic pulmonary edema. The procedure should be stopped, and diuretic treatment should be initiated. For patients with hypoxemia, mechanical ventilation with CPAP/BiPAP or endotracheal intubation may be required if oxygen support is needed.

14.1.2.6 Changes in Blood Components After TPE

Decreased Coagulation Factors: TPE with albumin or other non-plasma replacement fluids causes a predictable decrease in blood clotting factors, leading to a predisposition to bleeding. Immediately after a single plasma volume exchange, the prothrombin time (PT) may increase by 30%, and the activated partial thromboplastin time (aPTT) may double. These changes generally return to normal within 4 h [14, 52]. However, more pronounced and longer-lasting changes can occur when multiple exchanges are performed over a short period, such as three or more treatments per week [53]. If multiple TPE procedures are planned, baseline PT, aPTT, and fibrinogen levels should be checked before starting the procedure. This should be repeated daily or every other day. For patients at risk of bleeding, if a replacement fluid other than plasma is used, plasma should be administered for each liter or more of replacement fluid. Plasma should be given at the end of the procedure.

Decreased Immunoglobulin Levels: Repeated TPE with non-plasma replacement fluid can cause a decrease in the patient's immunoglobulin (Ig) levels. The need for monitoring serum IgG levels depends on several factors, including the frequency of exchange, the number of blood volumes exchanged per session, the patient's immune status, and the patient's ability to produce Ig. For patients undergoing aggressive TPE, such as two to three plasma volume exchanges per session and/or sessions performed every other day, a baseline IgG level should be obtained [54]. Intravenous Ig (IVIG; 100–400 mg/kg) can be administered to patients whose IgG level falls below 500 mg/dL and who have systemic infection or are at high risk of infection.

14.1.2.7 Removal of Pharmaceuticals with TPE

TPE may affect drug concentrations through direct removal or through plasma excretion of metabolizing enzymes. In general, all daily drug doses should be administered after the TPE session. Drugs with a very low volume of distribution (<0.2 L/kg) and high protein binding (>80%) are most likely eliminated by TPE [10]. This is also true for therapeutic antibodies. Rituximab, eculizumab, IVIG, and total parenteral nutrition fluids should be given after the TPE session.

14.1.2.8 Anaphylactoid Reaction Associated with ACEi Use

Rarely, flushing, hypotension, abdominal cramps (anaphylaxis-like), and other gastrointestinal symptoms have been reported during TPE in patients receiving ACEi. Since ACEi inhibit the breakdown of bradykinins, hypotension may occur if kinins are activated during apheresis in patients receiving these drugs. This has been most commonly reported with the use of hydrophilic, electronegative membranes, such as the polyacrylonitrile AN69 filter. This reaction is also associated with dextran sulfate systems, albumin replacement fluids, and Plasmaflo OP filters (polyethylene) [10]. In a study of 299 consecutive patients undergoing TPE, anaphylaxis-like symptoms occurred in all 14 patients receiving ACEi, but only in 7% of those not receiving ACEi [55]. Based on these observations, discontinuation of ACEi 24–48 h before TPE or switching to an angiotensin receptor blocker has been recommended if the patient can tolerate temporary drug discontinuation [16, 56].

14.1.3 Conclusion

TP is an extracorporeal therapy that removes pathogens from plasma. In clinical practice, it is important to manage the potential complications of this lifesaving treatment for various diseases. Especially in clinics without advanced apheresis centers, it is crucial for physicians to periodically update their knowledge to ensure the appropriate management of emergency complications during and after the procedure.

References

1. Altobelli C, Anastasio P, Cerrone A, Signoriello E, Lus G, Pluvio C, Perna AF, Capasso G, Simeoni M, Capolongo G. Therapeutic plasmapheresis: a revision of literature. Kidney Blood Press Res. 2022;48(1):66–78.
2. Ipe TS, Marques MB. Vascular access for therapeutic plasma exchange. Transfusion. 2018;58(Suppl 1):580–9.
3. Mortzell Henriksson M, Newman E, Witt V, Derfler K, Leitner G, Eloot S, et al. Adverse events in apheresis an update of the WAA registry data. Transfus Apher Sci. 2016;54(1):2–15.
4. Mokrzycki MH, Kaplan AA. Therapeutic plasma exchange: complications and management. Am J Kidney Dis. 1994;23:817.
5. Kaplan A. Complications of apheresis. Semin Dial. 2012;25:152.
6. Doggett BM, Session-Augustine N, Roig J, Strunk M, Valiyaparambil S, Sarode R, De Simone N. Single-needle: an effective alternative to dual-needle peripheral access in therapeutic plasma exchange. J Clin Apher. 2019;34:21–5.
7. Mustieles MJ, Acosta M, Cid J, Jiménez M, Mateo D, Andreu B, Alba C, Perea D, Lozano M. Peripheral venous access devices for apheresis: 16-gauge is not always needed. Transfusion. 2020;60:607–12.
8. Lemaire A, Parquet N, Galicier L, Boutboul D, Bertinchamp R, Malphettes M, Dumas G, Mariotte E, Peraldi MN, Souppart V, Schlemmer B, Azoulay E, Canet E. Plasma exchange in the intensive care unit: technical aspects and complications. J Clin Apher. 2017;32:405–12.
9. Alder BC, editor. Standards for cellular therapy services. 10th ed. Bethesda: AABB; 2021.
10. Cervantes CE, Bloch EM, Sperati CJ. Therapeutic plasma exchange: core curriculum 2023. Am J Kidney Dis. 2023;81(4):475–92.
11. Ward DM. Conventional apheresis therapies: a review. J Clin Apher. 2011;26:230–8.
12. Tohme JF, Bilezikian JP. Hypocalcemic emergencies. Endocrinol Metab Clin N Am. 1993;22:363.
13. McLeod BC, editor. Apheresis principles and practice. 2nd ed. AABB: Bethesda; 2003.
14. Kaplan AA, Halley SE. Plasma exchange with a rotating filter. Kidney Int. 1990;38:160.
15. Weinstein R. Prevention of citrate reactions during therapeutic plasma exchange by constant infusion of calcium gluconate with the return fluid. J Clin Apher. 1996;11:204.
16. Webb J, Andrzejewski C. Chapter 25: Therapeutic apheresis. In: John CS, Delaney M, Johnson ST, Katz LM, editors. Technical manual. 20th ed. Bethesda: AABB; 2020.
17. Pearl RG, Rosenthal MH. Metabolic alkalosis due to plasmapheresis. Am J Med. 1985;79:391.
18. Hafer C, Golla P, Gericke M, Eden G, Beutel G, Schmidt JJ, Schmidt BM, De Reys S, Kielstein JT. Membrane versus centrifuge-based therapeutic plasma exchange: a randomized prospective crossover study. Int Urol Nephrol. 2016;48:133–8.
19. Tutarel O, Golla P, Beutel G, Bauersachs J, David S, Schmidt BM, Lichtinghagen R, Kielstein JT. Therapeutic plasma exchange decreases levels of routinely used cardiac and inflammatory biomarkers. PLoS One. 2012;7:e38573.
20. Orlin JB, Berkman EM. Partial plasma exchange using albumin replacement: removal and recovery of normal plasma constituents. Blood. 1980;56:1055.
21. Goss GA, Weinstein R. Pentastarch as partial replacement fluid for therapeutic plasma exchange: effect on plasma proteins, adverse events during treatment, and serum ionized calcium. J Clin Apher. 1999;14:114.
22. Cid J, Carbassé G, Gamir M, Jiménez M, Arellano-Rodrigo E, Lozano M. Acid-base balance disturbances in plasma exchange depend on the replacement fluid used. Transfusion. 2015;55:2653–8.
23. Radhakrishnan M, Batra A, Periyavan S, Philip M, Anand V. Hydroxyethyl starch and kidney function: a retrospective study in patients undergoing therapeutic plasma exchange. J Clin Apher. 2018;33:278–82.

24. Huestis DW. Mortality in therapeutic haemapheresis. Lancet. 1983;1:1043.
25. Sutton DM, Nair RC, Rock G. Complications of plasma exchange. Transfusion. 1989;29:124.
26. Ring J, Messmer K. Incidence and severity of anaphylactoid reactions to colloid volume substitutes. Lancet. 1977;1:466.
27. Bambauer R, Jutzler GA, Albrecht D, et al. Indications of plasmapheresis and selection of different substitution solutions. Biomater Artif Cells Artif Organs. 1989;17:9.
28. Cardona V, Ansotegui IJ, Ebisawa M, et al. World allergy organization anaphylaxis guidance 2020. World Allergy Organ J. 2020;13:100472.
29. Shaker MS, Wallace DV, Golden DBK, et al. Anaphylaxis-a 2020 practice parameter update, systematic review, and grading of recommendations, assessment, development and evaluation (GRADE) analysis. J Allergy Clin Immunol. 2020;145:1082.
30. Brown SG, Blackman KE, Stenlake V, Heddle RJ. Insect sting anaphylaxis; prospective evaluation of treatment with intravenous adrenaline and volume resuscitation. Emerg Med J. 2004;21:149.
31. Perel P, Roberts I, Ker K. Colloids versus crystalloids for fluid resuscitation in critically ill patients. Cochrane Database Syst Rev. 2013;(2):CD000567.
32. Kawano T, Scheuermeyer FX, Stenstrom R, et al. Epinephrine use in older patients with anaphylaxis: clinical outcomes and cardiovascular complications. Resuscitation. 2017;112:53.
33. Simons KJ, Simons FE. Epinephrine and its use in anaphylaxis: current issues. Curr Opin Allergy Clin Immunol. 2010;10:354.
34. McLean-Tooke AP, Bethune CA, Fay AC, Spickett GP. Adrenaline in the treatment of anaphylaxis: what is the evidence? BMJ. 2003;327:1332.
35. Wheeler DW, Carter JJ, Murray LJ, et al. The effect of drug concentration expression on epinephrine dosing errors: a randomized trial. Ann Intern Med. 2008;148:11.
36. Apter AJ, Kaplan AA. An approach to immunologic reactions associated with plasma exchange. J Allergy Clin Immunol. 1992;90:119.
37. Cohn CS, Delaney M, Johnson ST, Katz LM, editors. Technical manual. 20th ed. Bethesda: AABB; 2020.
38. Roubinian N. TACO and TRALI: biology, risk factors, and prevention strategies. Hematology Am Soc Hematol Educ Program. 2018;2018(1):585–94.
39. Toy P, Popovsky MA, Abraham E, Ambruso DR, Holness LG, Kopko PM, McFarland JG, Nathens AB, Silliman CC, Stroncek D, National Heart, Lung and Blood Institute Working Group on TRALI. Transfusion-related acute lung injury: definition and review. Crit Care Med. 2005;33(4):721–6.
40. Skeate RC, Eastlund T. Distinguishing between transfusion related acute lung injury and transfusion associated circulatory overload. Curr Opin Hematol. 2007;14(6):682–7.
41. Kim KN, Kim DW, Jeong MA. The usefulness of a classification and regression tree algorithm for detecting perioperative transfusion-related pulmonary complications. Transfusion. 2015;55(11):2582–9.
42. Sachs UJ. Recent insights into the mechanism of transfusion-related acute lung injury. Curr Opin Hematol. 2011;18(6):436–42.
43. Toy P, Gajic O, Bacchetti P, Looney MR, Gropper MA, Hubmayr R, Lowell CA, Norris PJ, Murphy EL, Weiskopf RB, Wilson G, Koenigsberg M, Lee D, Schuller R, Wu P, Grimes B, Gandhi MJ, Winters JL, Mair D, Hirschler N, Sanchez Rosen R, Matthay MA, TRALI Study Group. Transfusion-related acute lung injury: incidence and risk factors. Blood. 2012;119(7):1757–67.
44. Gajic O, Rana R, Winters JL, et al. Transfusion-related acute lung injury in the critically ill: prospective nested case-control study. Am J Respir Crit Care Med. 2007;176:886.
45. Wallis JP. Transfusion-related acute lung injury (TRALI): presentation, epidemiology and treatment. Intensive Care Med. 2007;33(Suppl 1):S12.
46. Looney MR, Gropper MA, Matthay MA. Transfusion-related acute lung injury: a review. Chest. 2004;126:249.
47. Tang BM, Craig JC, Eslick GD, et al. Use of corticosteroids in acute lung injury and acute respiratory distress syndrome: a systematic review and meta-analysis. Crit Care Med. 2009;37:1594.
48. Tekin A. Infections transmitted by the transfusion of blood and blood products. Konuralp Tıp Dergisi. 2011;3(2):38–45.
49. Clifford L, Jia Q, Subramanian A, et al. Risk factors and clinical outcomes associated with perioperative transfusion-associated circulatory overload. Anesthesiology. 2017;126:409.
50. Popovsky MA, Moore SB. Diagnostic and pathogenetic considerations in transfusion-related acute lung injury. Transfusion. 1985;25:573.
51. Tobian AA, Sokoll LJ, Tisch DJ, et al. N-terminal pro-brain natriuretic peptide is a useful diagnostic marker for transfusion-associated circulatory overload. Transfusion. 2008;48:1143.
52. Chirnside A, Urbaniak SJ, Prowse CV, Keller AJ. Coagulation abnormalities following intensive plasma exchange on the cell separator. II. Effects on factors I, II, V, VII, VIII, IX, X and antithrombin III. Br J Haematol. 1981;48:627.
53. Gelabert A, Puig L, Maragall S, et al. Coagulation alterations during massive plasmapheresis. In: Sieberth HG, editor. Plasma exchange. Stuttgart: Schattauer Verlag; 1980. p. 71.
54. Kaplan AA. Towards a rational prescription of plasma exchange: the kinetics of immunoglobulin removal. Semin Dial. 1992;5:227.
55. Owen HG, Brecher ME. Atypical reactions associated with use of angiotensin-converting enzyme inhibitors and apheresis. Transfusion. 1994;34:891.
56. Perkins KA. Contraindication of angiotensin-converting enzyme (ACE) inhibitors for patients receiving therapeutic plasma exchanges. Nephrol Nurs J. 2008;35:571.

15 Complications of Therapeutic Plasma Exchange in Intoxication

Murat Özkale and Yasemin Özkale

15.1 Background

In neurological, hematological, renal, and autoimmune diseases with a known or suspected immune pathogenesis, therapeutic plasma exchange (TPE) is the primary mode of treatment. Many studies have reported complications of TPE in these disease groups; however, the use and complications of TPE in intoxication are not fully understood. Shemin et al. examined complications of 1727 TPE procedures in 174 patients (aged 9–87 years) and reported a complication rate of 36%. The most common TPE indication was thrombotic thrombocytopenic purpura (TTP), and the most common TPE complication was fever [1]. Another study reported complications of 1201 TPE procedures in 435 children (aged 3 months to 15 years) and found a complication rate of 12.7%. The most common TPE indication was intoxication (pesticide, animal toxin, plant toxin, and drug), and the most common complications were pruritus and urticaria [2]. Basic-Jukic et al. reported complications of 4857 TPE procedures in 509 patients, which included ten intoxication cases, and found a complication rate of 4.75%. The most common complications were paresthesias, hematoma at the puncture site, clotting, allergic reactions, and bleeding [3]. To the best of our knowledge, TPE for treating intoxication alone has been evaluated in only two studies: one by Dişel et al. involving adults and another by Özkale et al. involving children [4, 5]. Dişel et al. reviewed 42 patients (aged 17–83 years) who had undergone TPE due to a range of intoxications and observed that organophosphate intoxication was the most common indication. However, the authors did not report the complications of TPE [4]. On the other hand, Özkale et al. reported 14 children diagnosed with intoxication who underwent TPE, with indications ranging from multidrug intoxication to mercury poisoning [5]. Clinical improvement was observed after TPE in 13 of the 14 patients, and 1 patient with verapamil intoxication died. Özkale et al. noted mild allergic reactions in 1 of the 14 intoxicated patients [5]. Additionally, some case studies have reported the effectiveness of TPE for various types of intoxication, including amitriptyline, theophylline, carbamazepine, *Amanita phalloides* mushroom, diltiazem, verapamil, amlodipine, propranolol, L-thyroxine, and heavy metals such as mercury. However, complications of TPE were not mentioned in these studies [6–9].

M. Özkale (✉)
Department of Pediatric Intensive Care Unit, Faculty of Medicine, Dr. Turgut Noyan Teaching and Medical Research Center, Baskent University, Adana, Turkey

Y. Özkale
Department of Pediatric, Faculty of Medicine, Dr. Turgut Noyan Teaching and Medical Research Center, Baskent University, Adana, Turkey

I. Kozanoglu (ed.), *Problem Solving in Apheresis Medicine*,
https://doi.org/10.1007/978-3-031-74081-7_15

15.2 Physiological Background and Treatment Goals and Principles

Rapid reduction in the levels of toxic substances or drugs is the cornerstone of treating intoxication, and TPE is used achieve this goal. TPE involves the separation of blood into its component parts, either through centrifugation or filtration, followed by the removal of plasma and its replacement with an equal volume of fresh frozen plasma (FFP) or a combination of serum albumin and isotonic sodium chloride [10]. TPE can be considered as a treatment option in intoxication if the toxin to be removed (1) is too large for removal by other procedures, (2) has a comparatively prolonged half-life, (3) is acutely toxic and resistant to conventional therapy, and (4) has a high protein-binding affinity with a low volume of distribution. In addition, TPE can be considered in patients with drug intoxication, especially in those who do not exhibit clinical improvement despite supportive and antidotal treatments, have uncontrolled and ongoing toxidrome symptoms, have a poor clinical condition (low Glasgow Coma Scale), or have an unknown type and amount of the causative toxic substance [1–5]. Timely TPE treatment in patients with unknown intoxication who present in clinically poor condition can have a profound effect on the prognosis. TPE also offers benefits for toxin-induced complications such as hemolysis or TTP. For instance, in patients with drug-induced hemolysis, TPE removes products of red blood cell destruction and hemoglobin. In addition, plasma infusion itself (independent of the removal of toxic circulating compounds) has beneficial effects. For example, when plasma is used as a replacement fluid during TPE, it provides an opportunity to administer active cholinesterase in organophosphate poisoning [11].

15.3 Patient Education

TPE appears to be safe and effective in treating intoxication when performed by a trained team. The complication rates are much lower in recent years compared with earlier years, and most complications are minor, self-limiting, easily treatable, and not life-threatening. Minor complications of TPE include allergic reactions, symptomatic hypocalcemia, hypotension, infection, and complications related to catheter placement. Major complications include sepsis, anaphylaxis, shock, acute pulmonary edema, myocardial infarction, and death [1–5]. Recent studies have also shown very low mortality rates associated with TPE. The incidence of death related to TPE was found to be 0.05% in a meta-analysis [12].

15.4 Consideration

The medical history of patients, including the drugs they use, any history of allergies, and previous transfusion reactions, should be reviewed before TPE. In addition, baseline tests should include a complete blood count, immunoglobulin levels, coagulation tests (including fibrinogen), hepatic and renal function tests, and electrolyte levels, especially ionized calcium. If possible, patients should be closely monitored throughout the procedure. Vital signs, including blood pressure, respiratory rate, heart rate, and temperature, should be checked before and during TPE, e.g., every 10–15 min depending on the patient's hemodynamic status. If any signs or symptoms (e.g., dyspnea, seizures, chest pain, and hypotension) suggesting possible complications of TPE are detected, or if the patient's general status or hemodynamics deteriorates, the procedure should be discontinued, and symptoms should be investigated [13].

15.5 Pearls and Pitfalls Complication

The principles of TPE are the same for adults and children, but some technical differences exist in children, including the establishment of vascular access and volume distribution. However, improvements in techniques and the availability of various types of central venous catheters and ports have enhanced safety and encouraged the use of TPE in children in recent years [5]. Complications related to TPE are divided into two groups: vascular access (catheter)-related and procedure (TPE)-related complications.

15.6 Complications of TPE in Intoxication

1. **Complications Associated with Vascular Access:** Central or peripheral veins can be used for vascular access in patients. Most complications occur with the use of a peripheral venous catheter. While mechanical complications are largely operator-dependent and are usually detected at the time of catheter insertion (e.g., pneumothorax), infectious and thrombotic complications tend to occur later than mechanical complications [1–3]. Complications associated with vascular access and their prevention are summarized in Table 15.1.
2. **Complications Associated with Anticoagulants:** Anticoagulation for TPE aims to achieve a delicate balance between preventing circuit failure due to the loss of expensive blood components and preventing bleeding. Heparin and citrate are the most common anticoagulants, while epoprostenol can also be used when citrate is unavailable and heparin is contraindicated. Most TPE treatments performed with standard centrifugal devices use citrate anticoagulation. Although this technique can be modified for use with a membrane plasma separation (MPS) system, most MPS treatments are performed with heparin [1, 3, 10]. Complications associated with anticoagulants and their prevention are summarized in Table 15.2.
3. **Complications Associated with Replacement Fluid:** The patient's fluid volume removed by TPE must be replaced to prevent significant volume depletion. Albumin (5%), normal saline, a combination of albumin and normal saline, and FFP are the replacement fluids of choice for most conditions. The optimal choice often varies depending on the clinical setting. Adverse reactions are more common when FFP is used as the replacement fluid [1, 3, 10, 13–15]. Complications associated with replacement fluid are summarized in Table 15.3.
4. **Other Complications**

   Volume Overload: Increased intravascular volume prior to the procedure; underlying heart, kidney, or liver disease; rapid fluid shifts; and transfusion-associated circulatory overload can cause volume overload during the TPE procedure [1–3].

   Hypotension: Underlying heart, kidney, or liver disease, low intravascular volume before TPE, transfusion reactions, angiotensin-converting enzyme inhibitor (ACEi)-associated hypotension, membrane incompatibility with plasma membrane separation, and vasovagal reactions can cause hypotension during the TPE procedure [1–3].

   Removal of or Clinically Relevant Decrease in Certain Proteins or Medications: TPE with non-plasma replacement fluid produces a predictable decrease in blood coagula-

Table 15.1 Complications associated with vascular access

Vascular complications	Clinical findings	Prevention
• Peripheral veins • Indwelling intravascular catheters	• Infection, pain, nerve damage, thrombosis, perforation, dissecting hematomas, air embolism, and arteriovenous fistulas	• Optimal vein should be selected for accessibility, size, and location based on the number and length of procedures • An experienced team should insert the catheter and confirm placement radiologically prior to TPE • Coagulation parameters should be evaluated before removing the catheter

Table 15.2 Complications associated with anticoagulants

Anticoagulant type	Complications	Prevention
• Sodium citrate	• Hypocalcemia	• Evaluation of ionized calcium levels before and during TPE • Monitor electrocardiographic activity • Slowing the TPE rate • Pretreatment with administer prophylactic calcium (oral, intravenous push, or continuous infusion) as pretreatment
	• Metabolic alkalosis	• If there is underlying renal failure, hemodialysis may be preferred
	• Hypomagnesemia	• Evaluation of calcium and magnesium levels • Administration of magnesium sulfate in symptomatic patients
	• Hypokalemia	• Check potassium levels after TPE and treat if hypokalemia is present
	• Changes in parathyroid hormone levels	
• Heparin	• Bleeding	• Administration of protamine sulfate
	• Heparin-induced thrombocytopenia	• Discontinuation of all heparin exposure
	• Nonimmune (heparin-associated) thrombocytopenia	• Thrombocyte count should be monitored
	• Skin necrosis and local and systemic allergic reactions	• According to the patient's symptoms • Discontinue heparin treatment • Administration of antihistamines, epinephrine, glucocorticoids, or more aggressive treatment

Table 15.3 Complications associated with replacement fluid

Type of replacement fluid	Complications
• 5% albumin	• Dilutional coagulopathy • Loss of immunoglobulins
• Albumin-saline combination	• When colloid and crystalloid solutions are used in combination, the amount of colloid should not be less than 50% of the total infused. Using colloid and crystalloid solutions together with the colloid comprising less than 50% of the total infusion may lead to dilutional coagulopathy or insufficient oncotic pressure
• Saline	• Insufficient oncotic pressure, edema, and/or hypotension • Depletion of coagulation factors and immunoglobulins
• Fresh frozen plasma	• Anaphylactic reactions • Hives • Transfusion-related acute lung injury • Acute hemolytic transfusion • Infectious risks of plasma

tion factors, which may predispose the patient to bleeding, deplete immunoglobulins, and result in low-serum immunoglobulin G and other immunoglobulin levels, therapeutic monoclonal antibodies, and other medications [16–18].

References

1. Shemin D, Briggs D, Greenan M. Complications of therapeutic plasma exchange: a prospective study of 1,727 procedures. J Clin Apher. 2007;22(5):270–6.
2. Lu J, Zhang L, Xia C, Tao Y. Complications of therapeutic plasma exchange: a retrospective study of 1201

procedures in 435 children. Medicine (Baltimore). 2019;98(50):e18308.
3. Basic-Jukic N, Kes P, Glavas-Boras S, Brunetta B, Bubic-Filipi L, Puretic Z. Complications of therapeutic plasma exchange: experience with 4857 treatments. Ther Apher Dial. 2005;9(5):391–5.
4. Dişel NR, Akpınar AA, Sebe A, Karakoç E, Sürer S, Turhan FT, et al. Therapeutic plasma exchange in poisoning: 8 year's experience of a university hospital. Am J Emerg Med. 2015;33:1391–5.
5. Özkale M, Özkale Y. The role of therapeutic plasma exchange in the treatment of childhood intoxication: a single-center experience. Pediatr Crit Care Med. 2020;21:e988–95.
6. Tiftik N, Kiykim A, Altintas E, Sezer K, Doruk N, Sezgin O, et al. Therapeutic plasma exchange for multidrug intoxication: a case report. J Clin Apher. 2003;18:132–3.
7. Kolsal E, Tekin IO, Piskin E, Aydemir C, Akyuz M, Cabuk H, et al. Treatment of severe amitriptyline intoxication with plasmapheresis. J Clin Apher. 2009;24(1):21–4.
8. Kozanoglu I, Kahveci S, Asma S, Yeral M, Noyan A, Boga C, et al. Plasma-exchange treatment for severe carbamazepine intoxication: a case study. J Clin Apher. 2014;29(3):178–80.
9. Jander S, Bischoff J. Treatment of amanita phalloides poisoning: I. Retrospective evaluation of plasmapheresis in 21 patients. Therap Apher. 2000;4:303–7.
10. Ibrahim RB, Liu C, Cronin SM, Murphy BC, Cha R, Swerdlow P, et al. Drug removal by plasmapheresis: an evidence-based review. Pharmacotherapy. 2007;27(11):1529–49.
11. Madore F. Plasmapheresis in acute intoxication and poisoning. In: Critical care nephrology (third edition). https://doi.org/10.1016/B978-0-323-44942-7.00100-X.
12. Kaplan A. Complications of apheresis. Semin Dial. 2012;25:152–8.
13. Soares Ferreira Júnior A, Hodulik K, Barton KD, Onwuemene OA. Hemostatic effects of therapeutic plasma exchange: a concise review. J Clin Apher. 2022;37(3):292–312. https://doi.org/10.1002/jca.21973. Epub 2022 Feb 23
14. Tabor E. The epidemiology of virus transmission by plasma derivatives: clinical studies verifying the lack of transmission of hepatitis B and C viruses and HIV type 1. Transfusion. 1999;39:1160–8.
15. Walker RH, editor. Technical manual. 11th ed. Bethesda: American Association of Blood Banks; 1993.
16. Kaplan AA, Halley SE. Plasma exchange with a rotating filter. Kidney Int. 1990;38:160–6.
17. Chirnside A, Urbaniak SJ, Prowse CV, Keller AJ. Coagulation abnormalities following intensive plasma exchange on the cell separator. II. Effects on factors I, II, V, VII, VIII, IX, X and antithrombin III. Br J Haematol. 1981;48:627–34.
18. Gelabert A, Puig L, Maragall S, et al. Coagulation alterations during massive plasmapheresis. In: Sieberth HG, editor. Plasma exchange. Stuttgart: Schattauer Verlag; 1980. p. 71.

Complications During Apheresis in Patients with Sepsis

16

Sule Mine Bakanay Ozturk
and Ankara Bilkent Şehir Hastanesi

16.1 Introduction

Sepsis is defined as life-threatening organ dysfunction caused by a systemic inflammatory response to infection [1, 2]. Bacterial wall components, such as endotoxins or lipopolysaccharides, known as pathogen-associated molecular patterns (PAMPs) and damage-associated molecular patterns (DAMPs) released from injured host tissues, with subsequent release of both pro- and anti-inflammatory cytokines into the bloodstream, appear to play an important role in triggering this response [3]. Additionally, decreased ADAMTS13 (a disintegrin and metalloproteinase with thrombospondin motifs-13) enzyme activity and increased von Willebrand factor (vWF) multimers seem to play a role in coagulopathy, microvascular occlusion, and tissue ischemia.

Organ dysfunction in sepsis is evaluated using the Sequential Organ Failure Assessment (SOFA) scoring system. A SOFA score ≥2 indicates organ dysfunction. Septic shock is a subset of sepsis that is accompanied by circulatory and cellular abnormalities and has a high mortality rate. Septic shock is defined as the need for a vasopressor to maintain the mean arterial pressure >65 mmHg despite adequate fluid resuscitation, with a serum lactate level >2 mmol/L [1]. Sepsis may lead to septic shock, multiorgan failure (MOF), and death if not recognized early and treated promptly. Severe sepsis and septic shock account for about 10% of admissions to intensive care units (ICUs) and are among the leading causes of ICU mortality worldwide. Mortality associated with septic shock remains as high as 20–40%.

Conventional therapy for sepsis includes antibiotics, infection control with antimicrobials, and hemodynamic support, including intravenous (IV) fluid replacement, vasopressors, and mechanical ventilation. The latest guidelines for sepsis recommend renal replacement therapy if acute kidney injury develops. Despite advances in the treatment and supportive care of critically ill patients, there is still an unmet medical need for additional therapies in sepsis and septic shock [4].

In the last two decades, there has been growing interest in using extracorporeal therapies as adjuncts to the standard treatment for sepsis. Therapeutic plasma exchange (TPE) involves separating plasma from other components of blood, either by membrane filtration or centrifugation. The plasma is removed and replaced with a solution such as human albumin and/or plasma, or a combination of crystalloid/colloid solution

S. M. B. Ozturk (✉)
Ankara Yıldırım Beyazıt University, Faculty of Medicine, Ankara Bilkent City Hospital, Ankara, Turkey

A. B. Ş. Hastanesi
Bilkent City Hospital, Hematology Department, Oncology Tower, Ankara, Turkey

I. Kozanoglu (ed.), *Problem Solving in Apheresis Medicine*,
https://doi.org/10.1007/978-3-031-74081-7_16

Table 16.1 Effects of TPE on the levels of circulating factors in sepsis

Substances removed by TPE	Substances repleted by TPE
Bacterial toxins, PAMPs	Anticoagulant Antithrombin III ADAMTS13 Protein C
Activated complement, C3	
Procoagulant, ultralarge vWF	
Inflammatory cytokines DAMPs, cytokines, chemokines, CRP, procalcitonin, TNFα, IL-1β	Immunoglobulins IgG, M, A
Pro-permeability Angiopoietin-2, heparanase-1	Anti-permeability Angiopoietin-1, sTie-2, heparanase-2

TPE therapeutic plasma exchange; *PAMPs* pathogen-associated molecular patterns; *DAMPs* damage-associated molecular patterns; *CRP* C-reactive protein; *TNFα* tumor necrosis factor-α; *IL-1β* interleukin-1β; *ADAMTS13* a disintegrin and metalloproteinase with thrombospondin motifs-13; *sTie-2* a soluble receptor tyrosine kinase with immunoglobulin-like and epidermal growth factor-like domains

[5]. Vascular access is established by central venous insertion of an 11 Fr, double-lumen hemodialysis catheter. In sepsis, fresh frozen plasma (FFP) is the preferred replacement fluid, and 1–1.5 times the patient's plasma volume is exchanged within approximately 120 min. A centrifugal TPE device is generally used, and anticoagulation is achieved by regional citrate infusion. Plasma exchange has the potential to improve survival in sepsis by removing the excessive potentially harmful substances and replacing depleted protective factors with healthy donor plasma [6] (Table 16.1).

16.2 Efficacy of TPE in Sepsis

Various observational studies and randomized clinical trials (RCTs) have reported the efficacy of TPE in sepsis. In 2014, Rimmer et al. conducted a systemic review and meta-analysis to explore the efficacy and safety of plasma exchange in patients with sepsis and septic shock, identifying 4 randomized controlled trials that recruited a total of 194 patients [7]. After a short follow-up of 14 or 28 days, the use of TPE was associated with an insignificant reduction in all-cause mortality, which was mainly observed in adults but not in children [8–11]. The largest of these studies utilized one to two daily TPE sessions, resulting in a 28-day mortality rate of 33% compared to 54% in the control group ($p < 0.05$), which became nonsignificant ($p = 0.07$) when controlled for confounding factors [9].

Recently, Zhang et al. reported the results of another meta-analysis, which included a total of 390 patients from five trials, and found that TPE was associated with a significant reduction in all-cause mortality in adults [12–16]. In another trial involving patients with sepsis, 22 patients who received TPE were matched with 22 patients who received conventional therapy. No difference was found in the improvement rate of SOFA scores, 28-day mortality, or the incidence of new-onset organ failure. Moreover, TPE could marginally prolong ICU stay with no significant difference in time to discharge alive [17].

Stahl et al. performed a prospective randomized controlled trial in patients with septic shock and showed that a single session of TPE, started within 24 h after the onset of septic shock, led to hemodynamic stabilization and a reduction in norepinephrine dose within 6 h in 50% of patients who received TPE, compared to patients treated with standard care. This early hemodynamic stabilization was maintained 24 h after randomization and was accompanied by a reduction in blood lactate levels, indicating shock reversal in the TPE group [18, 19]. Similar positive effects were also observed in patients with severe COVID-19 disease who underwent one to five daily TPE sessions, with improved 28-day mortality in the TPE group ($p < 0.05$) [5].

Despite the benefits of TPE in patients with sepsis, there is still a paucity of evidence regarding its effect on survival. The 2023 American Society for Apheresis (ASFA) Guidelines stated that "the optimum role of apheresis therapy is not established; decision making should be individualized" and gave a weak recommendation based on high-quality evidence [5, 20]. Large, well-designed, definitive studies are needed to validate plasmapheresis as a treatment for sepsis.

16.3 Complications of TPE in Sepsis

Therapeutic plasma exchange is an invasive treatment requiring central venous access, and the use of FFP as a replacement fluid carries several potential adverse events. The total frequency of complications is reported as 5.8%. However, severe adverse events are rare, with the incidence of events requiring discontinuation of treatment being about 0.2–0.4%. Mortality is reported as 0.03–0.05%, primarily due to respiratory and cardiac complications. Complications related to vascular access, citrate toxicity, and the use of FFP as a replacement fluid are the main issues observed in the general patient population requiring TPE with FFP [21, 22]. Due to effective donor testing today, the transmission of infections (HIV, hepatitis, and others) is considered to be a rare complication.

There are several safety issues that should be considered when performing TPE in patients with sepsis. First, these patients are often already hemodynamically unstable, with most requiring hemodynamic support and mechanical ventilation. Introducing an extracorporeal therapy in this setting can be challenging. Second, in cases of sepsis with MOF, citrate metabolism may be prolonged, increasing the risk of citrate toxicity. Moreover, citrate-induced metabolic alkalosis mainly develops in patients with concurrent kidney failure. Patients with kidney failure who require TPE may need hemodialysis following the procedure to restore acid-base, electrolyte, and fluid balance as necessary. Additionally, it has been shown that TPE induces alterations in the immune system, including changes in lymphocyte number and distribution, changes in natural killer cell number and activity, increased T suppressor function, and a shift from Th2 to Th1 ratio [23]. Potential adverse effects of extracorporeal therapies on the immune system of septic patients, as well as interference with anticoagulation strategies, require further investigation. Another important safety issue when performing plasmapheresis in patients with sepsis is its impact on pharmacokinetics of medications, particularly antimicrobials, which are the mainstay of sepsis treatment.

Although there are important safety issues, such as plasma transfusion reactions, transfusion-related acute lung injury (TRALI), coagulopathy, vascular access complications, TPE has been a safe procedure for the treatment of septic patients [4]. In the studies presented so far, apart from reports of transient episodes of hypotension and allergic reactions to FFP, no severe adverse reactions to plasmapheresis treatment were reported [3]. The most common complications are paresthesias due to citrate-associated hypocalcemia, vascular access issues, hypotension, and urticaria [22]. In a retrospective study of 111 patients with sepsis/septic shock who underwent TPE or immunoadsorption, 14 patients (12.6%) had allergic reactions, 9 (8.1%) had hypocalcemia, 8 (7.2%) had a decrease in hemoglobin, while 63.9% had no complications. No procedure-related fatal complications were observed [24]. Although most reactions are mild to moderate, several side effects may be critical for patients with sepsis. Regular vital sign measurements, cardiac monitoring, and having emergency equipment nearby are essential precautions to increase the safety of TPE in patients with sepsis.

16.3.1 Citrate Toxicity

Sodium citrate is infused either as an extracorporeal system anticoagulant or present in the FFP as a replacement fluid. Citrate binds ionized calcium, leading to hypocalcemia, which occurs in up to 9% of procedures [21]. The symptoms of citrate-induced hypocalcemia include perioral and distal extremity paresthesias, the most common symptoms, as well as hypotension, QT interval prolongation, arrhythmias, and tetany in severe cases. In cases of sepsis with MOF, citrate metabolism may be prolonged, rendering septic patients prone to citrate toxicity. Moreover, patients with sepsis often have altered mental status and may not be able to communicate early symptoms of hypocalcemia. For this reason, cardiac monitoring and intraprocedural evaluation of Ca^{2+} levels are crucial for taking early precautions. The first action is to slow the exchange rate and reduce citrate infusion by substituting the citrate solution with a citrate-plus-heparin solution. Generally, prophylactic administration of 10 mL of 10% $CaCl_2$ intravenously over 15–30 min, beginning 15 min after starting TPE, is recommended. Since plasmapheresis lasts a long time, an additional 10 mL of $CaCl_2$ is administered 1 h into the treatment. If unresponsive and severe hypocalcemia develops during the procedure, 5–10 mL of 10% Ca gluconate is administered intravenously over 10–15 min. Calcium should not be added directly to plasma; a separate line should be used [21, 25].

Citrate-induced metabolic alkalosis primarily develops in patients with renal failure and may result in confusion, tremor, lightheadedness, and numbness. Hemodialysis is required to remove excess bicarbonate. If both TPE and hemodialysis are required on the same day, it is preferred to perform TPE first, allowing dialysis to correct citrate-induced metabolic alkalosis [26].

16.3.2 Allergic and Anaphylactic Reactions

Allergic reactions may occur when FFP is used as a replacement fluid. Anaphylactic reactions are characterized by fever, rigors, urticaria, wheezing, bronchospasm, hypotension, and cardiopulmonary collapse. Prevention of allergic and anaphylactic reactions requires following patient blood management guidelines for blood product use. If the patient is IgA-deficient, it is recommended to obtain plasma from IgA-deficient donors. If an IgA-deficient donor is unavailable, albumin can be used as a replacement fluid. Pretreatment with ephedrine, glucocorticoids, or diphenhydramine may be useful in patients with a known history of allergies. In cases where allergic or anaphylactic reactions occur, antihistamines (25–50 mg diphenhydramine IV) can be given for mild cases. If symptoms persist, glucocorticoids (100 mg methylprednisolone IV) may be administered. For severe reactions, 0.3–0.5 mL of 1:1000 SC epinephrine may be given and repeated every 15 min if necessary. In patients with known sensitivity to FFP, a prophylactic regimen of 50 mg prednisone 13, 7, and 1 h before treatment, 50 mg diphenhydramine 1 h before, and 25 mg ephedrine 1 h before treatment may be used [27].

In cases of suspected allergy, such as hives, urticaria, and pruritus, it is recommended to temporarily pause the procedure. The use of diphenhydramine ± glucocorticoids and closely monitoring for worsening symptoms are advised. The procedure can be restarted once the symptoms abate. Rarely, anaphylactoid symptoms, such as a burning sensation in the eyes, tearing, and periorbital edema, may develop immediately after the start of TPE due to ethylene oxide, which is used as a sterilizing agent. Clearing the tubes is recommended in cases of ethylene oxide toxicity [27, 28].

16.3.3 Transfusion-Related Acute Lung Injury (TRALI)

This complication develops as a result of leukoagglutination in the pulmonary circulation due to infused antibodies from the donor's plasma, which react with antigens on the recipient's leukocytes. TRALI is characterized by the sudden onset of hypoxic respiratory insufficiency, noncardiogenic pulmonary edema, and bilateral pulmonary infiltrates during or within several hours of plasma infusion. Management is mainly supportive, and intubation may be required. This condition may worsen the hemodynamics of septic patients. Paradoxically, plasmapheresis may help remove donor antibodies against the recipient's leukocytes [29].

16.3.4 Hypotension

The reported incidence of hypotension after plasmapheresis is 1.7%. A variety of conditions predispose patients to hypotension during plasmapheresis (Table 16.2). Patients may experience symptoms of hypotension such as vertigo, lightheadedness, nausea, extreme sweating, and

Table 16.2 Main complications of TPE in sepsis

Complication	Recommendations
Citrate toxicity Citrate-induced hypocalcemia Citrate-induced metabolic alkalosis	Cardiac monitoring and intraprocedural evaluation of Ca^{2+} levels, slowing citrate infusion rate, administration of prophylactic IV calcium Hemodialysis to remove excess bicarbonate
Anaphylactic/allergic reactions Fever, rigors, urticaria, wheezing, bronchospasm, hypotension, cardiopulmonary collapse, hives, urticaria, pruritus Ethylene oxide toxicity with burning sensation in the eyes, tearing, and periorbital edema Angiotensin-converting enzyme inhibitor (ACEi)-associated reaction and flushing due to accumulation of bradykinins	Follow the patient blood management guidelines for blood product use Obtain plasma from IgA-deficient donors if the patient is IgA-deficient Antihistamines, glucocorticoids, epinephrine Clearing the tubes, adequate priming of the filter Discontinue ACEi 24–48 h before procedure
Transfusion-related acute lung injury (TRALI)	Supportive treatment Intubation if required Plasmapheresis may help remove donor antibodies
Hypotension Hypovolemia, vasovagal, hypo-oncotic fluids, anaphylaxis, hypocalcemia, arrhythmia, TRALI, hemorrhage, ACEi-related, pulmonary embolism, cardiovascular collapse Membrane bioincompatibility with plasma membrane separation	Optimize volume status prior to apheresis Discontinue ACEi 24–48 h before procedure Stop the procedure Evaluate and manage the underlying cause Place the patient in Trendelenburg position IV fluid resuscitation Vasopressors Change the membrane or do not continue with plasmapheresis
Decreased exposure of medications Removal of antimicrobials with low volume of distribution and high protein binding	Therapeutic drug monitoring for ß-lactams, aminoglycosides, linezolid, teicoplanin, vancomycin, and voriconazole Administer monoclonal antibodies, total parenteral nutrition, IV immunoglobulins after plasmapheresis
Problems of vascular access Infection, pain, nerve damage, thrombosis, perforation, dissecting hematomas, air embolism, arteriovenous (AV) fistulas	Follow standards of practice for insertion and care of catheters Confirm placement radiologically prior to apheresis procedures Evaluate platelet count and coagulation parameters

tachycardia. In cases of documented hypotension, the procedure should be stopped, the patient should be placed in the Trendelenburg position, and saline or colloid bolus should be administered. Since patients in sepsis may already be confused or comatose, they may not be able to report their symptoms. Additionally, the underlying MOF and low intravascular volume before the procedure pose significant challenges in septic patients. For this reason, it is important to closely monitor blood pressure continuously during apheresis. It is recommended to optimize volume status prior to apheresis with IV fluids and to start vasopressors in a timely manner. If needed, increasing hemoglobin with red blood cell units is also recommended.

Transfusion reactions, angiotensin-converting enzyme inhibitor (ACEi)-associated reactions, and membrane incompatibility with plasma membrane separation are some rarer causes of hypotension. Since sepsis develops relatively acutely and it is important to start TPE early after diagnosis, for patients on ACEis, it may not be possible to stop the medication 24–48 h before procedure. However, it is better not to use any antihypertensive medication after the diagnosis of sepsis, as these patients are already prone to hypotension, and the possibility of bradykinin reactions should be considered. If plasma membrane separation is suspected as the cause of hypotension, it is recommended to change the membrane or switch to a therapy other than apheresis [27].

16.3.5 Impact of TPE on Medication Exposure in Patients with Sepsis

Sepsis-associated homeostatic alterations can affect drug distribution and clearance, raising concerns about the risk of suboptimal antimicrobial exposure in critically ill patients with sepsis. Administration of extracorporeal therapies introduces an additional pharmacokinetic (PK) compartment that may further influence antimicrobial exposure by altering the volume of distribution (Vd) and clearance of these drugs. Moreover, antimicrobials may be cleared through absorption or transmembrane removal during extracorporeal therapies.

During TPE, the removal of antimicrobials with low Vd and high protein binding (>80%) may be enhanced. A recent literature review found that ß-lactams (cefazolin and ceftriaxone) and liposomal amphotericin B are significantly removed via TPE. This may lead to treatment failure and the emergence of multidrug-resistant pathogens [30, 31]. For this reason, the 2021 Surviving Sepsis Campaign guidelines recommended administering empiric antimicrobials immediately after sepsis recognition and optimizing dosing strategies based on PK and pharmacodynamic principles to maximize pathogen killing and prevent drug toxicity [32].

In comparison with standard dosing regimens, several strategies have been proposed to improve antimicrobial exposure. Among them, the therapeutic drug monitoring (TDM) appears to be a promising tool, enabling real-time antimicrobial PK measurements at the bedside. This allows clinicians to adjust the antimicrobial dose according to the patient's evolving clinical condition and pathogen susceptibility. Chromatography-based TDM is a new approach that can be used in routine clinical practice. The recently published guidelines recommend TDM for dose titration of ß-lactams, aminoglycosides, linezolid, teicoplanin, vancomycin, and voriconazole [33]. Monoclonal antibodies, total parenteral nutrition, IV immunoglobulin, and some medications, such as cyclophosphamide, are most likely removed by plasma exchange and are recommended to be administered after TPE.

16.4 Conclusion

TPE using healthy donor plasma has the potential to improve survival in sepsis. Clinical studies have not reported major safety issues, except for cases of transient hypotension, citrate-induced hypocalcemia, allergic reactions to FFP, and vascular access problems. In critically ill patients, symptoms may be obscured, and adverse reactions to plasmapheresis may be underreported. There are, however, challenging safety issues regarding the use of TPE in patients with sepsis, such as hemodynamic instability and the presence of MOF, which may exacerbate adverse effects. Additionally, there is a risk of inadequate medication exposure due to removal via plasma exchange. There appears to be an unmet need for large RCTs to confirm the effect of TPE on survival and to further explore the complications of TPE in patients with sepsis.

References

1. Singer M, Deutschman CS, Seymour CW, Shankar-Hari M, Annane D, Bauer M, et al. The third international consensus definitions for sepsis and septic shock (Sepsis-3). JAMA. 2016;315(8):801–10. https://doi.org/10.1001/jama.2016.0287.
2. Rhodes A, Evans LE, Alhazzani W, Levy MM, Antonelli M, Ferrer R, et al. Surviving sepsis campaign: international guidelines for management of sepsis and septic shock: 2016. Intensive Care Med. 2017;43(3):304–77. https://doi.org/10.1007/s00134-017-4683-6.
3. Klinkmann G, Altrichter J, Reuter DA, Mitzner S. Therapeutic apheresis in sepsis. Ther Apher Dial. 2022;26(Suppl 1):64–72. https://doi.org/10.1111/1744-9987.13815.
4. Rimmer E. Therapeutic plasma exchange in septic shock: a pilot study. Transfus Apher Sci. 2020;59(6):102998. https://doi.org/10.1016/j.transci.2020.102998.
5. Connelly-Smith L, Alquist CR, Aqui NA, Hofmann JC, Klingel R, Onwuemene OA, et al. Guidelines on the use of therapeutic apheresis in clinical practice—evidence-based approach from the writing Committee of the American Society for apheresis: the ninth spe-

cial issue. J Clin Apher. 2023;38(2):77–278. https://doi.org/10.1002/jca.22043.

6. Stahl K, Wendel-Garcia PD, Bode C, David S. Unraveling the secret of re-balancing homeostasis in sepsis: a critical view on extracorporeal blood purification modalities. Intensive Care Med. 2022;48(1):130–2. https://doi.org/10.1007/s00134-021-06560-6.
7. Rimmer E, Houston BL, Kumar A, Abou-Setta AM, Friesen C, Marshall JC, et al. The efficacy and safety of plasma exchange in patients with sepsis and septic shock: a systematic review and meta-analysis. Crit Care. 2014;18(6):699. https://doi.org/10.1186/s13054-014-0699-2.
8. Reeves JH, Butt WW, Shann F, Layton JE, Stewart A, Waring PM, Presneill JJ. Continuous plasma filtration in sepsis syndrome. Plasma filtration in Sepsis Study Group. Crit Care Med. 1999;27(10):2096–104. https://doi.org/10.1097/00003246-199910000-00003.
9. Busund R, Koukline V, Utrobin U, Nedashkovsky E. Plasmapheresis in severe sepsis and septic shock: a prospective, randomised, controlled trial. Intensive Care Med. 2002;28(10):1434–9. https://doi.org/10.1007/s00134-002-1410-7.
10. Nguyen TC, Han YY, Kiss JE, Hall MW, Hassett AC, Jaffe R, et al. Intensive plasma exchange increases a disintegrin and metalloprotease with thrombospondin motifs-13 activity and reverses organ dysfunction in children with thrombocytopenia-associated multiple organ failure. Crit Care Med. 2008;36(10):2878–87. https://doi.org/10.1097/ccm.0b013e318186aa49.
11. Long EJ, Taylor A, Delzoppo C, Shann F, Pearson G, Buckley D, Butt W. A randomised controlled trial of plasma filtration in severe paediatric sepsis. Crit Care Resusc. 2013;15(3):198–204. Erratum in: Crit Care Resusc. 2016 Dec;18(4):289.
12. Keith PD, Wells AH, Hodges J, Fast SH, Adams A, Scott LK. The therapeutic efficacy of adjunct therapeutic plasma exchange for septic shock with multiple organ failure: a single-center experience. Crit Care. 2020;24(1):518. https://doi.org/10.1186/s13054-020-03241-6.
13. Khamis F, Al-Zakwani I, Al Hashmi S, Al Dowaiki S, Al Bahrani M, Pandak N, et al. Therapeutic plasma exchange in adults with severe COVID-19 infection. Int J Infect Dis. 2020;99:214–8. https://doi.org/10.1016/j.ijid.2020.06.064.
14. Sevketoglu E, Yildizdas D, Horoz OO, Kihtir HS, Kendirli T, Bayraktar S, Carcillo JA. Use of therapeutic plasma exchange in children with thrombocytopenia-associated multiple organ failure in the Turkish thrombocytopenia-associated multiple organ failure network. Pediatr Crit Care Med. 2014;15(8):e354–9. https://doi.org/10.1097/PCC.0000000000000227.
15. Fortenberry JD, Nguyen T, Grunwell JR, Aneja RK, Wheeler D, Hall M, et al. Therapeutic plasma exchange in children with thrombocytopenia-associated multiple organ failure: the thrombocytopenia-associated multiple organ failure network prospective experience. Crit Care Med. 2019;47(3):e173–81. https://doi.org/10.1097/CCM.0000000000003559.
16. Aygün F, Varol F, Durak C, Talip Petmezci M, Kacar A, Dursun H, et al. Evaluation of continuous renal replacement therapy and therapeutic plasma exchange, in severe sepsis or septic shock in critically ill children. Medicina (Kaunas). 2019;55(7):350. https://doi.org/10.3390/medicina55070350.
17. Luo X, Li X, Lai X, Ke L, Zhou J, Liu M, et al. Therapeutic plasma exchange in patients with sepsis: secondary analysis of a cluster-randomized controlled trial. J Clin Apher. 2023;38(1):55–62. https://doi.org/10.1002/jca.22027.
18. David S, Bode C, Putensen C, Welte T, Stahl K, EXCHANGE study group. Adjuvant therapeutic plasma exchange in septic shock. Intensive Care Med. 2021;47(3):352–4. https://doi.org/10.1007/s00134-020-06339-1.
19. Stahl K, Wand P, Seeliger B, Wendel-Garcia PD, Schmidt JJ, Schmidt BMW, et al. Clinical and biochemical endpoints and predictors of response to plasma exchange in septic shock: results from a randomized controlled trial. Crit Care. 2022;26(1):134. https://doi.org/10.1186/s13054-022-04003-2.
20. Putzu A, Schorer R, Lopez-Delgado JC, Cassina T, Landoni G. Blood purification and mortality in sepsis and septic shock: a systematic review and meta-analysis of randomized trials. Anesthesiology. 2019;131(3):580–93. https://doi.org/10.1097/ALN.0000000000002820.
21. Mokrzycki MH, Kaplan AA. Therapeutic plasma exchange: complications and management. Am J Kidney Dis. 1994;23(6):817–27. https://doi.org/10.1016/s0272-6386(12)80135-1.
22. Mörtzell Henriksson M, Newman E, Witt V, Derfler K, Leitner G, Eloot S, et al. Adverse events in apheresis: an update of the WAA registry data. Transfus Apher Sci. 2016;54(1):2–15. https://doi.org/10.1016/j.transci.2016.01.003.
23. Reeves HM, Winters JL. The mechanisms of action of plasma exchange. Br J Haematol. 2014;164(3):342–51. https://doi.org/10.1111/bjh.12629.
24. Aydin K, Korkmaz S, Erkurt MA, Sarici A, Ekinci O, Baysal NA, et al. Apheresis in patients with sepsis: a multicenter retrospective study. Transfus Apher Sci. 2021;60(5):103239. https://doi.org/10.1016/j.transci.2021.103239.
25. Kaplan AA, Halley SE. Plasma exchange with a rotating filter. Kidney Int. 1990;38(1):160–6. https://doi.org/10.1038/ki.1990.181.
26. Pearl RG, Rosenthal MH. Metabolic alkalosis due to plasmapheresis. Am J Med. 1985;79(3):391–3. https://doi.org/10.1016/0002-9343(85)90320-1.
27. Apter AJ, Kaplan AA. An approach to immunologic reactions associated with plasma exchange. J Allergy Clin Immunol. 1992;90(1):119–24. https://doi.org/10.1016/s0091-6749(06)80018-7.

28. Kaplan A. Complications of apheresis. Semin Dial. 2012;25(2):152–8. https://doi.org/10.1111/j.1525-139X.2011.01026.x.
29. Popovsky MA. Transfusion-related acute lung injury: incidence, pathogenesis and the role of multicomponent apheresis in its prevention. Transfus Med Hemother. 2008;35(2):76–9. https://doi.org/10.1159/000117811.
30. Cuttuli SL, Cascarano L, Lazzaro P, Tanzarella ES, Pintaudi G, Grieco DL, et al. Antimicrobial exposure in critically ill patients with sepsis-associated multi-organ dysfunction requiring extracorporeal organ support: a narrative review. Microorganisms. 2023;11(2):473. https://doi.org/10.3390/microorganisms11020473.
31. Bauer PR, Ostermann M, Russell L, Robba C, David S, Ferreyro BL, et al. Plasma exchange in the intensive care unit: a narrative review. Intensive Care Med. 2022;48(10):1382–96. https://doi.org/10.1007/s00134-022-06793-z.
32. Evans L, Rhodes A, Alhazzani W, Antonelli M, Coopersmith CM, French C, et al. Executive summary: surviving sepsis campaign: international guidelines for the Management of Sepsis and Septic Shock 2021. Crit Care Med. 2021;49(11):1974–82. https://doi.org/10.1097/CCM.0000000000005357. Erratum in: Crit Care Med. 2022 Apr 1;50(4):e413–e414.
33. Abdul-Aziz MH, Alffenaar JC, Bassetti M, Bracht H, Dimopoulos G, Marriott D, et al. Antimicrobial therapeutic drug monitoring in critically ill adult patients: a Position Paper. Intensive Care Med. 2020;46(6):1127–53. https://doi.org/10.1007/s00134-020-06050-1.

Part V

Problems During Red Cell Exchange Procedure

17 Managing Acute Complications of Sickle Cell Disease

Duygu Nurdan Avcı

17.1 Background

Sickle cell anaemia (SCA) is an autosomal recessive haemoglobinopathy caused by a single gene mutation. In this condition, hydrophilic glutamic acid is replaced by hydrophobic valine at the sixth amino acid position of the beta chain, leading to the formation of haemoglobin S (HbS). The HbS mutation causes the β1 and β2 chains in the haemoglobin molecule to bind to oxygen, forming a hydrophobic motif. This polymerisation disrupts erythrocyte structure and elasticity and triggers cellular dehydration [1]. The degree of polymerisation depends on the duration of deoxygenation and the intracellular levels of HbS and HbF [2]. HbS becomes inflexible and polymerises in the deoxygenated state, deforming the erythrocyte membrane. As a result, erythrocytes assume a sickle-like shape. Sickled erythrocytes, along with endothelial, leukocyte, and platelet activation, reduced plasma vasodilator nitric oxide, and increased vascular tone, lead to vaso-occlusion. The resulting tissue and organ ischaemia causes both acute and chronic complications in affected patients. Acute complications in SCA can lead to comorbidity and mortality if not managed correctly. Erythrocyte exchange (RBC exchange) is a crucial treatment option for managing these complications.

D. N. Avcı (✉)
Hematology Department, Baskent University School of Medicine, Ankara, Turkey

The primary aim of RBC exchange is to remove sickled erythrocytes using an apheresis device and to infuse erythrocyte suspensions prepared from healthy donors into the patient. Many current apheresis devices are equipped with automated technology. However, certain disadvantages remain, including the need for personnel experienced in apheresis procedures and blood exchange, the frequent requirement of a central venous catheter, and the risk of complications associated with blood product use. This chapter will discuss acute complications of SCA, treatments for these complications, and indications for RBC exchange.

17.2 Acute Complications

17.2.1 Acute Vaso-occlusive Crisis, Painful Episodes

The most prominent clinical manifestation of SCA is acute vaso-occlusive, painful episodes. These episodes are the primary reason for seeking emergency treatment and hospitalisation. Occlusion of the microvascular system leads to localised pain and inflammation. Although no specific cause is usually identified, factors such as infection, fever, acidosis, hypoxia, dehydration, sleep apnoea, and exposure to excessive heat or cold can trigger crises. The most common sites of pain are bones and the abdomen, which

I. Kozanoglu (ed.), *Problem Solving in Apheresis Medicine*,
https://doi.org/10.1007/978-3-031-74081-7_17

may present as symmetrical, asymmetrical, or migrating pain. Since dehydration is a significant triggering factor, fluid therapy is recommended regardless of the patient's hydration status [2]. For mild pain, the first-line treatment involves "non-opioid and adjunctive therapies". Second-line treatment includes "weak opioid, non-opioid, and adjunctive therapies", while third-line treatment for severe pain involves "strong opioid, non-opioid, and adjunctive therapies" [3]. In prolonged painful crises, simple erythrocyte transfusion or erythrocyte exchange transfusion may be administered to reduce HbS levels.

17.2.2 Acute Chest Syndrome

Acute chest syndrome (ACS) is the leading cause of mortality and the second most common reason for hospitalisation in SCA. The clinical findings of ACS include chest pain, cough, fever, hypoxia, respiratory distress, and new lesions on chest X-ray [4, 5]. All these findings do not need to be present simultaneously to make a diagnosis, and chest X-ray lesions typically appear 24–48 h after clinical symptoms. ACS is three times more common in children but tends to have a more severe course in adults. Fifty percent of patients present to the hospital with an acute pain crisis [6]. Causes include bacterial and viral infections, pulmonary embolism, and fat embolism. ACS often presents with fever, dyspnoea, and decreased oxygen saturation, usually associated with pneumonia. Infection may be the underlying cause of ACS or a complication of it. Chest pain is common and may be pleuritic due to pulmonary infarction. Radiological findings typically show multilobar infiltration. While the exact pathophysiology and causes of ACS remain unclear, treatment includes broad-spectrum antibiotics targeting infection and vaso-occlusion, as well as transfusion therapy. Antibiotic coverage should include S. pneumoniae (considering local resistance) and atypical pneumonia agents like C. pneumoniae and M. pneumoniae. All patients should receive thrombosis prophylaxis with low molecular weight heparin and nasal oxygen inhalation at 2–4 L/min. Simple transfusion or erythrocyte exchange should be performed to increase oxygenation by lowering HbS levels. Erythrocyte exchange is recommended for patients with severe symptoms [7].

17.2.3 Acute Stroke

Strokes in patients with SCA can present as ischaemic, haemorrhagic, and transient ischaemic attacks. Silent infarcts, which appear as areas of increased T2 signal abnormality, do not result in neurological deficits. Stasis and ischaemia caused by sickle cells contribute to stroke formation. Following a stroke, the HbS percentage is targeted to be reduced below 30% through simple transfusion or erythrocyte exchange. Studies indicate that patients who undergo erythrocyte exchange as the initial treatment show better response [8]. If these patients are only monitored clinically after the acute phase, the risk of recurrent stroke is 70% [9]. To prevent this, a chronic transfusion or regular erythrocyte exchange programme every 3 months should be initiated to maintain HbS levels below 30% [10]. Primary and secondary prevention of stroke is achieved through chronic transfusion. Bone marrow transplantation is an important alternative for patients at high risk of stroke who have compatible donors [11].

17.2.4 Priapism

Priapism is a painful erection condition that affects 30% of male patients with SCA and results from ischaemia. It is characterized by a rigid, painful corpus cavernosum following decreased or interrupted cavernosal blood flow. Treatment of priapism in adults and children includes aspiration of blood from the corpus cavernosum, followed by intracavernosal injection of sympathomimetics (1–3 mL, 100–500 μg/mL phenylephrine). Intravenous hydration and exchange transfusion may also be used, but aspiration and beta sympathomimetic treatment should not be delayed [12]. In recurrent cases, chronic transfusion therapy and surgical interventions such as "shunt" procedures may be required.

17.2.5 Acute Haematological Incidents

(a) Aplastic crisis: This condition is most commonly seen following Parvovirus B19 infection, which targets erythrocyte precursors. It presents as transient erythrocyte aplasia and usually resolves on its own with supportive care.
(b) Splenic sequestration: Signs of splenic sequestration include sudden splenic enlargement, a decrease in haemoglobin of 2 g or more, and increased erythropoiesis. Thrombocytopenia may also occur. This condition is usually observed in children aged 3 months to 5 years [13]. It can result in hypovolaemic shock and even death. Treatment involves careful blood transfusion. Since blood trapped in the spleen may re-enter the circulation after transfusion, the target haemoglobin level should remain below 8 g/dL. Splenic sequestration recurs in about half of cases, and long-term treatment options include chronic transfusion or splenectomy [14].

17.2.6 Hepatobiliary Complications

Cholelithiasis occurs as a result of chronic haemolysis and increased bilirubin production. The treatment is cholecystectomy, with laparoscopic methods being more commonly preferred today. Sickle cell collagenopathy develops due to hypoxia and dilation of the duct caused by sickling in the end arteries of the biliary arterial tree. Sickle cell hepatopathy results from intrahepatic sickling of erythrocytes. Treatment is limited to erythrocyte exchange and liver transplantation, and there is no conclusive evidence supporting these approaches. Acute hepatic crisis is of unknown aetiology, caused by decreased blood flow in the hepatic sinusoids. It presents with right upper quadrant pain, subfebrile fever, and vomiting, usually accompanied by mild to moderate elevation of liver enzymes and bilirubin. Treatment is conservative, and the condition usually resolves spontaneously. In severe cases, simple or partial erythrocyte exchange may be required. Hepatic sequestration crises are characterized by acute enlargement and pooling of blood in the liver. Reticulocyte and bilirubin levels increase, along with a rapid decrease in haemoglobin and haematocrit. Hydration and erythrocyte transfusion are recommended for treatment. Acute intrahepatic cholestasis develops due to obstruction of hepatic sinusoids, stasis, and ballooning of hepatocytes. Intrahepatic sickling and cholestasis can be reversed with early diagnosis, erythrocyte exchange, fresh frozen plasma, platelet transfusion, and plasmapheresis. Hepatitis B and C may occur as a result of transfusions in these patients [15].

17.2.7 Infections

The main reasons for increased susceptibility to infections are impaired spleen function, but defects in complement activation, micronutrient deficiencies, tissue ischaemia, and inflammation also contribute. Streptococcus pneumoniae, Haemophilus influenza type b, and non-typhoid *Salmonella* species are significant infections seen in these patients. Other common infectious agents include Mycoplasma, Klebsiella pneumoniae, and Yersinia enterocolitica, which cause pneumonia and ACS. Penicillin prophylaxis is recommended for these patients during the first months of life. Patients with SCA should be vaccinated against Streptococcus pneumoniae, Neisseria meningitidis, and Haemophilus influenza [16].

17.3 Treatments

The general approach in the management of acute complications of SCA includes controlling infections, transfusion therapies, preventing crisis recurrence, agents that increase HbF production, and chelation therapies.

Table 17.1 Indications for transfusion in patients with SCA

	Simple transfusion	Chronic simple transfusion	RBC exchange
Recommended cases	Symptomatic anaemia Acute neurological findings Acute chest syndrome Acute multiple organ failure pre-surgery Acute splenic or hepatic sequestration Sepsis and meningitis	Stroke prevention Recurrent acute chest syndrome or prevention of multiple organ failure Those with renal failure and anaemia who do not respond to erythropoietin treatment Pulmonary hypertension or chronic hypoxia Chronic heart failure	Acute neurological findings Severe acute chest syndrome Acute multiple organ failure Avoiding hypervolemia and hyperviscosity before surgery Reducing iron accumulation
Controversial cases		Recurrent episodes of severe painful seizures Non-healing leg ulcers recurrent priapism	Acute priapism

This table has been modified from reference number [17]

17.3.1 Transfusion Therapies

Transfusion therapy is used for both the treatment and prevention of disease-related complications. It can be performed as simple transfusion, chronic simple transfusion, partial transfusion, or exchange transfusion. Generally, it is recommended not to transfuse patients unless the haemoglobin level falls below 7 g/dL, and not to increase the haemoglobin level above 10 g/dL to avoid hyperviscosity. Erythrocyte subgroups should be checked in all newly diagnosed patients with SCA. Filtered products from donors who are not sickle cell carriers, and are at most 5 days old, should be used. Products with appropriate CcEe, Kell, and Kidd (JkA, JkB) antigens should be selected whenever possible [17]. Table 17.1 shows the transfusion recommendations for patients with SCA [17].

17.3.2 Exchange Transfusion

In acute complications of SCA, the decision to use RBC transfusion or manual/automated erythrocyte (RBC) exchange depends on the patient's clinical condition, as well as the centre's apheresis services and ability to obtain blood products quickly. RBC exchange offers more efficient and rapid removal of HbS without causing volume overload, maintaining the patient's isovolaemia. Complications of RBC exchange include central venous catheter thrombosis, bleeding, and hyperhaemolysis, a rare haemolytic reaction [18].

17.4 Erythrocyte Exchange Indications

The American Society for Apheresis (ASFA) classifies indications for therapeutic apheresis into four categories based on evidence [19]. Disorders for which apheresis therapy is recognised as first- or second-line treatment are included in Categories I and II, respectively. Category III includes disorders where the optimal role for apheresis treatment has not been established, and individualised treatment is required. Category IV includes disorders for which published evidence indicates or at least suggests that apheresis is ineffective or harmful. RBC exchange indications for SCA are divided into two subgroups: acute/non-acute and chronic [19, 20]. Table 17.2 shows the indications for RBC exchange transfusion in acute complications of SCA according to the 2019 ASFA Guidelines.

17.5 Technique and Mechanism of Action

RBC exchange requires special equipment and trained personnel. The primary aim of therapeutic RBC exchange is to remove abnormal (sickled) and excess red blood cells, replacing them with healthy donor red cells. Apheresis practitioners should calculate the target haematocrit (HCT) and the desired FCR (fraction of the patient's RBCs) remaining at the end of the

Table 17.2 The indications for RBC exchange transfusion in acute complications of SCA

Indication	Procedure	Recommendation	Category
Acute stroke	RBC exchange	Grade IC	I
Acute chest syndrome (severe)	RBC exchange	Grade IC	II
Other complications[a]	RBC exchange	Grade IIC	III

[a] Includes priapism, multiorgan failure, splenic/hepatic sequestration, and intrahepatic cholestasis

procedure, or the target volume to be replaced. In general, the aim is to reduce end-of-procedure HbS to <30%. The final HCT should be 30 ± 3% to avoid clinically significant hyperviscosity [19].

17.5.1 Blood Product Selection and Specifications

Rapid communication with blood banks or transfusion centres is important to meet the need for blood products in the management of acute complications. It is preferred that the erythrocyte suspensions (ES) planned for use are fresh (<7 days), leukocyte-free, sickling test negative, irradiated, and subgroup appropriate (C, E, and Kell) [21, 22].

17.5.2 Erythrocyte Exchange Process Technical Information

The primary aim of RBC exchange is to remove abnormal (sickled) and excess red blood cells and replace them with healthy donor red cells. Most current apheresis devices are fully automated and equipped with advanced microprocessor-based computer programmes [20, 22]. An apheresis device with a special software programme designed specifically for RBC exchange should be preferred [21]. When the patient's height, gender, body weight, and current HCT value are entered into the device, it can calculate the total blood volume and erythrocyte volume of the patient [23, 24]. In addition, important data, such as the target HCT level at the end of the procedure, the HCT of the replacement fluids, and the FCR, must be entered into the device. Based on this information, the apheresis device can calculate the volume of replacement fluid required to achieve the target HbS and HCT values.

In a standard RBC exchange procedure, when the total erythrocyte volume of the patient is replaced once, approximately 65% of the original circulating erythrocytes are removed (FCR, 35%). In other words, in a patient with a pre-procedure HbS level of 100%, if the erythrocyte volume is replaced once, the post-procedure HbS concentration decreases to approximately 35%. In a patient with twice the total erythrocyte mass, approximately 90% of the circulating erythrocytes are removed (FCR, 10%) [23, 24]. Citrate dextrose solution-A (ACD-A) or citrate phosphate dextrose should be used as the anticoagulant during the procedure. Increasing the inlet/ACD-A ratio is the correct approach to prevent citrate-related complications [23].

17.5.3 Vascular Route Selection

To perform apheresis, a suitable vascular access is required to ensure continuous blood flow at an adequate rate. However, peripheral venous access is not always sufficient, and many patients require a central venous catheter [25]. Another, less commonly used, minimally invasive method is the insertion of an intravenous catheter inserted into the peripheral radial artery for blood supply and peripheral venous return. Most patients require central venous catheterisation. This method can lead to complications such as catheter-related haematoma, infection, and thrombosis [26]. The most preferred method is subclavian catheter placement [25, 27]. Femoral catheter applications have a higher risk of complications. Central catheters should be removed as soon as possible due to the associated risks. Prolonged catheterisation increases the risk of thrombosis and infection [26].

17.5.4 Calculations

The patient's gender, height, weight, pre-procedure HbS, targeted end-of-procedure HbS, FCR, and the HCT value of the erythrocyte suspension used form the basis of the calculations required for the procedure. FCR is the percentage of the patient's original erythrocytes targeted to remain in circulation at the end of the procedure. It is calculated by the ratio of the patient's end-of-procedure targeted HbS value to the current HbS value. Total blood volume, total erythrocyte volume, FCR, and replacement volume are used to calculate the amount of erythrocyte suspension units to be used. Regardless of the target HCT and HbS in the exchange process, isovolaemic balance is maintained in the patient [23, 24].

17.6 Complications

The RBC exchange procedure is generally well tolerated. However, complications such as low blood pressure, dizziness, hypocalcaemia, nausea, and vomiting may rarely occur during the procedure. Hypocalcaemic reactions due to citrate used for anticoagulation may also occur. In patients with SCA, it may be necessary to use less citrate to avoid exposing them to citrate toxicity. To mitigate this, it is recommended to increase the inlet/ACD-A ratio [20, 28].

In addition to complications related to vascular access, particularly central venous catheter insertion, many complications related to the use of blood products can occur in these patients [26, 29]. The most common of these are iron accumulation, acute or delayed haemolytic transfusion reactions, transmission of transfusion-related infections, and allergic reactions [29].

17.7 Findings

Life-threatening acute complications, such as SCA-associated cerebral stroke, ACS, and multi-organ failure following acute vaso-occlusive crisis, have a poor prognosis if left untreated. The main goal of treatment is to increase tissue oxygenation. The most effective method to remove deoxygenated HbS is erythrocyte exchange. It is preferred over simple transfusion because it prevents iron accumulation, reduces the HbS level to below 30% at the end of the procedure, and avoids hyperviscosity [28]. To minimize procedure-related complications, it is important to closely monitor patients, use Rh- and subgroup-compatible blood, ensure continuity of staff in the apheresis unit, regularly train apheresis users, and perform periodic maintenance on apheresis devices [30].

References

1. Azar S, Wong TE. Sickle cell disease: a brief update. Med Clin North Am. 2017;101(2):375–93.
2. Uwaezuoke SN, Ayuk AC, Ndu IK, Eneh CI, Mbanefo NR, Ezenwosu OU. Vaso occlusive crisis in sickle cell disease: current paradigm on pain management. J Pain Res. 2018;11:3141–50.
3. Bunn HF. Pathogenesis and treatment of sickle cell disease. N Engl J Med. 1997;337:762–9.
4. Vichinsky EP, Styles LA, Colangelo LH, Wright EC, Castro O, Nickerson B. Acute chest syndrome in sickle cell disease: clinical presentation and course. Blood. 1997;89:1787–92.
5. Vichinsky EP, Neumayr LD, Earles AN, et al. Causes and outcomes of the acute chest syndrome in sickle cell disease. New Engl J Med. 2000;342:1855–65.
6. Bellet PS, Kalinyak KA, Shukla R, Gelfand MJ, Rucknagel DL. Incentive spirometry to prevent acute pulmonary complications in sickle cell diseases. New Engl J Med. 1995;333:699–703.
7. Novelli EM, Gladwin MT. Crises in sickle cell disease. Chest. 2016;149(4):1082–93.
8. Hulbert ML, Scothorn DJ, Panepinto JA, et al. Exchange blood transfusion compared with simple transfusion for first overt stroke is associated with a lower risk of subsequent stroke: a retrospective cohort study of 137 children with sickle cell anemia. J Pediatr. 2006;149(5):710–2.
9. Powars D, Wilson B, Imbus C, Pegelow C, Allen J. The natural history of stroke in sickle cell disease. Am J Med. 1978;65:461–71.
10. Aygun B, McMurray MA, Schultz WH, et al. Chronic transfusion practice for children with sickle cell anemia and stroke. Br J Haematol. 2009;145:524–8.
11. Webb J, Kwiatkowski JL. Stroke in patients with sickle cell disease. Expert Rev Hematol. 2013;6(3):301–16.
12. Anele UA, Morrison BF, Burnett AL. Molecular pathophysiology of priapism: emerging targets. Curr Drug Targets. 2015;16(5):474–83.
13. Topley JM, Rogers DW, Stevens MCG, Serjeant GR. Acute splenic sequestration and hypersplenism in

the first five years in homozygous sickle cell disease. Arch Dis Childhood. 1981;56:765–9.
14. Kinney TR, Ware RE, Schultz WH, Filston HC. Long-term management of splenic sequestration in children with sickle cell disease. J Pediatr. 1990;117:194–9.
15. Issa H, Al-Salem AH. Hepatobiliary manifestations of sickle cell anemia. Gastroenterology Res. 2010;3(1):1–8.
16. Sobota A, Sabharwal V, Fonebi G, Steinberg M. Howwe prevent and manage infection in sickle cell disease. Br J Haematol. 2015;170(6):757–67.
17. Turkish Hematology Society guide. 1st ed. Galenos Ankara; 2022.
18. Padmanabhan A, Connelly-Smith L, Aqui N, Balogun RA, Klingel R, Meyer E, Pham HP, Schneiderman J, Witt V, Wu Y, Zantek ND, Dunbar NM, Schwartz GEJ. Guidelines on the use of therapeutic apheresis in clinical practice—evidence-based approach from the writing Committee of the American Society for apheresis: the eighth special issue. J Clin Apher. 2019;34(3):171–354.
19. Biller E, Zhao Y, Berg M, et al. Red blood cell exchange in patients with sickle cell disease-indications and management: a review and consensus report by the therapeutic apheresis subsection of the AABB. Transfusion. 2018;58:1965–72.
20. Kozanoglu I, Ozdogu H. Use of red blood cell exchange for treating acute complications of sickle cell disease. Transfus Apher Sci. 2018;57:23–6.
21. Kozanoglu I, Boga C, Ozdogu H, Sezgin N, Kizilkilic E, Kural M. Automated red cell exchange procedures in patients with sickle cell disease. Transfus Apher Sci. 2007;36:305–12.
22. Shaz B, Schwartz J. Clinical application. In: Linz W, Crookston K, Duvall D, Kong B, Jones H, Sabin S, editors. Principles of apheresis technology. 4th ed. Vancouver: American Society for Apheresis; 2010. p. 27–35.
23. Tekin Turhan F, Karadamar M, Güvenç B. Terapötik Eritrosit değişiminde endikasyona özel işlem yaklaşımları. Turkiye Klinikleri J Hematol-Special Topics. 2015;8(1):9–26.
24. McLeod BC. Red cell exchange. In: Crookston K, Eder A, King K, Kiss J, Sarode R, Winters JL, editors. Therapeutic apheresis: a physician's handbook. 1st ed. Bethesda: AABB; 2005. p. 115–33.
25. Kalantari K. The choice of vascular access for therapeutic apheresis. J Clin Apher. 2012;27:153–9.
26. Yeral M, Boga C, Oguzkurt L, Asma S, Kasar M, Kozanoglu I. Short-term central venous catheter complications in patients with sickle cell disease who undergo apheresis. J Thromb Thrombolysis. 2014;37(2):97–101.
27. Jeng MR, Feusner J, Skibola C, Vichinsky E. Central venous catheter complications in sickle cell disease. Am J Hematol. 2002;69:103–8.
28. Davis BA, Allard S, Porter JB, et al. Guidelines on red cell transfusion in sickle cell disease. Part II: indications for transfusion. Br J Haematol. 2017;176:192–209.
29. Chou ST. Transfusion therapy for sickle cell disease: a balancing act. Hematol Am Soc Hematol Educ Program. 2013;2013:439–46.
30. Tsitsikas DA, Orebayo F, Agapidou A, et al. Distinct patterns of response to transfusion therapy for different chronic complications of sickle cell disease: a useful insight. Transfus Apher Sci. 2017;56:713–6.

Part VI

Risk Evaluation in Double Filtration Plasmapheresis

Basic Principles of Double-Filtration Plasmapheresis

18

Ilknur Kozanoğlu

18.1 Background

Therapeutic plasma exchange (TPE) is the process of removing large volumes of patient plasma using an apheresis device and replacing it with appropriate replacement fluids. TPE is typically used to remove plasma that may contain harmful substances associated with a disease, such as monoclonal immunoglobulins (paraproteins), autoantibodies, immunocomplexes, lipids, and toxins [1–3]. The removal of immunocomplexes from plasma through plasma exchange is recognized as useful adjunctive therapy when other treatment approaches are inadequate. Monoclonal immunoglobulins increase plasma viscosity and may cause cardiovascular, respiratory, and central nervous system symptoms, renal failure, acute tubular necrosis in severe cases, and bleeding problems. Correcting these life-threatening organ failures due to hyperviscosity in a short time is possible with TPE [1–4]. Various poisons, drugs, and toxins can be removed from the patient's plasma by plasma exchange [5]. Some toxic substances cannot cross the dialysis membrane due to their molecular size or their binding to plasma proteins. Various fluids are used to replace the plasma removed during the TPE procedure [1–6]. The purpose of replacement fluids is to maintain intravascular volume, as well as to restore important plasma proteins, maintain colloid osmotic pressure, balance electrolytes, and replace trace elements. The fluid to be used is usually determined by the patient's albumin level, coagulation profile, and underlying disease. The first fluid used is 5% albumin, which is the basic replacement fluid. Today, it is the standard replacement fluid in most centers. Since it is hyperoncotic, it may lead to dilutional anemia. In standard practice at many centers, 5% albumin solution constitutes at least 60% of the replacement fluid, although 100% replacement with 5% albumin is not expected. Hypotensive attacks and pyrogenic reactions may develop depending on the factors it contains. Fresh frozen plasma (FFP) is preferred, especially in thrombotic thrombocytopenic purpura (TTP) and related diseases [7]. TPE is less likely to cause dilutional anemia than albumin, but the risk of allergic reactions and transfusion-related infection is higher [7]. Long-term use is limited due to the development of antibodies against plasma components [1–6].

I. Kozanoğlu (✉)
Adana Adult BMT Center, Baskent University, Adana, Türkiye

Acibadem Labmed Medical Laboratories, Hematology Laboratories, Istanbul, Türkiye
e-mail: ilknur.kozanoglu@acibademlabmed.com.tr

I. Kozanoglu (ed.), *Problem Solving in Apheresis Medicine*,
https://doi.org/10.1007/978-3-031-74081-7_18

Cascade filtration (CF) is a therapeutic plasma treatment performed through extracorporeal circulation, based on the principle of removing pathogens from plasma in a semi-selective manner [8–10]. Double filtration plasmapheresis (DFPP) was historically used for blood group-incompatible renal transplantation. Very few studies are available worldwide regarding its efficiency in removing specific plasma components and its safety. This chapter will review the basic principles of cascade filtration, the devices and filters used, the diseases in which the procedure is useful, and the complications associated with the procedure.

18.2 Technical Principles

DFPP is a method of selective plasmapheresis, pioneered by Agishi et al. in Japan in the 1980s, for desensitization in blood group-incompatible renal transplantation [10]. Over time, it has been used for various indications. In this procedure, the first filter, called the "plasma separator," separates plasma from cellular components, similar to membrane filtration. Filtered plasma passes through a second filter, called "plasma fractionator," which allows smaller molecules to pass back into circulation and discards molecules larger than the pore size of the fractionator [8–10].

The plasma is separated from its cellular components by filtration through a primary membrane plasma separator. Primary membrane plasma separation can be performed using a highly permeable filter and standard dialysis equipment or two blood pumps. First, a membrane must be selected that is biocompatible and has a pore size that allows the passage of all plasma constituents, including electrolytes, albumin, fibrinogen, and immunoglobulins, while retaining white blood cells, red blood cells (RBCs), and platelets. The shear rate of blood must be sufficiently high to prevent cellular components from being drawn to the surface of the membrane as plasma leaves the blood channel [11, 12]. This can be monitored with transmembrane pressure to avoid RBC lysis and membrane plugging, as well as by monitoring the hematocrit for RBC fraction. There are two different types of primary membrane plasma separators: flat membrane and hollow fiber plasma membranes for DFFP [8–11].

The separated plasma passes through a second fractionating filter. The content of the fractionated plasma determines which plasma components are removed and which are returned to the patient. The selectivity of DFPP is determined by three factors. The first is the size of the molecule to be filtered, which is determined by the filter pore diameter. If the permeability threshold of the filter is smaller than the pathogen causing the disease, the plasma passing through the filter during the process is free of the pathogen [8–10]. Other factors affecting selectivity include the rate at which plasma enters and exits the fraction. Molecules confined to the intravascular space, such as IgM or low-density lipoprotein cholesterol, are cleared safely in two sessions, while other substances are cleared more effectively with stable clearance rates over treatments following the first two sessions. Substances with larger volumes of distribution, such as IgG or IgA, are cleared most effectively with four or more sessions. DFPP has several advantages over other modalities [8–10]. The procedure is completely autologous, with disease-causing pathogenic molecules removed and essential proteins returned to the patient. As with plasma exchange, it does not carry the complications associated with fluid overload or the risks of viral and bacterial contamination from plasma infusion from a different organism. In this procedure, albumin or therapeutic donor plasma is not administered externally. A typical extracorporeal circuit used in DFFP shown in Fig. 18.1 [7, 10].

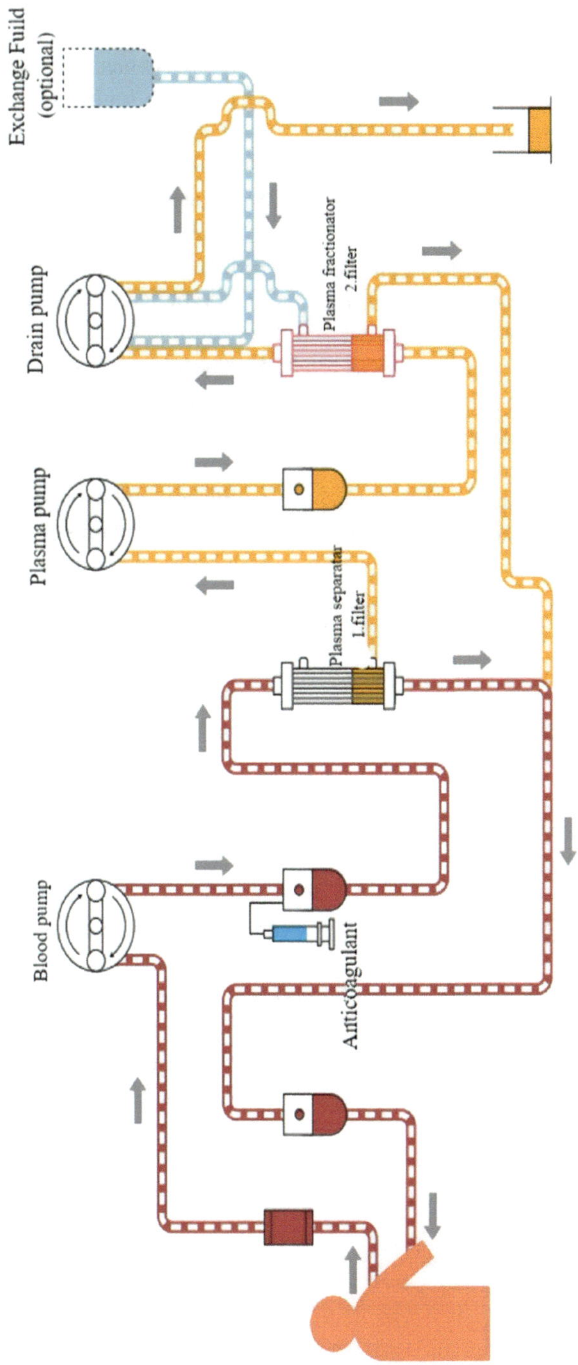

Fig. 18.1 Extracorporeal circulation circuit for DFPP. (Adapted from Hitit Medical [12])

18.3 Indications for DFFP

DFPP can be used for the elimination of autoantibodies, immune complexes, or lipoproteins. The term *rheopheresis* refers to DFPP performed using a plasma filter with a medium mean pore size in the treatment of microcirculatory disorders. In principle, plasma filtration can also be performed after centrifugal plasma separation [7].

There are defined and globally recognized treatment protocols for disease groups for which double filtration is indicated. DFPP can be applied for both acute and chronic diseases. In the case of acute diseases, DFPP is usually performed as TPE with five to ten consecutive sessions of 1–2 h. For chronic diseases, it is performed several times a year, depending on the underlying disease and the patient's condition [7, 10]. DFPP can be used instead of plasma exchange when the target substance to be removed is larger than IgG. In Japan, National Health Insurance covers DFPP treatment for more than 20 diseases. The list below shows the disease groups for which DFPP is commonly used [7, 10]:

1. **Metabolic Disorders**
   - Familial hypercholesterolemia
2. **Rheumatic Disorders**
   - Systemic lupus erythematosus
   - Rheumatoid arthritis
   - Malignant rheumatoid arthritis
   - Kawasaki disease
3. **Hematologic Disorders**
   - Severe blood-type incompatible
   - Thrombotic thrombocytopenic purpura
   - Immune thrombocytopenic purpura
   - Macroglobulinemia
   - Hyperviscosity syndromes
   - Hemophilia with inhibitor
4. **Nephrologic Disorders**
   - Anti-glomerular basement membrane (GBM) antibody-mediated rapidly progressive glomerulonephritis (RPGN)
   - Antineutrophil cytoplasmic antibody (ANCA)-mediated RPGN
   - Focal segmental glomerulosclerosis (FSGS)
5. **Neurological Disorders**
   - Myasthenia gravis
   - Guillain–Barré syndrome
   - Chronic inflammatory demyelinating polyradiculoneuropathy
   - Multiple sclerosis
6. **Dermatologic Disorders**
   - Pemphigus vulgaris
   - Pemphigoid
   - Toxic epidermal necrolysis
   - Stevens–Johnson syndrome
7. **Hepatic Disorders**
   - Chronic hepatitis C
   - Acute hepatic failure
   - Postoperative hepatic failure
8. **Other Indications**
   - Age-related macular degeneration (dry)
   - Sudden hearing loss

The American Society for Apheresis (ASFA) defines DFPP as a filter-based therapeutic procedure that removes pathogenic substances from separated plasma based on their size, which is primarily determined by molecular weight and three-dimensional configuration (e.g., autoantibodies, immune complexes, lipoproteins, etc.), using plasma filters with different pore sizes [7].

Currently, the filtration devices necessary for DFPP treatment are not licensed in the USA but are available in Europe, Canada, and Asia. Nevertheless, DFPP is given more importance in the ninth edition of the ASFA (Table 18.1).

Table 18.1 Category and grade recommendations for DFPP by ASFA

Disease/condition	Indication	Procedure	Category	Grade
Age-related macular degeneration	Dry, high risk	DFPP	III	2B
Atopic dermatitis, recalcitrant	–	ECP/IA/TPE/DFPP	III	2B
Cryoglobulinemia	Severe/symptomatic	TPE/DFPP	II	2A
Myasthenia gravis	Acute, short-term treatment	TPE/DFPP/IA	I	1B
Myasthenia gravis	Long-term treatment	TPE/DFPP/IA	II	2B
Pemphigus vulgaris	Severe	TPE	III	2B
Pemphigus vulgaris	Severe	IA/DFPP/ECP	III	2C
Sudden sensorineural hearing loss	–	LA/DFPP/TPE	III	2A

Abbreviations: *ASFA* American Society for Apheresis; *DFPP* double-filtration plasmapheresis; *ECP* extracorporeal photopheresis; *IA* immune absorption; *TPE* therapeutic plasma exchange; *LA* lipid apheresis

18.4 Complications of DFPP

DFPP removes high molecular weight molecules semi-selectively, thereby minimizing albumin loss, the need for substitution fluids, and associated hemodynamic fluctuations. However, complications related to DFPP have rarely been reported. The most common complications associated with DFPP include hemolysis, hypotension, and catheter-related issues. In one study, hemolysis, by far the most common complication of DFPP, occurred in 20% of the procedures [13–15].

Hemolysis is a complication unique to membrane filtration, which does not occur in the centrifugation method [16]. Increasing transmembrane pressure leads to deterioration of plasma flux, sieving, and hemolysis [16, 17].

Hypotension is a potential complication of all procedures involving extracorporeal circulation, including TPE, DFPP, and immunoadsorption plasmapheresis. The incidence of hypotension related to the plasmapheresis procedure in one study of 2502 DFPP sessions (3.3%) is similar to that reported previously for 13,107 plasma exchange sessions (1.7%) [18, 19]. Volume and protein depletion are the most likely causes of hypotension [19, 20]. The plasma fractionators (Evaflux 4 A or Cascadeflo-1770) with a pore size of 30–37 nm have sieving coefficients of 0.9 for albumin (MW 67,000), 0.4 for immunoglobulin G (MW 160,000), and 0.3 for IgM (MW 950,000) [21–24].

18.5 Conclusion

Filtration plasmapheresis is a system that removes plasma components from the patient's blood with the help of a filter, depending on their size [7, 10]. In this process, plasma is separated from the blood in the first stage. In the second stage, non-selective filters are used. The most important feature of these filters is their pore diameters [24]. During the process, high molecular weight substances, such as immunoglobulins and coagulation proteins, are not completely removed as in conventional plasma exchange. In addition, albumin is not completely removed as in conventional plasma exchange; only a certain amount of albumin is removed, depending on the type of membrane used. Therefore, albumin loss is reduced [11]. As a result, the volume of plasma processed can be much higher compared to conventional plasma exchange.

In summary, the number of diseases treated with DFPP has been increasing in recent years. DFPP was first reported in Japan in 1980 and has been used for over 40 years in Japan and many other countries as a safe and established treatment modality for many drug-resistant or refractory diseases [10].

References

1. Cervantes CE, Bloch EM, Sperati CJ. Therapeutic plasma exchange: core curriculum 2023. Am J Kidney Dis. 2023;81(4):475–92.

2. Kennedy MS, Domen RE. Therapeutic apheresis. Applications and future directions. Vox Sang. 1983;45(4):261–77.
3. Madore F, Lazarus JM, Brady HR. Therapeutic plasma exchange in renal diseases. J Am Soc Nephrol. 1996;7(3):367–86.
4. Rock G, Buskard NA. Therapeutic plasmapheresis. Curr Opin Hematol. 1996;3(6):504–10.
5. Kale-Pradhan PB, Woo MH. A review of the effects of plasmapheresis on drug clearance. Pharmacotherapy. 1997;17(4):684–95.
6. Kaplan AA. Therapeutic plasma exchange for the treatment of rapidly progressive glomerulonephritis. Ther Apher. 1997;1(3):255–9.
7. Connelly-Smith L, Alquist CR, Aqui NA, Hofmann JC, Klingel R, Onwuemene OA, Patriquin CJ, Pham HP, Sanchez AP, Schneiderman J, Witt V, Zantek ND, Dunbar NM. Guidelines on the use of therapeutic apheresis in clinical practice—evidence-based approach from the writing committee of the American Society for apheresis: the ninth special issue. J Clin Apher. 2023;38(2):77–278.
8. Siami FS, Siami GA. Plasmapheresis by using secondary membrane filters: twelve years of experience. ASAIO J. 2000;46:383–8.
9. Agishi T, Kaneko I, Hasuo Y, Sanaka T, Sudo N, Hayasaka Y, et al. DFPP utilizing new membrane technology. J Jpn Soc Dial Ther. 1981;14:61–5.
10. Hirano R, Namazuda K, Hirata N. Double filtration plasmapheresis: review of current clinical applications. Ther Apher Dial. 2021;25(2):145–51.
11. Lyu R, Chen W, Hsieh S. Plasma exchange versus DFPP in the treatment of Guillain-Barre syndrome. Ther Apher Dial. 2002;6:163–6.
12. Hitit Medikal Terapötik Aferez Eğitici Rehberi. 2019. https://www.hititmedical.com/pdf/egitim_rehberleri.pdf.
13. Nishi S, Hasegawa S, Gejyo F, Saito K, Nakagawa Y, Takahashi K. The safety measures for double filtration plasma apheresis (DFPP) before ABO-incompatible kidney transplantation. Int Congr Ser. 2006;1292:91–5.
14. Yeh JH, Chiu HC. Coagulation abnormalities in serial double-filtration plasmapheresis. J Clin Apher. 2001;16:139–42.
15. Yeh JH, Chen WH, Chiu HC. Complications of double-filtration plasmapheresis. Transfusion. 2004;44:1621–5.
16. Fok WW, Wu SC, Hsiao NY, Chen TW, Huang TP. Hemolysis in plasmapheresis. Acta Nephrol. 1996;10:16–21.
17. Mokrzycki MH, Kaplan AA. Therapeutic plasma exchange: complications and management. Am J Kidney Dis. 1994;23:817–27.
18. McLeod BC, Sniecinski I, Ciavarella D, et al. Frequency of immediate adverse effects associated with therapeutic apheresis. Transfusion. 1999;39:282–8.
19. Rodnitzky RL, Goeken JA. Complications of plasma exchange in neurological patients. Arch Neurol. 1982;39:350–4.
20. Vucic S, Davies L. Safety of plasmapheresis in the treatment of neurological disease. Aust NZ J Med. 1998;28:301–5.
21. Sprenger KG, Rasche H, Franz HE. Membrane plasma separation: complications and monitoring. Artif Organs. 1984;8:360–3.
22. Couriel D, Weinstein R. Complications of therapeutic plasma exchange: a recent assessment. J Clin Apheresis. 1994;9:1–5.
23. Wu MJ, Shu KH, Cheng CH, Lian JD. Complications of membrane-filtration plasma exchange. Chung Hua I Hsueh Tsa Chih (Taipei). 1997;60:147–54.
24. Sueoka A. Present status of apheresis technologies. 2. Membrane plasma fractionator. Ther Apher. 1996;1:135–46.

Comparison of Double-Filtration Plasmapheresis and Plasma Exchange

19

Ilknur Kozanoğlu, Osman Sahin, and Cem Kis

19.1 Introduction

Therapeutic plasma exchange (TPE), also known as plasmapheresis, is a treatment modality that has been in use for about 80 years, with techniques undergoing constant changes and advancements [1]. The primary goal of plasmapheresis-based treatment modalities is to remove immune complexes, protein-bound toxins, autoantibodies, high-molecular-weight solutes, and protein-bound solutes; the clinical effect of this removal is usually faster than that achieved with immunosuppressive therapy [1, 2]. TPE involves separating the plasma from the formed elements of the patient's blood for therapeutic purposes and replacing it with artificial plasma or crystalloid or colloid solutions with similar physical properties (e.g. pH and viscosity) to those of the removed plasma. Indications for plasmapheresis include the replacement of deficient plasma factors, removal of inflammatory mediators, enhancement of immune regulation, and regulation of reticuloendothelial system function. TPE is a form of therapeutic apheresis used as primary or adjunctive treatment in many diseases, including haematologic, neurologic, oncologic, rheumatologic, immunologic, renal, endocrine, toxicologic, and dermatologic conditions [1–3].

In plasma exchange procedures, plasma can be replaced with a colloid solution (e.g. albumin and/or plasma) or a combination of crystalloid and colloid solutions. In one volume of TPE, 150 g of plasma protein (consisting of 110 g of albumin and 40 g of globulin and other proteins) is removed. Most plasma proteins removed by TPE have important physiological functions; therefore, plasmapheresis has the potential to alter normal physiology. Although 125 g of albumin is replaced when albumin is used as the replacement fluid, other important plasma components, such as immunoglobulins and coagulation factors, are not replaced. Some studies have shown that drug clearance is affected due to the removal of drugs during TPE, and effective plasma dose adjustment may not be achievable [1–3].

In addition, the replacement fluids used in TPE may cause undesirable effects. When plasma is used, plasma proteins can be replaced; however, complications such as infectious disease, allergic reactions, anaphylaxis, and transfusion-related acute lung injury may occur. If the infusion rate is too high, the citrate in the plasma may lead to ionised hypocalcaemia. When albumin is used as a replacement fluid, it may bind to free

I. Kozanoğlu (✉)
Adana Adult BMT Center, Baskent University, Adana, Türkiye

Acibadem Labmed Medical Laboratories, Hematology Laboratories, Istanbul, Türkiye
e-mail: ilknur.kozanoglu@acibademlabmed.com.tr

O. Sahin · C. Kis
Division of Hematology, Department of Internal Medicine, Faculty of Medicine, Baskent University, Ankara, Turkey

I. Kozanoglu (ed.), *Problem Solving in Apheresis Medicine*,
https://doi.org/10.1007/978-3-031-74081-7_19

calcium and contribute to ionised hypocalcaemia. Moreover, reactions to albumin, including hypotensive, febrile, and anaphylactic reactions, may occur. When hydroxyethyl starch is used, complications may include anaphylactic reactions and persistent pruritus due to skin deposition [1–6].

To avoid these adverse effects of TPE, methods have been developed to selectively remove pathological components from plasma and return it to the patient as 'cleaned' plasma. This approach minimises the removal of desirable substances and helps prevent complications associated with replacement fluids. These techniques vary in their degree of selectivity [7, 8]. They can be highly selective (removing only antibodies directed against a specific antigen), relatively selective (removing only immunoglobulins or lipoproteins), or minimally selective (removing substances above a certain size) [7, 8].

The American Society for Apheresis (ASFA) defines double-filtration plasmapheresis (DFPP) as a filter-based therapeutic procedure that uses plasma filters with different pore sizes to remove pathogenic substances from separated plasma, based on the size of the substances, which is mainly determined by molecular weight and three-dimensional configuration (e.g. autoantibodies, immune complexes, and lipoproteins) [9].

The filtration devices necessary for DFPP are not licensed in the United States but are available in Europe, Canada, and Asia. However, DFPP is given increased importance in the ninth edition of the ASFA Guidelines [9].

Filtration plasmapheresis removes plasma components from the patient's blood using a filter appropriate for the size of the plasma components. In this system, plasma is separated from the blood in the first stage, and nonselective filters are applied in the second stage. The pore diameter of these filters is a critical feature. During filtration, high-molecular-weight substances, such as immunoglobulins and coagulation proteins, are not entirely removed, as they are in conventional plasma exchange [7–9]. In addition, albumin is not completely removed, as it is in conventional plasma exchange; instead, albumin removal occurs at a controlled rate, depending on the membrane type used. Consequently, less albumin is lost, and the volume of plasma processed can be significantly higher than that in conventional plasma exchange [7–10].

Filtration plasmapheresis systems are used to treat groups of diseases similar to those treated with TPE. Research has demonstrated effective removal of autoantibodies and clinical improvement in some of these diseases. Filtration plasmapheresis procedures have been applied to remove anti-A and anti-B antibodies to enable ABO-compatible kidney transplantation, to treat haemolytic disease of the foetus and newborn in pregnant women, and to address hyperviscosity in both Waldenström's macroglobulinaemia and multiple myeloma [11–16].

No randomised controlled studies have compared plasmapheresis with filtration plasmapheresis, except in Guillain-Barré syndrome. In a randomised study by Lyu et al., 39 patients with acute Guillain-Barré syndrome underwent plasma exchange, and 63 patients underwent double cascade filtration. Patients who underwent plasma exchange in the early phase showed better clinical response rates. No difference was observed in the later phase, although filtration procedures reportedly had fewer complications [14].

During DFPP, waste plasma is deposited in the secondary filter. As waste plasma accumulates, the pressure triggers a flush to remove it from the filter. At this point, a specialised nurse or technician determines whether fluid replacement is necessary [7–18].

Apheresis consultant physicians should play an active role in determining which procedure is appropriate for each patient. The choice between plasma exchange and double cascade filtration should be guided by the following criteria (Table 19.1):

1. **Haemodynamic status of the patient:** Patients with haemodynamic instability, cardiac, or renal insufficiency should be managed cautiously. Patient age and any additional health conditions should also be considered.

Table 19.1 Comparison of the advantages and disadvantages of filtration plasmapheresis systems compared with conventional plasma exchange

Advantages	Disadvantages
Removes only the substance of interest, preserving normal or beneficial plasma components	May not effectively remove pathological substances when the disease pathophysiology is unknown or unclear
No need for replacement fluid, minimising transfusion reactions and reducing the risk of disease transmission	Exposes the patient's blood to biologically active columns and materials, which may trigger reactions
Avoids replacement fluid-related costs	Expensive to use, with limited reimbursement options
Some systems do not require separation of whole blood into plasma and cellular components (e.g. haemoperfusion systems)	Devices required for operation in some systems can be quite complex
Some systems remove more pathological substances than plasma exchange	
Causes minimal loss of albumin	

2. **Disease diagnosis:** Plasma exchange is preferred for diseases such as thrombotic thrombocytopenic purpura and haemolytic uraemic syndrome. However, for prolonging graft life in transplant patients with panel-reactive antibody-positive humoral rejection, filtration procedures are preferred to minimise antigen exposure. In patients with familial hyperlipidaemia or elevated low-density lipoprotein, filtration systems may be chosen to reduce unnecessary plasma use. For cases requiring bilirubin removal, filtration plasmapheresis with bilirubin columns is recommended [7, 8]. This approach helps preserve beneficial plasma components such as proteins and clotting factors, which is also advantageous for patients with liver failure and hypoalbuminaemia (Table 19.1).
3. **Bleeding and coagulation issues:** In patients with bleeding diathesis undergoing plasma exchange, fresh frozen plasma should be used as the replacement fluid (Table 19.1). When filtration is selected, close monitoring of plasma fibrinogen level is essential. A minimum interval of 24–48 h between filtration sessions is advised to support fibrinogen synthesis (Table 19.1) [7, 8].
4. **Need for rapid response:** Although plasma exchange procedures generally produce faster responses, filtration plasmapheresis may be more effective in removing cytokines in patients with sepsis. Disease- and patient-specific decisions may be required in such cases [7, 8].
5. **Need for replacement fluids:** The advantage of minimal or no replacement fluids in the filtration process is significant. Filtration techniques may be preferred in patients who have an allergy to one of the replacement fluids. Although fresh frozen plasma used in plasma exchange procedures has been found to be free from microbiological contamination, the inherent risk of infection remains a serious concern [19]. The use of large volumes of fresh frozen plasma, especially in patients requiring multiple apheresis sessions, may increase the risk of infection. In addition, difficulties in obtaining replacement fluids and reimbursement challenges are important factors that may lead patients to prefer filtration plasmapheresis (Table 19.1).
6. **Reimbursement issues:** Both procedures face reimbursement challenges for necessary sets or replacement fluids, placing physicians and patients in difficult situations (Table 19.1). For example, filtration plasmapheresis procedures are associated with reimbursement problems in the United States [9, 12, 19–21].

Apheresis techniques are advancing rapidly. Mastering these techniques may provide new hope for the effective treatment of certain diseases. Plasma exchange procedures have been used for many years to treat various conditions. However, filtration plasmapheresis procedures have been increasingly used for a growing number of patients and indications in recent years, with their popularity rising quickly. Plasma exchange involves the removal of plasma from the patient using a plasmapheresis device, separating the plasma, and returning the formed elements along with the replacement fluid [19]. As most high-molecular-weight solutes are returned to the patient with albumin, the need for replacement fluid is reduced. Immunoadsorption, on the other hand, removes only immunoglobulins from plasma without requiring replacement fluid and without depleting clotting factors and complement. Treatment decisions should be made after evaluating various factors, such as the patient's diagnosis, age, performance status, risk of complications, and bleeding or coagulation issues. Few clinical studies have focused on the superiority of each technique over the other. Randomised controlled clinical trials are needed to determine which procedure is more effective for each disease [19–21].

References

1. Cervantes CE, Bloch EM, Sperati CJ. Therapeutic plasma exchange: core curriculum 2023. Am J Kidney Dis. 2023;81(4):475–92.
2. Kennedy MS, Domen RE. Therapeutic apheresis. Applications and future directions. Vox Sang. 1983;45(4):261–77.
3. Volkin RL, Starz TW, Winkelstein A, Shadduck RK, Lewis JH, Hasiba U, et al. Changes in coagulation factors, complement, immunoglobulins, and immune complex concentrations with plasma exchange. Transfusion. 1982;22(1):54–8.
4. Wing EJ, Bruns FJ, Fraley DS, Segel DP, Adler S. Infectious complications with plasmapheresis in rapidly progressive glomerulonephritis. JAMA. 1980;244(21):2423–6.
5. Shermin D, Briggs D, Greenan M. Complication of therapeutic plasma exchange: a prospective study of 1727 procedures. J Clin Apher. 2007;22(5):270–6.
6. Askari S, Nollet K, Debol SM, Brunstein CG, Eastlund T. Transfusion-related acute lung injury during plasma exchange: suspecting the unsuspected. J Clin Apher. 2002;17(2):93–6.
7. Agishi T, Kaneko I, Hasuo Y, Sanaka T, Sudo N, Hayasaka Y, et al. DFPP utilizing new membrane technology. J Jpn Soc Dial Ther. 1981;14:61–5.
8. Hirano R, Namazuda K, Hirata N. Double filtration plasmapheresis: review of current clinical applications. Ther Apher Dial. 2021;25(2):145–51.
9. Connelly-Smith L, Alquist CR, Aqui NA, Hofmann JC, Klingel R, Onwuemene OA, Patriquin CJ, Pham HP, Sanchez AP, Schneiderman J, Witt V, Zantek ND, Dunbar NM. Guidelines on the use of therapeutic apheresis in clinical practice—evidence-based approach from the writing Committee of the American Society for apheresis: the ninth special issue. J Clin Apher. 2023;38(2):77–278.
10. Kawasumi. https://www.sb-kawasumi.jp/e/business/plasmapheresis.html.
11. Kumlien G, Ullström L, Losvall A, Persson LG, Tydén G. Clinical experience with a new apheresis filter that specifically depletes ABO blood group antibodies. Transfusion. 2006;46(9):1568–75.
12. Siami GA, Siami FS. Membrane plasmapheresis in the United States: a review over the last 20 years. Ther Apher. 2001;5(4):315–20.
13. Thalgahagoda S, Webb NJ, Roberts D, Birch A, Milford DV, Tavakoli A, et al. Successful ABO incompatible renal transplantation following rituximab and DFPP after failed immunoadsorption. Pediatr Transplant. 2014;18(3):74–6.
14. Lyu R, Chen W, Hsieh S. Plasma exchange versus DFPP in the treatment of Guillain-Barre syndrome. Ther Apher Dial. 2002;6:163–6.
15. Otsubo S, Tanabe K, Shinmura H, Ishikawa N, Tokumoto T, Hattori M, et al. Effect of posttransplant double filtration plasmapheresis on recurrent focal and segmental glomerulosclerosis in renal transplant recipients. Ther Apher Dial. 2004;8(4):299–304.
16. Jiang X, Feng J, Ye Y. Double-filtration plasmapheresis for treatment of acute renal failure in a multiple myeloma patient. Ther Apher Dial. 2014;18(3):318–9.
17. Mineshima M, Yokoi R, Horibe K, Eguchi K, Kaneko I, Agishi T, et al. Effects of operating conditions on selectivity of plasma fractionator in double filtration plasmapheresis. Ther Apher. 2001;5(6):444–8.
18. Yeh JH, Chen WH, Chui HC, Bai CH. Clearance studies subsequent sessions of double filtration plasmapheresis. Artif Organs. 2006;30(2):111–4.
19. Nakaji S, Yamamoto T. Membranes for therapeutic apheresis. Ther Apher. 2002;6(4):267–70.
20. Wu MJ, Shu KH, Cheng CH, Lian JD. Complications of membrane-filtration plasma exchange. Chung Hua I Hsueh Tsa Chih (Taipei). 1997;60:147–54.
21. Sueoka A. Present status of apheresis technologies. 2. Membrane plasma fractionator. Ther Apher. 1996;1:135–46.

Part VII

Problems During Extracorporeal Photopheresis (ECP)

Extracorporeal Photopheresis in Patients with Acute Graft-Versus-Host Disease

20

Hakan Ozdogu and Çigdem Gereklioglu

20.1 Background

Graft-versus-host disease (GvHD), a severe complication of allogeneic hematopoietic stem cell transplantation, is categorized as either acute (aGvHD) or chronic (cGvHD). Despite current prophylaxis strategies, aGvHD occurs in 50% of patients (Grades 3–4) and is severe in 14% of cases, with a mortality rate of 36% [1].

Corticosteroids are the preferred first-line therapy for both aGvHD and cGvHD. Approximately 60% of patients with aGvHD do not respond to first-line therapy or show recurrence after an initial response. These patients are diagnosed with steroid-refractory (SR)-GvHD; the 6-month survival rate in such cases is approximately 50%, and the overall survival rate is only 5–30% [2].

Extracorporeal photopheresis (ECP), mechanistic target of rapamycin (mTOR) inhibitors, and mycophenolate mofetil are the most commonly administered treatments for SR-GvHD. In May 2019, the US Food and Drug Administration (FDA) approved the Janus kinase (JAK) 1/2 inhibitor ruxolitinib for adult and pediatric patients aged ≥12 years with Grades 2–4 SR-aGvHD, based on an open-label, single-arm, multicenter study involving 49 patients (REACH1). The FDA later approved ruxolitinib for SR-cGvHD in September 2021, based on the results of the REACH3 study.

Many second-line treatment options have been investigated. However, these treatments usually cannot control GvHD activity and have various side effects (e.g., increased risk of infection, disease recurrence, and severe systemic immunosuppression), along with unacceptable late effects. ECP has become an important treatment option for SR-GvHD because it does not lead to systemic immunosuppression; it also has significant efficacy and an excellent safety profile.

Although corticosteroids are first-line treatments for both aGvHD and cGvHD, there is no standard second-line treatment approach. The second-line treatment applied usually depends on institutional policies, clinician preference, ease of application, treatment availability, and patient preference [1, 3–6]. ECP is typically used in combination with corticosteroids or other immunosuppressive drugs. Since it is difficult to evaluate the efficacy of ECP in such cases, the response to ECP has been evaluated based on the ability to taper other immunosuppressive drugs (with a particular focus on steroid-preserving effects) and clinical developments [7–14].

Despite the available data, there remains a lack of clarity regarding which sequence should be applied in the treatment of SR/steroid-

H. Ozdogu (✉)
Hematology Department, Baskent University School of Medicine, Ankara, Turkey

Ç. Gereklioglu
Family Medicine of Çukurova University School of Medicine, Adana, Turkey

I. Kozanoglu (ed.), *Problem Solving in Apheresis Medicine*,
https://doi.org/10.1007/978-3-031-74081-7_20

dependent patients, which combinations of ECP with other possible anti-GvHD therapies can be used, which administration and tapering schedules are optimal, and how treatment responses can be evaluated.

20.2 Technique and Mechanism of Action

ECP involves isolation of the patient's mononuclear cells by apheresis, followed by ex vivo exposure of these cells to UVA and 8-methoxypsoralen (8-MOP), and then transfusion of the modified leukocytes back into the patient [11, 15–17]. This process has no known immunosuppressive effect and leads to immune tolerance by increasing the number of regulatory T cells (Tregs) [11, 15–18].

Although ECP received FDA approval in 1988 and more than two million procedures have been performed thus far, its mechanism of action is not clearly understood. Its efficacy is presumably related mainly to the apoptosis of lymphocytes and differentiation of dendritic cells. Initial studies assumed that ECP initiated apoptosis in lymphoid cells due to the covalent binding of 8-MOP to DNA, leading to cell cycle blockade [19, 20]. Further studies focused on the increased differentiation of intensely immature dendritic cells [21], triggered by contact with extracorporeal surfaces and platelets in the tubing and centrifuge chamber of the device [22].

Dendritic cells are master regulators that govern antigen-specific T-cell immunity and T-cell tolerance; thus, they are central and critical components of the ECP immunotherapeutic response. Indeed, ECP is regarded as a dendritic antigen-presenting cell-based therapy [23]. The cytokine profile in peripheral blood is modified after reinfusion of cells treated with 8-MOP and UVA, shifting from proinflammatory to anti-inflammatory cytokine production [24]. During ECP, T cells are also activated, leading to the formation of Tregs, which play a crucial role in downregulating immune reactions. In patients with aGvHD, a significantly greater number of Tregs may be detected in the peripheral blood [25].

Gatza et al. further showed that the injection of ECP-treated splenocytes from mice developing GvHD triggered IL-10-producing Tregs, which could reverse the experimental condition [26]. Overall, recent data have suggested that ECP triggers immune tolerance. However, Treg production does not fully explain the ability of ECP to selectively target pathogenetic T cells in the cutaneous T-cell lymphoma environment [27]. Although ECP has been suggested to induce an antitumor response toward tumoral T cells [20], the mechanism underlying the action of ECP remains obscure. A better understanding of this mechanism would help optimize treatment regimens. Novel ECP applications have the potential for efficacy in patients with aGvHD [11].

20.3 ECP/Prophylaxis

There have been a limited number of studies regarding the prophylactic role of ECP in GvHD, the ECP procedure as a component of the conditioning regimen, and GvHD prophylaxis after hematopoietic stem-cell transplantation. The first evaluation by Miller et al. (2004) integrated ECP into a reduced-intensity conditioning regimen, along with pentostatin and low-dose total body irradiation (600 cGy). Although 9% of the patients developed Grade 2 or higher aGvHD, 43% developed cGvHD, and 12% exhibited generalized disease. However, most patients had received multiple therapies and had comorbid conditions [28]. Michallet et al. conducted a prospective multicenter phase II study of prophylactic ECP after the reduced-intensity conditioning regimen and showed promising results, with cumulative incidence rates of 15% for aGvHD and 22% for cGvHD [29]. In conclusion, the use of ECP for aGvHD prophylaxis has not been introduced as a routine procedure. Further studies are needed to determine its efficacy.

20.4 First-Line Therapy for Acute GvHD

The rate of non-relapse mortality is high, and overall survival is shorter in patients with failure of first-line (steroid) therapy [30]. There have been few studies, and only limited evidence is available regarding the use of ECP as first-line therapy to improve the outcomes of first-line therapy in aGvHD; these studies were mostly retrospective and observational in nature [32–34]. Therefore, sufficient evidence is not available to support the addition of ECP to corticosteroid treatment or the use of ECP alone in the treatment of pre-GvHD.

20.5 Treatment of ECP/Steroid-Refractory Acute GvHD

Although corticosteroids continue to be the first-line therapy for aGvHD, there are various second-line treatment options, and none has demonstrated significant advantages over the others. No standardized treatment options are currently available. There have been no randomized controlled studies of the efficacy of ECP in SR-aGvHD. However, prospective studies have shown high response rates in aGvHD [11, 31–37]. Considering that the studies were not uniform, interpretation of the results is limited. General response rates varied between 52% and 100% in SR-aGvHD, with rates of 66–100% for the skin, 40–83% for the gastrointestinal tract, and 27–71% for the liver.

Second-line treatment options for GvHD should be evaluated in cases of steroid dependency and steroid intolerance. However, no criteria have been defined for adding a novel treatment or switching to another treatment modality during the use of second-line or further treatments. According to real-world clinical data, the 2-year overall survival rate is 25% in patients with SR Grade 3 and Grade 4 lower gastrointestinal tract GvHD [38].

Ruxolitinib is the first drug approved by the FDA (2019) to treat SR-aGvHD. The combination of ruxolitinib and ECP was used in 18 patients with lower gastrointestinal tract GvHD. In this retrospective study, Modemann et al. observed a complete response rate of 44% and a 2-year survival rate of 56% among patients with poor prognosis [39]. In a meta-analysis of SR-aGvHD, response rates were reportedly 86% in the skin, 60% in the liver, and 68% in the gastrointestinal tract [40]. Despite the promising results, prospective and randomized studies are needed to provide insights into unknown aspects, such as the role and effectiveness of combination therapies, ECP, ruxolitinib, and other anti-GvHD therapies.

20.6 Treatment Scheme of ECP in Acute GvHD

The recommendations for ECP in aGvHD by the TECP group Task Force are as follows:

- One cycle consists of 2 consecutive days of treatment.
- The duration of treatment should be a minimum of 8 consecutive weeks, with one cycle per week.
- Response to treatment should be evaluated after 8 weeks. If a complete response is achieved, treatment should be reduced to one cycle per 2 weeks and then terminated.
- If partial response is achieved, weekly treatment should continue, along with weekly evaluations.
- The procedure should be stopped unless further responses are achieved.
- The response may require additional time in cases of lower gastrointestinal tract GvHD, and the treatment period may be prolonged. In cases of Grade 3–4 aGvHD, the addition of other agents that may act more rapidly should be considered (Table 20.1).

Table 20.1 ECP indications and schedule for aGvHD treatment in current guidelines

ASFA (2019)	**Indication:** Salvage treatment after failure of first-line therapy **Schedule:** One cycle (two to three treatments) performed weekly until disease response and then tapered to every other week before stopping
European Dermatology Forum (2020)	**Indication:** aGvHD with no response to first-line corticosteroid therapy **Schedule:** One cycle (two to three treatments) every week until achievement of complete response and no benefit of maintenance. Assess weekly
Nordic ECP Quality Group (2020)	**Indication:** Steroid-refractory, steroid-dependent, or steroid-intolerant aGvHD **Schedule:** One sequence (one treatment on 2 consecutive days) weekly for 4 weeks. Assess treatment response at 4-week intervals **If complete response is achieved:** Steroid-refractory aGvHD: Two more sequences of ECP and then stop Steroid-dependent/steroid-intolerant aGvHD: Taper ECP over 1–2 weeks **If partial response is achieved:** Continue weekly ECP **If no change or progressive disease:** Consider additional or alternative treatment options
Turkish ECP (TECP) Group [48]	**Indication:** Steroid-refractory, steroid-dependent, or steroid-intolerant aGvHD **Schedule:** One cycle consists of 2 consecutive days of treatment. Duration of treatment should be a minimum of 8 consecutive weeks with one cycle per week. Treatment response should be assessed after 8 weeks **If complete response is achieved:** Taper with two more administrations once every 2 weeks and then stop **If partial response is achieved:** Continue weekly treatment and assess weekly. Treatment should be stopped when no further response is observed. Treatment should be stopped in cases with stable disease, progressive disease, or no response **Lower gastrointestinal GvHD:** Response may require additional time, and the treatment duration may be extended. In the presence of Grade 3–4 aGvHD, the inclusion of therapeutic agents with more rapid effects should be considered

aGvHD acute graft-versus-host disease; *ECP* extracorporeal photopheresis; *GvHD* graft-versus-host disease

20.7 ECP/Adverse Effects

Complication rates are low, and the severity is mild, particularly in patients who do not require a central venous catheter. Complications consist of hypotension, mild anemia, and mild thrombocytopenia [16, 41, 42]. Due to increased photosensitivity, patients are advised to take protective measures against UVA exposure for the skin and eyes for 24–48 h after the procedure [43]. ECP is contraindicated in patients with sensitivity to psoralen products, known photosensitivity, a risk of retinal damage, pregnancy, hemodynamic instability, respiratory instability, low leukocyte count (<1 × 10^9/L despite granulocyte colony-stimulating factor), low platelet count (<20 × 10^9/L), uncontrolled infection, and active bleeding [3, 44–46]. Other adverse effects are mostly associated with volume shifts causing hypotension, which can be managed by pausing the procedure and/or administering fluids. Transient fevers up to 38–39 °C have been observed at 6–8 h after reinfusion of treated mononuclear cells [47].

In conclusion, ECP has a very good safety profile. It does not cause systemic immunosuppression and does not adversely affect the graft-versus-leukemia effect. No increased risk of disease recurrence or opportunistic infections associated with ECP and no World Health Organization Grade 3–4 side effects have been reported.

References

1. Greinix HT, Eikema DJ, Koster L, et al. Improved outcome of patients with graft-versus-host disease after allogeneic hematopoietic cell transplantation for hematologic malignancies over time: an EBMT mega-file study. Haematologica. 2022;107:1054–63. https://doi.org/10.3324/haematol.2020.265769.
2. Socie G, Milpied N, Yakoub-Agha I, et al. Long-term follow-up of a phase 3 clinical trial of inolimomab for the treatment of primary steroid refractory aGVHD. Blood Adv. 2019;3:184–6.
3. Penack O, Marchetti M, Ruutu T, et al. Prophylaxis and management of graft versus host disease after stem-cell transplantation for haematological malignancies: updated consensus recommendations of the European Society for Blood and Marrow Transplantation.

Lancet Haematol. 2020;7(2):e157–67. https://doi.org/10.1016/S2352-3026(19)30256-X.
4. Martin PJ, Rizzo JD, Wingard JR, et al. First- and second-line systemic treatment of acute graft-versus-host disease: recommendations of the American Society of Blood and Marrow Transplantation. Biol Blood Marrow Transplant. 2012;18(8):1150–63. https://doi.org/10.1016/j.bbmt.2012.04.005.
5. Dignan FL, Clark A, Amrolia P, et al. Diagnosis and management of acute graft-versus-host disease. Br J Haematol. 2012;18(8):1150–63. https://doi.org/10.1111/j.1365-2141.2012.09129.x.
6. Malard F, Huang XJ, Sim JPY. Treatment and unmet needs in steroid-refractory acute graft-versus-host disease. Leukemia. 2020;34(5):1229–40. https://doi.org/10.1038/s41375-020-0804-2.
7. Sarantopoulos S, Cardones AR, Sullivan KM. How I treat refractory chronic graft-versus-host disease. Blood. 2019;133(11):1191–200. https://doi.org/10.1182/blood-2018-04-785899.
8. Besnier DP, Chabannes D, Mah'e B, et al. Treatment of graft-versus-host disease by extracorporeal photochemotherapy: a pilot study. Transplantation. 1997;64(1):49–54.
9. Greinix HT, Volc-Platzer B, Rabitsch W, et al. Successful use of extracorporeal photochemotherapy in the treatment of severe acute and chronic graft-versus-host disease. Blood. 1998;92(9):3098–104.
10. Schwartz J, Padmanabhan A, Aqui N, et al. Guidelines on the use of therapeutic apheresis in clinical practice—evidence_ based approach from the writing Committee of the American Society for apheresis: the seventh special issue. J Clin Apher. 2016;31(3):149–62. https://doi.org/10.1002/jca.21470.
11. Perfetti P, Carlier P, Strada P, et al. Extracorporeal photopheresis for the treatment of steroid-refractory acute GVHD. Bone Marrow Transplant. 2008;42:609–17. https://doi.org/10.1038/bmt.2008.221.
12. Zhang H, Chen R, Cheng J, et al. Systematic review and meta-analysis of prospective studies for ECP treatment in patients with steroid-refractory acute GVHD. Patient Prefer Adherence. 2015;17:105–11. https://doi.org/10.2147/PPA.S76563.
13. Malagola M, Cancelli V, Skert C, et al. Extracorporeal photopheresis for treatment of acute and chronic graft versus host disease: an Italian multicentric retrospective analysis on 94 patients on behalf of the gruppo Italiano trapianto di midollo osseo. Transplantation. 2016;100(12):e147–55. https://doi.org/10.1097/TP.0000000000001466.
14. Ward DM. Extracorporeal photopheresis: how, when, and why. J Clin Apher. 2011;26(5):276–85. https://doi.org/10.1002/jca.20300.
15. Greinix HT, Volc-Platzer B, Knobler RM. Extracorporeal photochemotherapy in the treatment of severe graft-versus-host disease. Leuk Lymphoma. 2000;36(5–6):425–34.
16. Knobler R, Berlin G, Calzavara-Pinton P, et al. Guidelines on the use of extracorporeal photopheresis. J Eur Acad Dermatol Venereol. 2014;28(Suppl 1):1–37. https://doi.org/10.1111/jdv.12311.
17. Zhang H, Chen R, Cheng J, et al. Systematic review and meta-analysis of prospective studies for ECP treatment in patients with steroid-refractory acute GVHD. Patient Prefer Adherence. 2015;9:105–11.
18. Budde H, Kolb S, Salinas Tejedor L, et al. Modified extracorporeal photopheresis with cells from a healthy donor for acute graft-versus-host disease in a mouse model. PLoS One. 2014;9(8):e105896.
19. Bladon J, Taylor PC. Extracorporeal photopheresis induces apoptosis in the lymphocytes of cutaneous T-cell lymphoma and graft-versus-host disease patients. Br J Haematol. 1999;107(4):707–11.
20. Gerber A, Bohne M, Rasch J, et al. Investigation of annexin V binding to lymphocytes after extracorporeal photoimmunotherapy as an early marker of apoptosis. Dermatology. 2000;201(2):111–7.
21. Durazzo TS, Tigelaar RE, Filler R, et al. Induction of monocyte- to-dendritic cell maturation by extracorporeal photochemotherapy: initiation via direct platelet signaling. Transfus Apher Sci. 2014;50(3):370–8.
22. Spisek R, Gasova Z, Bartunkova J. Maturationstate of dendritic cells during the extracorporeal photopheresis and its relevance for the treatment of chronic graft-versus-host disease. Transfusion. 2006;46(1):55–65.
23. Edelson R, Wu Y, Schneiderman J. American council on ECP (ACE): why now? J Clin Apher. 2018;33(4):464–8.
24. Vowels BR, Cassin M, Boufal MH, et al. Extracorporeal photochemotherapy induces the production of tumor necrosis factor-alpha by monocytes: implications for the treatment of cutaneous T-cell lymphoma and systemic sclerosis. J Invest Dermatol. 1992;98(5):686–92.
25. Biagi E, Di Biaso I, Leoni V, et al. Extracorporeal photochemotherapy is accompanied by increasing levels of circulating CD4+CD25+GITR+Foxp3+CD62L+ functional regulatory T-cells in patients with graft-versus-host disease. Transplantation. 2007;84(1):31–9.
26. Gatza E, Rogers CE, Clouthier SG, et al. Extracorporeal photopheresis reverses experimental graft-versus host disease through regulatory T cells. Blood. 2008;112(4):1515–21.
27. Hannani D. Extracorporeal photopheresis: tolerogenic or immunogenic cell death? BeBeyond current dogma. Front Immunol. 2015;6:349.
28. Shaughnessy PJ, Bolwell BJ, van Besien K, et al. Extracorporeal photopheresis for the prevention of acute GVHD in patients undergoing standard myeloablative conditioning and allogeneic hematopoietic stem cell transplantation. Bone Marrow Transplant. 2010;45(6):1068–76.
29. Michallet M, Sobh M, Garban F, et al. Extracorporeal photopheresis for GVHD prophylaxis after reduced-intensity conditioning allogeneic hematopoietic stem cell transplantation: a prospective multicenter phase 2 study. Leuk Lymphoma. 2018;59(2):372–80.

30. Martin PJ, Nelson BJ, Appelbaum FR, et al. Evaluation of a CD5-specific immunotoxin for treatment of acute graft-versus-host disease after allogeneic marrow transplantation. Blood. 1996;88:824–30.
31. Salvaneschi L, Perotti C, Zecca M, et al. Extracorporeal photochemotherapy for treatment of acute and chronic GVHD in childhood. Transfusion. 2001;41(10):1299–305. https://doi.org/10.1046/j.1537-2995.2001.41101299.x.
32. Garban F, Drillat P, Makowski C, et al. Extracorporeal chemo phototherapy for the treatment of graft-versus-host disease: hematologic consequences of short-term, intensive courses. Haematologica. 2005;90(8):1096–101.
33. Greinix HT, Knobler RM, Worel N, et al. The effect of intensified extracorporeal photochemotherapy on long-term survival in patients with severe acute graft-versus-host disease. Haematologica. 2006;91(3):405–58.
34. Kanold J, Merlin E, Halle P, et al. Photopheresis in pediatric graft-versus-host disease after allogeneic marrow transplantation: clinical practice guidelines based on field experience and review of the literature. Transfusion. 2007;47(12):2276–89. https://doi.org/10.1111/j.1537-2995.2007.01469.x.
35. Calore E, Cal'o A, Tridello G, et al. Extracorporeal photochemotherapy may improve outcome in children with acute GVHD. Bone Marrow Transplant. 2008;42(6):421–5. https://doi.org/10.1038/bmt.2008.174.
36. Sakellari I, Gavriilaki E, Batsis I, et al. Favorable impact of extracorporeal photopheresis in acute and chronic graft versus host disease: prospective single-center study. J Clin Apher. 2018;33(6):654–60. https://doi.org/10.1002/jca.21660.
37. Abu-Dalle I, Reljic T, Nishihori T, et al. Extracorporeal photopheresis in steroid-refractory acute or chronic graft-versus-host disease: results of a systematic review of prospective studies. Biol Blood Marrow Transplant. 2014;20:1677–86. https://doi.org/10.1016/j.bbmt.2014.05.017.
38. Modemann F, Ayuk F, Wolschke C, et al. Ruxolitinib plus extracorporeal photopheresis (ECP) for steroid refractory acute graft-versus-host disease of lower GI-tract after allogeneic stem cell transplantation leads to increased regulatory T cell level. Bone Marrow Transplant. 2020;55:2286–93. https://doi.org/10.1038/s41409-020-0952-z.
39. Al Alfred A, Taylor PC, Dignan F, et al. The role of extracorporeal photopheresis in the management of cutaneous T-cell lymphoma, graft-versus-host disease and organ transplant rejection: a consensus statement update from the UK Photopheresis society. Br J Haematol. 2017;177(2):287–310. https://doi.org/10.1111/bjh.14537.
40. Jagasia M, Scheid C, Soci'e G, Ayuk FA, et al. Randomized controlled study of ECP with methoxsalen as first-line treatment of patients with moderate to severe cGVHD. Blood Adv. 2019;3:2218–29. https://doi.org/10.1182/bloodadvances.2019000145.
41. Mokrzycki MH, Balogun RA, et al. Therapeutic apheresis: a review of complications and recommendations for prevention and management. J Clin Apher. 2011;26(5):243–8. https://doi.org/10.1002/jca.20303.
42. Henriksson MM, Newman E, Witt V, et al. Adverse events in apheresis: an update of the WAA registry data. Transfus Apher Sci. 2016;54(1):2–15. https://doi.org/10.1016/j.transci.2016.01.003.
43. Shelat SG. Practical considerations for planning a therapeutic apheresis procedure. Am J Med. 2010;123:777–84. https://doi.org/10.1016/j.amjmed.2010.01.022.
44. Knobler R, Arenberger P, Arun A, Assaf C, Bagot M, Berlin G, et al. European dermatology forum—updated guidelines on the use of extracorporeal photopheresis 2020—part 1. J Eur Acad Dermatol Venereol. 2020;34(12):2693–716. https://doi.org/10.1111/jdv.16890.
45. McLeod BC, Sniecinski I, Ciavarella D, et al. Frequency of immediate adverse effects associated with therapeutic apheresis. Transfusion. 1999;39(3):282–8. https://doi.org/10.1046/j.1537-2995.1999.39399219285.x.
46. Das-Gupta E, Dignan F, Shaw B, et al. Extracorporeal photopheresis for treatment of adults and children with acute GVHD: UK consensus statement and review of published literature. Bone Marrow Transplant. 2014;49(10):1251–8. https://doi.org/10.1038/bmt.2014.106.
47. Choi J, Foss FM. Photopheresis. In: McLeod BC, Weinstein R, Winters JL, Szczepiorkowski AM, editors. Apheresis: principles and practice. 3rd ed. Bethesda, MD: AABB Press; 2010. p. 615.
48. Kaynar L, Tekgunduz E, Kozanoglu I, et al. Extracorporeal photopheresis in the treatment of acute and chronic graft-versus-host disease: a position statement from the Turkish Society of Apheresis (TSA). Transfus Apher Sci. 2022;61:103373.

21 Extracorporeal Photopheresis in Patients with Chronic Graft-Versus-Host Disease

Leylagül Kaynar and Yaşa Gül Mutlu

21.1 Background

Despite significant advances in targeted therapy, immunotherapy, and other cellular therapy options, allogeneic stem cell transplantation remains the only curative treatment option for various benign and malignant disorders. Graft-versus-host disease (GvHD) continues to pose a significant barrier to the success of allogeneic hematopoietic stem cell transplantation and is a primary cause of non-relapse mortality and significant morbidity.

GvHD is classified into two distinct entities with different clinical features and underlying pathophysiology: acute GvHD (aGvHD) and chronic GvHD (cGvHD). An overlap syndrome, characterized by features of both aGvHD and cGvHD, is also recognized [1]. cGvHD occurs in approximately 50% of cases, with incidence increasing with advanced age [2]. Diagnosis of cGvHD is based on the National Institutes of Health (NIH) consensus criteria, which encompass diverse clinical, pathological, and laboratory parameters, as well as the time of onset [1]. cGvHD has unique clinical manifestations, including sclerodermatous skin changes, bronchiolitis obliterans, and ocular involvement; however, it can mimic various autoimmune disorders [3].

Complex dysregulated adaptive and innate immune responses are involved in the development of cGvHD, a multifaceted condition with a complex pathophysiology comprising three biological phases: [1] early inflammation due to tissue damage, [2] thymic injury and T- and B-cell dysregulation, and [3] aberrant tissue repair and fibrosis [4]. These phases can overlap and may not occur sequentially or at all [4]. During the initial phase, host tissue damaged caused by pretransplant conditioning leads to the release of inflammatory cytokines, activating antigen-presenting cells and donor alloreactive T cells [5]. This process results in cytotoxicity to host cells and damage to the thymus and secondary lymphoid organs, predisposing patients to cGvHD [5]. In the second phase, thymic injury permits the emergence of auto- and alloreactive T-cell populations, resulting in a loss of central and peripheral tolerance as well as impaired regulatory T- (Treg) and B-cell function [6]. Tregs play a crucial role in controlling GvHD by suppressing the activation and proliferation of alloreactive T cells [7]. Recent studies have emphasized the importance of Tregs in mitigating the severity of GvHD and have explored the potential of Treg-based therapies [8]. Donor T follicular helper (Tfh) cells expand and promote donor B-cell survival, differentiation, and anti-host immunoglobulin production, further contributing

L. Kaynar (✉) · Y. G. Mutlu
Department of Hematology, School of Medicine, Istanbul Medipol University, Istanbul, Türkiye
e-mail: leylagul.kaynar@medipol.edu.tr

I. Kozanoglu (ed.), *Problem Solving in Apheresis Medicine*,
https://doi.org/10.1007/978-3-031-74081-7_21

to the pathogenesis of cGvHD [9]. Chronic inflammation is maintained by Th17 cells escaping immune regulation, highlighting the importance of a balanced Treg/Th17 ratio in controlling GvHD progression [10]. The third phase involves aberrant tissue repair, with IL-17 and CSF-1-dependent activated macrophages producing transforming growth factor (TGF)-β and platelet-derived growth factor alpha, resulting in fibroblast activation and cGvHD manifestations such as scleroderma or bronchiolitis obliterans [11].

Patients with mild cGvHD may be treated with local therapies, such as topical steroids, based on the organ or site affected [12]. While corticosteroids, typically 0.5–1 mg/kg/day, are the standard first-line treatment for moderate and severe cGvHD, there is no evidence supporting any benefit of combination therapies in the front-line setting [13]. A response to corticosteroid treatment alone is observed in only half of the patients undergoing this therapy. More than 50% of patients require further treatment within 2 years; however, there is no standardized approach for second-line therapy [12].

The US Food and Drug Administration (FDA) has approved three distinct therapies for cGvHD. The first agent to receive regulatory clearance was ibrutinib, a Bruton's tyrosine kinase (BTK) inhibitor traditionally indicated for the treatment of B-cell malignancies. Ibrutinib is approved for cGvHD patients who have demonstrated an inadequate response to one or more prior lines of systemic therapy. Belumosudil, an orally available selective Rho-associated coiled-coil-containing protein kinase 2 (ROCK2) inhibitor, is the second targeted therapy approved by the FDA for cGvHD. Belumosudil is indicated for patients who have received at least two prior lines of therapy. The third and most recent agent, ruxolitinib, is approved for use in cGvHD patients who have failed to respond one or two lines of prior systemic therapy.

Various agents with different mechanisms of action, such as rituximab, imatinib, sirolimus, abatacept, and etanercept, constitute second-line treatment options used in clinical practice. Extracorporeal photopheresis (ECP) is used in the second and subsequent lines, either in combination with or as an alternative to other agents, in steroid-resistant or steroid-intolerant patients. Despite novel FDA-approved therapies for patients with steroid-resistant/steroid-dependent cGvHD, the choice of which agent to use as a secondary option and the effectiveness of combined therapies have yet to be conclusively determined. Therefore, second-line treatment preferences are generally based on institutional standard operating procedures, physician preference and practice, availability, cost of treatment, and patient preference.

21.2 Extracorporeal Photopheresis Technique and Mechanism of Action

ECP has emerged as a significant therapeutic modality in the field of immunomodulation since its development in the late twentieth century. ECP was first introduced in the early 1990s as a novel therapeutic approach for the treatment of cutaneous T-cell lymphoma (CTCL) [14]. The therapy's efficacy in treating CTCL was well-established, leading to its exploration in other medical conditions involving immune dysregulation. Before ECP became an option for the treatment of GvHD, it was known that photochemotherapy (PUVA) had been successfully used in patients with cGvHD involving skin and oral manifestations [15]. In the late 1980s and early 1990s, patients suffering from cGvHD were treated with methoxsalen and PUVA, as reported in a case series [16]. In this series, patients were treated with methoxsalen orally and later exposed to ultraviolet A (UVA) radiation, either locally or as a total body irradiation, after a 1–2-h interval. The question remained whether the skin lesions improved due to a local effect and/or systemic effects. There was evidence that skin biopsies performed after treatment showed a reduction in lymphohistiocytic cells and immune-histologic changes, such as a significant reduction in CD3+ T cells. However, at that time, immune effects were not proven by controls. In 1994, a patient with cGvHD of skin manifestations, refractory to corticosteroids, cyclosporine, and PUVA therapy, was successfully treated with ECP for the first time in the literature [17]. Within a few years, in the late 1990s, ECP became a therapeutic option for GvHD, leading to a response rate of up to 60% in patients who had failed corticosteroid therapy [18, 19]. After ECP demonstrated promising results in cGVHD, its effectiveness in aGvHD was also established [20, 21].

ECP conventionally involves three main steps, and the entire procedure takes around 2–4 h. The procedure starts with the collection and separation of white blood cells (WBCs) from the patient through an automated leukapheresis procedure. In the second phase, the collected cells are treated with 8-methoxypsoralen (8-MOP) to make them photosensitive to UVA radiation. Before infusion, the collected cells are exposed to UVA light with a wavelength of 320–400 nm. Finally, the treated cells are reinfused into the patient. Currently, there are two different techniques: "off-line" and "in-line," depending on the type of device or system used. The in-line system is a closed system where the entire procedure, from collection to infusion, is completed within the closed system and performed sequentially. Conversely, in the "off-line" technique, target cells are collected by an apheresis device, treated with 8-MOP externally, irradiated by an external UVA light device, and then reinfused into the patient. The in-line technique has the advantage of reducing the risk of infection and infusion errors [22].

Both approaches have their own benefits. The "off-line" technique provides superior lymphocyte collection efficiency, leading to a higher cellular yield. Despite processing and irradiating higher cell numbers in ECP, a proportional increase in therapeutic response has not yet been observed [23]. The "off-line" approach is more suitable for pediatric patients due to the larger extracorporeal volume required by the "in-line" system. In-line ECP is fast and highly automated, allowing for precise control over infusion volumes and rates, thus minimizing the risk of dosing and infusion errors. As a completely closed system, there is no risk of potential contamination throughout the process [24].

The mechanism of action of ECP has yet to be fully understood. Patient-derived, collected WBCs are treated with 8-MOP. 8-MOP rapidly enters the nuclei of cells, and without UVA exposure, it is biologically inert. After exposure to UVA irradiation, 8-MOP becomes activated and binds to pyrimidine bases of DNA, cross-linking DNA strands and causing apoptosis [23]. Several potential mechanisms of action have been proposed, starting with the hypothesis of immunomodulation by the reinfused apoptotic cells. Studies have shown that DNA damage induced by UV radiation can promote immunotolerance by activating Tregs [24, 25]. It has been shown that Tregs play a crucial role in the setting of hematopoietic stem cell transplantation, and GvHD is associated with reduced levels of Tregs [26, 27].

Furthermore, infused ECP products produce a significant number of anti-inflammatory cytokines, such as IL-10 and TGF-β [28]. Given that 10% of leukocytes are treated with 8-MOP plus UVA during each ECP procedure, it is unlikely that these few apoptotic cells are responsible for all clinical efficacies. Another mechanism of action to consider is the maturation of monocytes to dendritic cells facilitated by ECP [25]. This mechanism has been demonstrated in several diseases treated with ECP [26]. Moreover, the exposure of monocytes and dendritic cells exposure to the plastic tubing set surface also promotes the differentiation and maturation of these cells, mediated via activated platelet signaling [29]. A more recent hypothesis involves tissue-resident memory T (TRM) cells. It has been shown that, apart from circulating immune cells, TRMs can survive after conditioning regimens, and these cells are involved in GvHD [30]. These cells can migrate to GvHD-involved tissues, and during this migration process, they might become targetable by ECP. Despite the aforementioned facts and results from the studies, the precise mechanism of action of ECP still needs to be fully explained, making an era of ongoing research.

21.3 ECP in Prophylaxis

ECP is well-established as a therapeutic option in the setting of GvHD. However, given the lack of evidence, the prophylactic use of ECP in allogeneic transplantation is not part of any standard GvHD prophylaxis regimen. ECP may be a rational option for reducing the incidence of GvHD, given its favorable safety profile. Several small, non-randomized phase II studies have shown the benefit of prophylactic ECP use, with lower GvHD rates and mortality compared to historical controls [27, 28]. A prospective multicenter phase II study showed that the cumulative incidence of cGvHD in patients treated with ECP for GvHD prophylaxis after reduced-intensity conditioning allogeneic hematopoietic stem cell transplantation was 22%, and overall survival was 84% at 2 years [28]. The cumulative incidence of aGvHD ≥ grade II in the same cohort was 15% within 100 days. Another study examining the role of prophylactic ECP in myeloablative conditioning showed that ECP for the prevention of aGvHD was very effective, with overall survival significantly higher in this group compared to historical controls (83% vs. 67%, respectively, with a relative risk of 0.44). Although cGvHD was not a primary endpoint in this study, the 1-year cumulative incidence of cGvHD in patients who were evaluable was 38% [27]. Recently, the first randomized study on this matter has been published. The study enrolled 157 patients with hematologic malignancies undergoing their first allogeneic hematopoietic stem cell transplantation and randomized them into two groups: 76 patients in the intervention group, who were treated with prophylactic ECP after engraftment, and 81 patients in the control group [29]. There was no difference in the incidence of either aGvHD or cGvHD between the two groups. In addition, no differences were observed between the groups in terms of GvHD-free, recurrence-free survival, event-free survival, overall survival, and non-recurrence mortality. Despite the supportive results of previous non-randomized studies, the evidence from the above-mentioned randomized controlled trial suggests that there is no rationale for using ECP in the setting of GvHD prophylaxis.

21.4 First-Line Therapy for cGvHD

In cGvHD, similar to aGvHD, corticosteroids are used as a first-line therapy. However, approximately half of the patients do not respond to this treatment modality or, conversely, become steroid-dependent or refractory, requiring second-line therapies [13]. No standard algorithm for the selection of second-line treatment currently exists [30]. The role of ECP as a first-line therapy for cGvHD is supported by limited data. Recently, a phase I pilot study evaluated the efficacy of first-line ECP treatment in moderate to severe cGvHD. The study randomized 60 patients into two arms: one arm received conventional treatment alone, while the other arm received conventional treatment in addition to ECP. The study results showed that the conventional treatment plus ECP arm had encouraging outcomes without a decline in patients' quality of life. At week 28, the conventional arm had an overall response rate (ORR) of 74.1%, compared to 60.9% in the conventional plus ECP arm [31].

There is no available data superior to corticosteroids in the frontline setting so far. Moreover, the current literature does not provide sufficient evidence to support the addition of ECP to corticosteroid therapy or its use alone in the treatment of cGvHD as a frontline therapy [32].

21.5 Treatment of ECP/Steroid-Refractory cGvHD

While there is no standard treatment approach for steroid-resistant, steroid-dependent, and steroid-intolerant cGvHD patients, two FDA-approved agents, ruxolitinib and ibrutinib, are available for cGvHD treatment [33, 34]. However, the treatment algorithm for steroid-refractory cGvHD remains unclear according to current guidelines. Despite this, these agents have become common second-line treatments in clinical practice. ECP is considered one of the second or more advanced treatment alternatives [13, 35, 36]. Several randomized controlled, prospective, and retrospective studies are available in the literature regarding the use of ECP in steroid-refractory cGvHD [37–45]. Due to changes in staging and response assessment of cGvHD according to NIH criteria, interpreting response rates between studies is challenging. Nonetheless, ECP has shown an ORR of around 30–80% in these studies. The main advantage of ECP is steroid-sparing effect, which has been reported by several investigators. In a prospective, randomized multicenter phase II study conducted by Flowers et al., conventional treatment alone ($n = 47$) or conventional treatment plus ECP therapy ($n = 48$) was applied to cases with skin GvHD that could not be controlled with standard corticosteroid therapy. As a result, at the end of the third month, the addition of ECP to conventional therapy showed a steroid dose-reducing effect [46]. Among the 29 patients who did not respond adequately in the control group and could not reduce their steroid dose (non-ECP), ECP was later applied, resulting in a response rate of 42–100% (complete and partial) in extracutaneous cGvHD after week 24, with the highest response in the oral mucosa at 70% [47]. Another encouraging result came from a prospective study by Foss et al., which reported that steroid sparing or discontinuation was possible in 80% of patients treated with ECP [39]. Dignan et al. reported similar results, with 77% of patients who completed 6 months of ECP treatment achieving corticosteroid dose reduction [43]. Since there is no evidence of a superior therapy in the first-line setting for cGvHD, corticosteroids remain a mandatory option for frontline therapy and are therefore widely used. The steroid-sparing effect of ECP is crucial for patients who are candidates for long-term steroid use due to adverse effects.

ECP, as an emerging significant therapeutic modality, has several issues that need to be addressed. First, steroid resistance and dependence should be properly defined. The Turkish ECP (TECP) group, established under the Turkish Society of Apheresis, recently published a position statement on ECP in aGvHD and cGvHD. The recommendations by TECP for ECP use in cGvHD and the definitions of steroid resistance and dependence are outlined below.

ECP therapy can be administered as a second-line or subsequent treatment for patients with steroid-resistant, steroid-dependent, and steroid-intolerant cGvHD, as described below:

1. Steroid-resistant cGvHD: progression despite prednisone at ≥1 mg/kg/day for 1 week.
2. Steroid-dependent aGvHD: Inability to reduce prednisone dose below 0.25 mg/kg/day after two failed attempts made 8 weeks apart or stable GvHD on ≥0.5 mg/kg/day of prednisone for 1–2 months.
3. Steroid-intolerant aGvHD: Intolerance to steroids at the dose required for treatment due to serious side effects.

In addition to numerous observational, prospective, and retrospective studies, the excellent safety profile of ECP and its lack of effect on the graft-versus-leukemia effect support the early use of ECP in post-steroid cGvHD treatments [48–50].

21.6 Treatment Scheme of ECP in cGvHD

ECP is commonly used alone or in combination with other treatment modalities in the setting of cGvHD. In a meta-analysis by Malik et al., the pooled response rates were reported as 74% in the skin, 68% in the liver, 60% in the eyes, 72% in the mouth, 48% in the lungs, 53% in the gastrointestinal system, and 64% in the musculoskeletal system [51].

Neither guidelines nor studies evaluating ECP treatment in the presence of cGvHD provide a clear determination of the most efficient treatment schedule. The recommendations in the guidelines and in studies vary regarding the intensity of ECP treatment at the beginning. One cycle is defined as two procedures on consecutive days in most schedules. In the literature, the frequency of cycles or procedures varies, with treatment either weekly or every 2–3 weeks. The duration of ECP is not standardized, and the recommendation for the intensity of the procedures in the guidelines is based on the response obtained [52–55]. The effect of ECP in cGvHD seems to be slow; therefore, it is recommended in the guidelines to assess the response after 2–3 months. Treatment schedules and management according to current guidelines are detailed in Table 21.1.

Table 21.1 Indications and treatment schedules for ECP in cGvHD according to recent guidelines[a]

The UK Photopheresis Society (2017) [53]
Indication: Steroid-refractory, steroid-dependent, or steroid-intolerant GvHD **Schedule:** One cycle (two treatments on consecutive days) every 2 weeks After completion of the initial six uninterrupted treatment cycles, assess to determine the further treatment **If partial response is achieved:** Taper 4-weekly treatment and continue until maximal response
ASFA[b] (2019) [56]
Indication: Second-line therapy of cutaneous and non-cutaneous cGvHD (level of evidence cII), either as monotherapy or in conjunction with other therapies **Schedule:** One cycle (two treatments) weekly for 4 weeks (or consider biweekly if treating only mucocutaneous cGvHD) and then one cycle every 2 weeks or for at least 8 weeks (assess at 2–3 monthly intervals). Continue to maximum response every 2–4 weeks with taper
European Dermatology Forum (2020) [55]
Indication: Second-line therapy in patients with steroid-dependent, steroid-intolerant, or steroid-resistant cGvHD and those with recurrent infections or a high-risk relapse of their underlying disease **Schedule:** Weekly one cycle (two treatments) for the first 3 months or until GvHD stabilizes, followed by one cycle twice per month and tapered depending on clinical response. If cGvHD progresses, a change in the treatment strategy should be considered Serial quality of life assessments, in addition to clinical response criteria, are recommended
Nordic ECP Quality Group (2020) [54]
Indication: Steroid-refractory, steroid-dependent, or steroid-intolerant cGvHD **Schedule:** One sequence (one treatment on 2 consecutive days) every second week for 12 weeks. Assess treatment response at 3 months **If complete response is achieved:** Stop ECP **If partial response, minimal response, or mixed response is achieved:** Reduce frequency to every 2 weeks **Progressive disease:** Stop ECP and/or consider additional or other treatment options
Turkish ECP (TECP) Group (2022) [54]
Indication: As a second-line or following lines of therapy for steroid-refractory, steroid-dependent, or steroid-intolerant cGvHD **Schedule:** One cycle weekly (biweekly if treating only mucocutaneous cGvHD) for the first 2–3 months, followed by one cycle twice per month for 2 months, and then tapered depending on clinical response Assesses the treatment response every 2–3 months **If complete response is achieved:** Stop ECP **If partial response is achieved:** Continue until achieving maximum response **Progressive/mixed or stable disease:** Stop treatment or add additional agents

[a] This table has been modified from reference number [32]
[b] The 2023 ASFA Guidelines proposed a general treatment scheme that typically involves one cycle extending up to 3 months, with the frequency of treatment being once a week or once every 2 weeks for disease stabilization. Thereafter, the frequency is reduced to one cycle every 2–4 weeks [57]

21.7 Considerations and Patient Groups to Be Cautioned for ECP

ECP requires long-term patient commitment. Therefore, there are clinical and practical factors that should be addressed before starting treatment, such as the patient's proximity to the hospital and the ability to maintain safe and suitable vascular access. Vascular access should be efficient to allow successful procedures over a long period; therefore, permanent venous access devices are recommended, especially for patients with inefficient peripheral venous access. Other clinical variables that should be assessed include hemodynamic and respiratory instability, uncontrolled infection, pregnancy, sensitivity to psoralen products, known photosensitivity, aphakia (which carries an increased risk of retinal damage), and active bleeding. Pretreatment blood tests vary depending on the patient's clinical status. However, most centers perform a complete blood count and assess electrolytes, including calcium, magnesium, and potassium, particularly when ACD-A is used as an anticoagulant. Generally, at least 1×10^9/L cells (WBC) in the peripheral blood are required to start ECP, and granulocyte-colony stimulating factor (G-CSF) support may be required for patients who do not have enough cells in their peripheral blood. Regarding platelet count, patients with a low platelet count (<20 × 109/L despite platelet transfusion support) should be approached with caution [54]. However, in patients with low hematocrit, platelet, and leucocyte counts, as well as those with low body weight, apheresis may be performed after taking the necessary precautions [33, 54].

21.8 ECP/Adverse Effects

The most important caveats about other immunosuppressive therapies currently available for the treatment of cGvHD are immunosuppression-induced opportunistic infections, organ toxicities, and underlying disease relapse. ECP does not cause immunosuppression or interfere with the graft-versus-leukemia effect; thus, it is quite safe for patients who have high-risk features of disease relapse [34]. Adverse effects in 13,871 ECP procedures were reported by the World Apheresis Association over a 17-year period, with a 5.4% rate for first treatments and 1.2% for subsequent procedures [46]. Furthermore, the severe adverse effect rate was 0.04%, and no ECP-related deaths were reported. Adverse reactions might occur either due to leukapheresis procedure, such as issues with the extracorporeal circuit, citrate toxicity, mild thrombocytopenia, and anemia, or psoralen-induced adverse events, such as skin redness, itchiness, or light sensitivity. Therefore, it is recommended that patients take measures to protect their skin and eyes from UVA rays for 24–48 h after the procedure due to increased photosensitivity [47]. Rarely, fever, tiredness, and hematuria might occur after reinfusion of ECP products due to the infusion of red blood cells post-exposure to 8-MOP [58].

21.9 Conclusion

Despite allogeneic stem cell transplantation being the only curative option for many diseases, GvHD causes significant mortality and morbidity in the majority of cases. In recent years, two FDA-approved agents, ruxolitinib and ibrutinib, have been widely used in the treatment of steroid-refractory GvHD. However, there is no consensus on the optimal treatment of steroid-refractory cGvHD in the guidelines. ECP is featured as a reasonable alternative in the guidelines, but its technical nature and the requirement for specialized experience that is not readily available at all centers makes it difficult to access. Another issue that it is also a long-term therapy that requires patient adherence. Despite these challenges, ECP remains a preferred treatment method for steroid-resistant GvHD due to its high response rates, lack of generalized immunosuppression, absence of increased risk of infection and relapse, and lack of serious complications.

References

1. Jagasia MH, Greinix HT, Arora M, Williams KM, Wolff D, Cowen EW, et al. National Institutes of Health consensus development project on criteria for clinical trials in chronic graft-versus-host disease: I. The 2014 diagnosis and staging working group report. Biol Blood Marrow Transplant. 2015;21(3):389–401. e1
2. Bhatt VR, Wang T, Chen K, Kitko CL, MacMillan ML, Pidala JA, et al. Chronic graft-versus-host disease, nonrelapse mortality, and disease relapse in older versus younger adults undergoing matched allogeneic peripheral blood hematopoietic cell transplantation: a Center for International Blood and Marrow Transplant Research Analysis. Transplant Cell Ther. 2022;28(1):34–42.
3. Socie G, Ritz J. Current issues in chronic graft-versus-host disease. Blood. 2014;124(3):374–84.
4. Zeiser R, Blazar BR. Pathophysiology of chronic graft-versus-host disease and therapeutic targets. N Engl J Med. 2017;377(26):2565–79.
5. Shlomchik WD. Graft-versus-host disease. Nat Rev Immunol. 2007;7(5):340–52.
6. Bleakley M, Riddell SR. Molecules and mechanisms of the graft-versus-leukaemia effect. Nat Rev Cancer. 2004;4(5):371–80.
7. Sakaguchi S, Miyara M, Costantino CM, Hafler DA. FOXP3+ regulatory T cells in the human immune system. Nat Rev Immunol. 2010;10(7):490–500.
8. Koreth J, Matsuoka K, Kim HT, McDonough SM, Bindra B, Alyea EP 3rd, et al. Interleukin-2 and regulatory T cells in graft-versus-host disease. N Engl J Med. 2011;365(22):2055–66.
9. Forcade E, Kim HT, Cutler C, Wang K, Alho AC, Nikiforow S, et al. Circulating T follicular helper cells with increased function during chronic graft-versus-host disease. Blood. 2016;127(20):2489–97.

10. Noval Rivas M, Chatila TA. Regulatory T cells in allergic diseases. J Allergy Clin Immunol. 2016;138(3):639–52.
11. MacDonald KP, Hill GR, Blazar BR. Chronic graft-versus-host disease: biological insights from preclinical and clinical studies. Blood. 2017;129(1):13–21.
12. Flowers ME, Martin PJ. How we treat chronic graft-versus-host disease. Blood. 2015;125(4):606–15.
13. Penack O, Marchetti M, Ruutu T, Aljurf M, Bacigalupo A, Bonifazi F, et al. Prophylaxis and management of graft versus host disease after stem-cell transplantation for haematological malignancies: updated consensus recommendations of the European Society for Blood and Marrow Transplantation. Lancet Haematol. 2020;7(2):e157–e67.
14. Edelson R, Berger C, Gasparro F, Jegasothy B, Heald P, Wintroub B, et al. Treatment of cutaneous T-cell lymphoma by extracorporeal photochemotherapy. Preliminary results. N Engl J Med. 1987;316(6):297–303.
15. Volc-Platzer B, Honigsmann H, Hinterberger W, Wolff K. Photochemotherapy improves chronic cutaneous graft-versus-host disease. J Am Acad Dermatol. 1990;23(2 Pt 1):220–8.
16. Hymes SR, Morison WL, Farmer ER, Walters LL, Tutschka PJ, Santos GW. Methoxsalen and ultraviolet A radiation in treatment of chronic cutaneous graft-versus-host reaction. J Am Acad Dermatol. 1985;12(1 Pt 1):30–7.
17. Owsianowski M, Gollnick H, Siegert W, Schwerdtfeger R, Orfanos CE. Successful treatment of chronic graft-versus-host disease with extracorporeal photopheresis. Bone Marrow Transplant. 1994;14(5):845–8.
18. Greinix HT, Volc-Platzer B, Rabitsch W, Gmeinhart B, Guevara-Pineda C, Kalhs P, et al. Successful use of extracorporeal photochemotherapy in the treatment of severe acute and chronic graft-versus-host disease. Blood. 1998;92(9):3098–104.
19. Besnier DP, Chabannes D, Mahe B, Mussini JM, Baranger TA, Muller JY, et al. Treatment of graft-versus-host disease by extracorporeal photochemotherapy: a pilot study. Transplantation. 1997;64(1):49–54.
20. Greinix HT, Volc-Platzer B, Knobler RM. Extracorporeal photochemotherapy in the treatment of severe graft-versus-host disease. Leuk Lymphoma. 2000;36(5–6):425–34.
21. Salvaneschi L, Perotti C, Zecca M, Bernuzzi S, Viarengo G, Giorgiani G, et al. Extracorporeal photochemotherapy for treatment of acute and chronic GVHD in childhood. Transfusion. 2001;41(10):1299–305.
22. Dunbar NM, Raval JS, Johnson A, Abikoff CM, Adamski J, Cooling LL, et al. Extracorporeal photopheresis practice patterns: an international survey by the ASFA ECP subcommittee. J Clin Apher. 2017;32(4):215–23.
23. Piccirillo N, Putzulu R, Massini G, Di Giovanni A, Giammarco S, Metafuni E, et al. Inline and offline extracorporeal photopheresis: device performance, cell yields and clinical response. J Clin Apher. 2021;36(1):118–26.
24. Helmberg W, Sipurzynski S, Groselje-Strehle A, Greinix H, Schlenke P. Does offline beat inline treatment: investigation into extracorporeal Photopheresis. Transfus Med Hemother. 2020;47(3):198–204.
25. Durazzo TS, Tigelaar RE, Filler R, Hayday A, Girardi M, Edelson RL. Induction of monocyte-to-dendritic cell maturation by extracorporeal photochemotherapy: initiation via direct platelet signaling. Transfus Apher Sci. 2014;50(3):370–8.
26. Atta M, Papanicolaou N, Tsirigotis P. The role of extracorporeal photopheresis in the treatment of cutaneous T-cell lymphomas. Transfus Apher Sci. 2012;46(2):195–202.
27. Shaughnessy PJ, Bolwell BJ, van Besien K, Mistrik M, Grigg A, Dodds A, et al. Extracorporeal photopheresis for the prevention of acute GVHD in patients undergoing standard myeloablative conditioning and allogeneic hematopoietic stem cell transplantation. Bone Marrow Transplant. 2010;45(6):1068–76.
28. Michallet M, Sobh M, Garban F, Bulabois CE, Yakoub-Agha I, Coiteux V, et al. Extracorporeal photopheresis for GVHD prophylaxis after reduced intensity conditioning allogeneic hematopoietic stem cell transplantation: a prospective multicenter phase 2 study. Leuk Lymphoma. 2018;59(2):372–80.
29. Ali MM, Gedde-Dahl T, Osnes LT, Perrier F, Veierod MB, Tjonnfjord GE, et al. Extracorporeal photopheresis as graft-versus-host disease prophylaxis: a randomized controlled trial. Transplant Cell Ther. 2023;29:364.e1.
30. Holtzman NG, Pavletic SZ. The clinical landscape of chronic graft-versus-host disease management in 2021. Br J Haematol. 2022;196(4):830–48.
31. Jagasia M, Scheid C, Socie G, Ayuk FA, Tischer J, Donato ML, et al. Randomized controlled study of ECP with methoxsalen as first-line treatment of patients with moderate to severe cGVHD. Blood Adv. 2019;3(14):2218–29.
32. Kaynar L, Tekgunduz E, Kozanoglu I, Ozkan HA, Aksu S, Ozkalemkas F, et al. Extracorporeal photopheresis in the treatment of acute and chronic graft-versus-host disease: a position statement from the Turkish Society of Apheresis (TSA). Transfus Apher Sci. 2022;61(1):103373.
33. McLeod BC, Sniecinski I, Ciavarella D, Owen H, Price TH, Randels MJ, et al. Frequency of immediate adverse effects associated with therapeutic apheresis. Transfusion. 1999;39(3):282–8.
34. Knobler R, Berlin G, Calzavara-Pinton P, Greinix H, Jaksch P, Laroche L, et al. Guidelines on the use of extracorporeal photopheresis. J Eur Acad Dermatol Venereol. 2014;28 Suppl 1(Suppl 1):1–37.
35. Wolff D, Schleuning M, von Harsdorf S, Bacher U, Gerbitz A, Stadler M, et al. Consensus conference on clinical practice in chronic GVHD: second-line treatment of chronic graft-versus-host disease. Biol Blood Marrow Transplant. 2011;17(1):1–17.
36. Abu-Dalle I, Reljic T, Nishihori T, Antar A, Bazarbachi A, Djulbegovic B, et al. Extracorporeal

photopheresis in steroid-refractory acute or chronic graft-versus-host disease: results of a systematic review of prospective studies. Biol Blood Marrow Transplant. 2014;20(11):1677–86.
37. Flowers ME, Apperley JF, van Besien K, Elmaagacli A, Grigg A, Reddy V, et al. A multicenter prospective phase 2 randomized study of extracorporeal photopheresis for treatment of chronic graft-versus-host disease. Blood. 2008;112(7):2667–74.
38. Greinix HT, van Besien K, Elmaagacli AH, Hillen U, Grigg A, Knobler R, et al. Progressive improvement in cutaneous and extracutaneous chronic graft-versus-host disease after a 24-week course of extracorporeal photopheresis—results of a crossover randomized study. Biol Blood Marrow Transplant. 2011;17(12):1775–82.
39. Foss FM, DiVenuti GM, Chin K, Sprague K, Grodman H, Klein A, et al. Prospective study of extracorporeal photopheresis in steroid-refractory or steroid-resistant extensive chronic graft-versus-host disease: analysis of response and survival incorporating prognostic factors. Bone Marrow Transplant. 2005;35(12):1187–93.
40. Dignan FL, Aguilar S, Scarisbrick JJ, Shaw BE, Potter MN, Cavenagh J, et al. Impact of extracorporeal photopheresis on skin scores and quality of life in patients with steroid-refractory chronic GVHD. Bone Marrow Transplant. 2014;49(5):704–8.
41. Del Fante C, Scudeller L, Viarengo G, Bernasconi P, Perotti C. Response and survival of patients with chronic graft-versus-host disease treated by extracorporeal photochemotherapy: a retrospective study according to classical and National Institutes of Health classifications. Transfusion. 2012;52(9):2007–15.
42. Couriel DR, Hosing C, Saliba R, Shpall EJ, Anderlini P, Rhodes B, et al. Extracorporeal photochemotherapy for the treatment of steroid-resistant chronic GVHD. Blood. 2006;107(8):3074–80.
43. Dignan FL, Greenblatt D, Cox M, Cavenagh J, Oakervee H, Apperley JF, et al. Efficacy of bimonthly extracorporeal photopheresis in refractory chronic mucocutaneous GVHD. Bone Marrow Transplant. 2012;47(6):824–30.
44. Nygaard M, Karlsmark T, Andersen NS, Schjodt IM, Petersen SL, Friis LS, et al. Longitudinal follow-up of response status and concomitant immunosuppression in patients treated with extracorporeal photopheresis for chronic graft versus host disease. Bone Marrow Transplant. 2019;54(1):35–43.
45. Apisarnthanarax N, Donato M, Korbling M, Couriel D, Gajewski J, Giralt S, et al. Extracorporeal photopheresis therapy in the management of steroid-refractory or steroid-dependent cutaneous chronic graft-versus-host disease after allogeneic stem cell transplantation: feasibility and results. Bone Marrow Transplant. 2003;31(6):459–65.
46. Blaha M, Gasova Z, Berlin G, Audzijoniene J, Griskevicius A, Dykes J, et al. Analysis of extracorporeal photopheresis within the frame of the WAA register. Transfus Apher Sci. 2021;60(5):103172.
47. Arora S, Setia R. Extracorporeal photopheresis: review of technical aspects. Asian J Transfus Sci. 2017;11(2):81–6.
48. Kanold J, Merlin E, Halle P, Paillard C, Marabelle A, Rapatel C, et al. Photopheresis in pediatric graft-versus-host disease after allogeneic marrow transplantation: clinical practice guidelines based on field experience and review of the literature. Transfusion. 2007;47(12):2276–89.
49. Greinix HT, Socie G, Bacigalupo A, Holler E, Edinger MG, Apperley JF, et al. Assessing the potential role of photopheresis in hematopoietic stem cell transplant. Bone Marrow Transplant. 2006;38(4):265–73.
50. Kanold J, Messina C, Halle P, Locatelli F, Lanino E, Cesaro S, et al. Update on extracorporeal photochemotherapy for graft-versus-host disease treatment. Bone Marrow Transplant. 2005;35(Suppl 1):S69–71.
51. Malik MI, Litzow M, Hogan W, Patnaik M, Murad MH, Prokop LJ, et al. Extracorporeal photopheresis for chronic graft-versus-host disease: a systematic review and meta-analysis. Blood Res. 2014;49(2):100–6.
52. Schwartz J, Padmanabhan A, Aqui N, Balogun RA, Connelly-Smith L, Delaney M, et al. Guidelines on the use of therapeutic apheresis in clinical practice-evidence-based approach from the writing Committee of the American Society for apheresis: the seventh special issue. J Clin Apher. 2016;31(3):149–62.
53. Alfred A, Taylor PC, Dignan F, El-Ghariani K, Griffin J, Gennery AR, et al. The role of extracorporeal photopheresis in the management of cutaneous T-cell lymphoma, graft-versus-host disease and organ transplant rejection: a consensus statement update from the UK Photopheresis society. Br J Haematol. 2017;177(2):287–310.
54. Nygaard M, Wichert S, Berlin G, Toss F. Extracorporeal photopheresis for graft-vs-host disease: a literature review and treatment guidelines proposed by the Nordic ECP quality group. Eur J Haematol. 2020;104(5):361–75.
55. Knobler R, Arenberger P, Arun A, Assaf C, Bagot M, Berlin G, et al. European dermatology forum—updated guidelines on the use of extracorporeal photopheresis 2020—part 1. J Eur Acad Dermatol Venereol. 2020;34(12):2693–716.
56. Padmanabhan A, Connelly-Smith L, Aqui N, Balogun RA, Klingel R, Meyer E, et al. Guidelines on the use of therapeutic apheresis in clinical practice—evidence-based approach from the writing Committee of the American Society for apheresis: the eighth special issue. J Clin Apher. 2019;34(3):171–354.
57. Connelly-Smith L, Alquist CR, Aqui NA, Hofmann JC, Klingel R, Onwuemene OA, et al. Guidelines on the use of therapeutic apheresis in clinical practice—evidence-based approach from the writing Committee of the American Society for apheresis: the ninth special issue. J Clin Apher. 2023;38(2):77–278.
58. Vieyra-Garcia PA, Wolf P. Extracorporeal photopheresis: a case of immunotherapy ahead of its time. Transfus Med Hemother. 2020;47(3):226–35.

Part VIII

What Should to Talk About for Apheresis at the Future

Quality Control Principles in Apheresis

22

Songül Tepebaşı and İlknur Kozanoğlu

22.1 Facility and Infrastructure

The apheresis unit should have sufficient physical space, infrastructure, and equipment to support its operations. The unit's layout and design must enable safe evaluation of donors and patient, as well as procedures that prevent contamination and mix-ups. Clear routes for fast and smooth transport to the intensive care unit and emergency services should be established in advance. Environmental controls should be implemented to minimize risk to patients and donors. Systems should be in place to monitor and record temperature, humidity, microbiological air quality, asepsis procedures, cleaning records, and waste removal processes [1–6].

S. Tepebaşı (✉)
Baskent University Adana Dr. Turgut Noyan Research and Medical Center, Quality Manager of Adult Bone Marrow Transplantation Center, Adana, Turkey

EBMT Quality Management Group, Maastricht, The Netherlands

İ. Kozanoğlu
Adana Adult BMT Center, Baskent University, Adana, Türkiye

Acibadem Labmed Medical Laboratories, Hematology Laboratories, Istanbul, Türkiye
e-mail: kozanoglu@baskent.edu.tr

22.2 Personnel and Job Description

Staff organization and collaboration are essential for achieving successful outcomes [5]. To ensure uninterrupted service, it is important to define the roles of key personnel. A sufficient number of trained and competent personnel should be assigned to the unit, with staffing levels based on the unit's activities.

Defining backup personnel, in addition to key personnel, is crucial to avoid interruption in activities [1–9].

The roles of personnel in the organizational chart of cellular therapy centers must be clearly defined in advance. Job descriptions should be written in a clear and understandable manner, so that employees can readily understand their responsibilities without needing to interpret beyond the written text [7].

22.3 Education and Qualifications

All employees working in therapeutic apheresis (TA) must continually develop to keep up with new treatment options. To support this, personnel knowledge and skills should be enhanced through ongoing training, while employee competencies are regularly assessed and documented. Effective employee performance reflects the quality and

I. Kozanoglu (ed.), *Problem Solving in Apheresis Medicine*,
https://doi.org/10.1007/978-3-031-74081-7_22

relevance of their training, alignment with job requirements, and the overall system's effectiveness in achieving expected outcomes [1–7]. Various methods can be used to assess employee qualifications for specific roles, including evaluation tables based on observation or electronic monitoring systems [8].

22.4 Device Maintenance and Controls

To achieve optimal efficiency from all devices used in the unit, the technical specifications of each device must meet required standards, and a sufficient number of devices should be available. New or recently repaired devices should be validated before use. Device settings and technical features can change over time or with usage, which may affect performance even if the device initially meets required conditions. Therefore, devices should be calibrated periodically, and procedures should be in place for addressing any issues. The qualifications of personnel performing maintenance and calibration should also be clearly defined [9–11].

22.5 Equipment

The purpose of inventory management is to ensure that consumables and reagent supplies needed for services are readily available on site. For effective stock management, there should be an up-to-date inventory of drugs, consumables, and kits used in all critical operations. All items in this inventory must be traceable. Critical stock levels should be established for essential materials, with expiration controls in place and visual alerts for critical and minimum stock levels. To prevent shortages, especially of critical drugs, minimum levels should be clearly defined. It is recommended to document shared responsibilities with the purchasing unit to ensure the timely and high-quality procurement of devices, materials, and consumables for operational processes [12–15].

22.6 Validation

All critical processes, measurements, services, environmental factors, and materials must be validated before use. The purpose of the validation process is to assess and document the functionality and performance of each procedure [13, 14].

Changes in tools and equipment, particularly modifications in applied processes, may negatively impact performance, quality, and service. In such cases, re-validation is required, and the new method is implemented only after compliance is confirmed. The Validation Master Plan should define each procedure requiring validation, specify who will conduct it, describe the method, and outline how results will be analyzed. Each validation study should be clear, understandable, acceptable, and thoroughly documented [13, 14].

22.7 Quality Management

22.7.1 Documentation

Documentation is one of the most important cornerstones of an effective quality management system (QMS). The QMS should ensure that work is standardized and that all stages are traceable, including those related to quality control and quality assurance, such as coding, patient/donor suitability, and procedures.

The QMS should include documentation such as standard operating procedures (SOPs), guidelines, training materials, reference manuals, report forms, and patient/donor records. SOPs should be written to outline the necessary steps for writing, approving, implementing, updating, archiving, and destroying the SOP (SOP for SOP). Before SOPs are implemented, training should be conducted, proficiency documented, and training repeated with each revision [5, 6, 16, 17].

22.7.2 Risk Management

It is essential to define how to determine the preventive, corrective, and control measures needed to identify hazards related to cellular therapies and to prioritize risks. Another important aspect of risk analysis is understanding the risks and deciding on methods to mitigate them. Four ways to respond to identified risks are described as follows [18–20]:

1. Avoiding or terminating the risk: Some risks can only be reduced to an acceptable level by terminating the activity.
2. Transferring the risk: It is possible to transfer some risks to others, such as through insurance or service level agreements.
3. Tolerating or bearing the risk: The risk can be tolerated by making adjustments, taking into account the potential benefits gained [18–20].

Events that seriously affect occupational health and safety, such as fire, flash, or explosion, should trigger reassessment, even if they do not result in a work-related accident or disease [18–20].

22.7.3 Audit

Auditing is an essential element of quality management. Audits are conducted to assess the effectiveness of the QMS and to determine whether changes or improvements are necessary. If the system is not meeting the desired level, audits should be conducted more frequently to improve the system [10, 21].

22.7.4 Adverse Events and Corrective and Preventive Actions

To identify factors that compromise patient, donor, product, or employee safety and to implement necessary corrections, all errors, accidents, and side effects associated with stem cell transplantation should be recorded, investigated, and addressed with preventive measures [10, 22, 23].

Necessary data should be collected to minimize risks and ensure that all process steps in the treatment processes are properly executed. A system should be established to inform, research, and record side effects and adverse events, and all employees should use this system. The quality manager should monitor the efficiency of the process and ensure proper documentation [10, 22, 23].

22.7.5 Emergency/Disaster

TA should have an emergency plan linked to national disaster preparedness and response plans to avoid confusion, prevent duplication of efforts, and optimize resource use [24].

In case of emergency, written instructions should outline the steps personnel must follow in the event of deviations. Duties related to emergency/disaster procedures should be documented, and personnel should receive training on their responsibilities. In collaboration with occupational safety experts, warning signs should be placed in necessary areas, and personal protective equipment should be used [24].

22.7.6 Continuous Quality Improvement

The goal of all arrangements is to ensure continuous improvement within the unit. To achieve this, it is essential to identify what needs improvement, determine who will be affected by the changes, and establish how ideas for improvement will be evaluated, planned, and implemented. Additionally, the effectiveness of these changes should be measured and audited.

22.8 Policies and Procedures

22.8.1 Patient and Donor Evaluation

All activities carried out in the unit must comply with European Union directives, laws, regulations, international standards, and guidelines [1–6]. In all procedures, the patient and donor should be informed, and their consent must be obtained. Before the procedure, evaluations should be made regarding the indication for the procedure, order content, patient and donor identification information, personnel, devices, equipment, drugs, and materials. All medical information about the patient or donor should be reviewed and recorded. Procedures should be performed by competent personnel under the supervision and control of a physician [1–6].

22.9 Traceability

Traceability refers to documenting who, when, at what time, with which device, for how long, with which order, and by whom, for all activities carried out in the unit, from start to finish or vice versa. Ensuring traceability facilitates compliance with rules and standards, reduces risk, and allows for better control of operations. This improves connectivity and coherence between processes [1–6].

At least, for cellular treatments, the following should be documented and traceable: patient/donor consent, orders, pretreatment preparation, medical observation and intervention during the procedure, adverse events occurring during the procedure, and who performed each action, when, and which device was used.

This includes tracking all records related to the patient and donor, obtaining necessary reports, entering laboratory results, creating special warnings and markings based on those results, and managing the content of the products collected from the patients and donors, as well as the required reports for product transfer and safe execution of all these processes.

22.10 Records

Accurate and complete documentation of patient files, including information about the patient's arrival and the procedures performed by all health professionals involved, helps the physician quickly identify the patient and begin effective treatment without delay. Accurate and complete data is essential for the implementation, development, and effectiveness of treatments. Therefore, data management activities should begin concurrently with quality activities in the unit. Properly recorded and archived comprehensive data assists physicians in making more accurate decisions regarding patients/donors and protects them from potential risks [25–29]. Data should be archived in accordance with directives, laws, regulations, and international standards. If data is to be destroyed, the responsible party and method of destruction should be clearly defined [1–6, 27–29].

22.11 Conclusion

To achieve successful treatment outcomes, all stages, including long-term follow-up of the patient and donor, must be planned and organized in accordance with internationally accepted standards from the patient's admission to the unit. The most effective way to ensure the safe and appropriate use of TA treatments, including cellular therapy products, is to standardize and control each step in the process.

References

1. Directive 2004/23/EC of the European Parliament and of the Council of 31 March 2004 on setting standards of quality and safety for the donation, procurement, testing, processing, preservation, storage and distribution of human tissues and cells.
2. Commission Directive 2006/17/EC of 8 February 2006 implementing Directive 2004/23/EC of the European Parliament and of the Council as regards certain technical requirements for the donation, procurement and testing of human tissues and cells.
3. Commission Directive 2006/86/EC of 24 October 2006 implementing Directive 2004/23/EC of the European Parliament and of the Council as regards traceability requirements, notification of serious adverse reactions and events and certain technical requirements for the coding, processing, preservation, storage and distribution of human tissues and cells.
4. Directive 2001/83/EC of the European Parliament and of the Council of 6 November 2001 on the Community code relating to medicinal products for human use.
5. FACT-JACIE. Standards for haematopoietic progenitor cell collection, processing and transplantation. 8th ed. 2021.
6. International standards for therapeutic apheresis units (TAU). 3 th ed. 2018.

7. Tepebası S, Kozanoglu I. Personnel requirements including job descriptions. In: Aljurt M, Snowden J, Hayden P, Orchard KH, McGrath E, editors. Quality management and accreditation in hematopoietic stem cell transplantation and cellular therapy. The JACIE guide. Switzerland: Springer; 2021. p. 53–60.
8. Kozanoglu I, Tepebası S. Training programme. In: Aljurt M, Snowden J, Hayden P, Orchard KH, McGrath E, editors. Quality management and accreditation in hematopoietic stem cell transplantation and cellular therapy. The JACIE guide. Switzerland: Springer; 2021. p. 157–64.
9. Kovancı A. Toplam Kalite Yönetimi. 1. Baskı. İstanbul: Sistem Yayıncılık; 2001. p. 15.
10. Boga C, Kozanoglu I. JACIE accreditation from the perspective of an accredited centre. Bone Marrow Transplant. 2017;52(9):1352.
11. Van Der Gouw L. Tracking and traceability. In: Aljurt M, Snowden J, Hayden P, Orchard KH, McGrath E, editors. Quality management and accreditation in hematopoietic stem cell transplantation and cellular therapy. The JACIE guide. Switzerland.: Springer; 2021. p. 83–8.
12. Monteleone R, Klarmann D. Qualification and validation. In: Aljurt M, Snowden J, Hayden P, Orchard KH, McGrath E, editors. Quality management and accreditation in hematopoietic stem cell transplantation and cellular therapy. The JACIE guide. Switzerland: Springer; 2021. p. 35–43.
13. EudraLex. EU guidelines for good manufacturing practice for medicinal products for human and veterinary use Annex 15: qualification and validation. Vol. 4. http://academy.gmp-compliance.org/guidemgr/fles/2015-10_annex15.pdf.
14. EudraLex. The rules governing medicinal products in the European Union. Vol 4. Good manufacturing practice medicinal products for human and veterinary use Annex 11: computerized systems. http://academy.gmp-compliance.org/guidemgr/fles/annex11_01-2011_en.pdf.
15. Villar OL. Process indicators. In: Aljurt M, Snowden J, Hayden P, Orchard KH, McGrath E, editors. Quality management and accreditation in hematopoietic stem cell transplantation and cellular therapy. The JACIE guide. Switzerland: Springer; 2021. p. 99–107.
16. JACIE. A practical guide to implement quality management in a stem cell transplantation programme. Quality management guide. 1st ed. 2008.
17. Aljurf M, et al. Quality management and accreditation in hematopoietic stem cell transplantation and cellular therapy: the JACIE guide. Cham, CH: Springer; 2021.
18. Vives J, Amposta J. Risk management. In: Aljurt M, Snowden J, Hayden P, Orchard KH, McGrath E, editors. Quality management and accreditation in hematopoietic stem cell transplantation and cellular therapy. The JACIE guide. Switzerland: Springer; 2021. p. 165–77.
19. Schneider CK, Salmikangas P, Jilma B, Flamion B, Todorova LR, Paphitou A, et al. Challenges with advanced therapy medicinal products and how to meet them. Nat Rev Drug Discov. 2010;9(3):195–201.
20. Fischbach MA, Bluestone JA, Lim WA. Cell-based therapeutics: the next pillar of medicine. Sci Transl Med. 2013;5(179):179–86.
21. López-Villar O, Dolva J. Audits. In: Aljurt M, Snowden J, Hayden P, Orchard KH, McGrath E, editors. Quality management and accreditation in hematopoietic stem cell transplantation and cellular therapy. The JACIE guide. Switzerland: Springer; 2021. p. 25–35.
22. Huynh P, Monteleone R. Adverse events and corrective and protective actions. In: Aljurt M, Snowden J, Hayden P, Orchard KH, McGrath E, editors. Quality management and accreditation in hematopoietic stem cell transplantation and cellular therapy. The JACIE guide. Switzerland: Springer; 2021. p. 89–99.
23. World Health Organization (WHO). Disaster preparedness and response: World Health Organization regional office for Europe; 2009. http://www.preventionweb.net/files/10464_NPmeetingAstanaWHOPPT.pdf. Accessed 11 Dec 2016.
24. Abrahams J. Disaster risk management for health overview. Geneva: World Health Organization; 2011.
25. Lo STT, Chan EYY, Chan GKW, et al. Health emergency and disaster risk management (Health-EDRM): developing the research field within the Sendai framework paradigm. Int J Disaster Risk Sci. 2017;8:145.
26. Ngo E, Patel N, Chandrasekaran K, Tajik AJ, Paterick TE. The importance of the medical record: a critical professional responsibility. J Med Pract Manage. 2016;31(5):305–8.
27. Huston JL. The need for mandatory clinical recording standards. Clin Med J R Coll Physicians London. 2004;4(3):255–7.
28. Mô Dang V, François P, Batailler P, et al. Medical record-keeping and patient perception of hospital care quality. Int J Health Care Qual Assur. 2014;27(6):531–43.
29. Carpenter I, Ram MB, Croft GP, Williams JG, Carpenter I. Medical records and record-keeping standards. Clin Med (Lond). 2007;7(4):328–31.

Current Developments and Research in Apheresis

23

Robert W. Maitta

23.1 Background

The 1960s marked a pivotal era of activism for a fairer society and the advent of technological advances in medicine that would transform the treatment landscape. Among the groundbreaking technologies developed during this time was the first apheresis platform. Initially conceived by IBM engineer George T. Judson in close collaboration with Dr. Emil Freireich at the National Cancer Institute, the first blood cell separator based on centrifugation was developed. This early apheresis machine made it possible, for the first time, to separate leukocytes from venous blood based on their density, allowing the selective collection of cells while simultaneously returning all other blood components to the donor [1]. It soon became apparent that the machine's ability to segregate blood components by density could facilitate the separation of not only leukocytes but also erythrocytes, plasma, and platelets. This breakthrough paved the way for apheresis to be used in treating diseases where patients could benefit from the removal of specific blood components. This innovation set in motion a series of developments that established apheresis as a therapeutic approach for many antibody-mediated diseases and hemoglobinopathies. Additionally, it enabled the collection of hematopoietic stem cells and cells used in cell therapy product manufacturing.

In the ensuing decades, apheresis has become a first-line or adjuvant therapy for an increasing number of disease presentations. Guidelines by the American Society for Apheresis (ASFA), a professional society dedicated to apheresis, are updated every few years based on the latest evidence in the medical literature [2]. In general, procedures can be classified as those that remove a specific blood component—leukocytapheresis (leukocyte depletion/collection), lymphocytapheresis (lymphocyte removal), granulocytapheresis (granulocyte collection), thrombocytapheresis (platelet depletion/collection), erythrocytapheresis (red blood cell collections), plasmapheresis (plasma collection), and hematopoietic progenitor stem cell (HPC) collection—or as procedures that exchange a blood component, such as red cell exchange (RCE) and therapeutic plasma exchange (TPE) [3]. Thanks to the ability of these machines to selectively remove specific blood components, their use has expanded to blood collection centers. In countries like the United States (US), apheresis donations now represent a growing proportion of blood component collections. A notable example is the increased proportion of platelet units derived from single donors (SDP) collected

R. W. Maitta (✉)
Department of Pathology, University Hospitals Cleveland Medical Center and Case Western Reserve University School of Medicine, Cleveland, OH, USA
e-mail: robert.maitta@case.edu

I. Kozanoglu (ed.), *Problem Solving in Apheresis Medicine*,
https://doi.org/10.1007/978-3-031-74081-7_23

through apheresis in the US and other industrialized nations.

With regard to hardware, apheresis platforms can be classified into two broad categories: those that rely on centrifugal forces for component segregation and those that operate using membrane filtration [4]. Technological advances in newer machines have made them increasingly sophisticated, with modern platforms providing extensive real-time information. This data enables operators to troubleshoot issues, fine-tune procedures for improved efficiency, and, most importantly, safeguard against potential adverse events.

Additionally, a small but constant flow of literature highlights the use of apheresis in an expanding range of diseases, keeping centrifugal apheresis technology a focus of active research. Given that the majority of apheresis studies involve centrifugal machines, this chapter will concentrate on these platforms.

23.2 HPC Collections

As mentioned earlier, the original goal of apheresis technology was to separate leukocytes from peripheral blood. It is therefore unsurprising that HPC collections from peripheral blood stem cells (PBSC) has seen significant growth. The use of these cells for transplantation and, more recently, the use of lymphocytes in manufacturing cellular therapies has prompted the ASFA to issue recommendations aimed at standardizing cell collection, whether for therapeutic, commercial, or research purposes. ASFA proposes guidance to improve leukocytapheresis across various stages, including onboarding, pre-collection, collection, and post-collection. These recommendations consider protocol feasibility, patient/donor safety throughout the process, and quality assurance measures to ensure the potency, purity, and safety of the collected product [5]. Similarly, accrediting agencies have published standards for product collection; however, discussion of these standards is beyond the scope of this text.

PBSC collections aim to obtain sufficient numbers of $CD34^+$ cells for transplantation. Currently, $CD34^+$ cell counts are measured either on the day of collection or the day prior to determine the donor's readiness for the procedure. This test relies on flow cytometry, which requires trained technologists and specialized equipment, often resulting in delays while awaiting results. New hematology analyzers offer a faster alternative to flow cytometry for determining the optimal timing for collection. These analyzers, equipped with HPC count capabilities, can provide rapid, accurate, and predictive results, enabling successful collections even when large cell collection targets are required [6]. Since these counts can be obtained alongside complete blood counts before collection, this approach offers a quick and cost-effective method for evaluating cell counts in advance.

PBSC collections from patients mobilized for several days with granulocyte colony-stimulating factor (G-CSF) are considered the standard of care for obtaining cells for stem cell transplantation [7]. PBSC collections are among the safest apheresis procedures, with large studies reporting only a few, mostly mild, adverse events [8–10]. However, achieving a successful collection requires a multidisciplinary approach to ensure not only the desired cell yield but, more importantly, the minimization of potential adverse events, regardless of whether the collection occurs in an autologous or allogeneic setting [11]. This approach begins with the mobilization regimen and includes a comprehensive evaluation of all relevant laboratory variables that may impact the stability of the subject during the collection process. It is important to acknowledge that invasive procedures such as apheresis carry inherent risks, starting with the placement of central venous access for the procedure. Despite these risks, PBSC collections can be made safer by carefully adjusting collection parameters to meet the desired cell yield [11]. Therefore, once a patient or donor has been thoroughly evaluated and deemed suitable for PBSC collection, preparations for apheresis must begin. These preparations aim to maximize the likelihood of achieving the cell target while addressing factors that directly affect the safety of the collection process.

Apheresis systems have inherent technical limitations, as they were not designed for use in small-frame patients. Adverse events are rare in apheresis, particularly in the context of donations, where they are infrequent and mostly associated with hypocalcemia. These events are more commonly observed in petite, older female patients and individuals with small blood volumes [12]. Patients with a small frame or low body mass index often present challenges, and this is especially true for young children. A primary difficulty in pediatric cases is the lower extracorporeal volume (ECV) tolerance in young children. Because the ECV (the volume of blood outside the body during the procedure) can represent a significant proportion of a child's total blood volume, especially in smaller patients, additional and thorough preparation is required to ensure safety. Furthermore, peripheral access in young children is often inadequate, as their veins may not support the high pressures and velocities needed for collections, necessitating the placement of central venous access. Other factors complicating pediatric collections include lower tolerance to electrolyte and fluid shifts due to smaller physiological reserves, slower responses to such shifts, and the challenge of remaining calm throughout the procedure to avoid triggering pressure alarms. These issues collectively make pediatric collections more challenging than adult collections [13, 14]. For the youngest patients, sedation is often employed to address these challenges [15].

Taking appropriate preparatory steps increases procedure safety while minimizing complications [16–18]. Interestingly, among children, adverse events have mostly been encountered in older pediatric patients, with severity ranging from moderate (54.5%) to severe (27.3%). These events fall into three main categories: hypocalcemia due to citrate effects, central access-related difficulties such as bleeding or thrombosis, and technical issues related to platform alarms [19]. In addition to hypocalcemia, hypovolemic shock and, in rare cases, hypervolemic cardiac overload have been reported [20]. In the rarest instances, significant hypotension, infection, and even death have been documented [21]. The frequency of these adverse events increases when more than one procedure is needed or when collections are prolonged. Therefore, it is important to limit collections to the time required to achieve the goal or to as few procedures as possible [19]. Fortunately, modern apheresis systems can perform collections more quickly and efficiently, even when running at lower speeds, as is often the case with younger pediatric patients [22–25]. This efficiency reduces the need for significantly longer procedures, thereby minimizing adverse events and the need for "large-volume collections." This is particularly important for patients with lower peripheral $CD34^+$ counts, who otherwise would require multiple days of collections with much longer procedures [26, 27].

Regarding vascular access, there is a desire in the field to minimize the use of central catheters, not only to decrease line placement-associated adverse events but also to reduce costs. However, it should be noted that peripheral access will rarely allow procedures to be performed at higher velocities, process larger volumes of blood, or allow for consecutive-day collections once veins have been used for apheresis. This means that collections such as those for chimeric antigen receptor (CAR) T-cell therapy manufacturing, which require a single-day collection, can be attempted peripherally. However, repeated collections to achieve a specific $CD34^+$ count will likely require central line placement to maintain high velocity and process a greater volume of blood to achieve the desired cell yield. This topic has been reviewed in the literature, which shows that for single or short-duration procedures, either peripheral access or central catheters can be used. However, in settings where multiple procedures are needed, such as therapeutic apheresis and PBSC collections, implantable ports, arteriovenous fistulas, central catheters, or tunneled catheters may be necessary [28]. Of note, the vasculature of young children has a greater propensity for vascular collapse under the stress of negative pressures generated by apheresis platforms. Since small veins require large-bore needles for apheresis, the placement of central lines often becomes unavoidable [29]. Therefore, the majority of young children requiring apheresis procedures will need central venous access, which explains the reported rates of adverse events related to line placement and location, such as asymptomatic thrombosis, in this population [30, 31].

The main form of anticoagulation approved for use with apheresis platforms is Anticoagulant Citrate Dextrose Solution, Solution A (ACD-A). Young children have a higher sensitivity to ACD-A, which, through its effect of chelating calcium, can cause hypocalcemia that may go unnoticed during a procedure because young children are unable to verbalize symptoms, especially when sedated [15, 17]. This lower tolerance is due to their limited calcium reserve capacity, requiring calcium supplementation during the procedure. Thankfully, new apheresis systems, through their higher efficiency, lead to fewer calcium losses since shorter procedures require less anticoagulation [32]. Therefore, the anticipatory/preparatory phase of collections should aim to optimize ionized calcium levels to prevent potential adverse events and closely monitor calcium levels during the procedure [33].

In patients with anemia or those who, because of their small size, can be particularly susceptible to changes in hematocrit during a procedure, the platform will require a blood prime to proceed. Blood priming consists of running a unit of red blood cells (RBCs) through the tubing and system so that the ECV does not result in a change in the patient's hematocrit at the start of the collection. Blood priming does not have a significant effect on the collection yield (dilutional effect) since only a few mL from the priming unit may enter the patient's circulation [13]. In addition, to address fluid shifts in small-weight patients/donors, an added element of safety in apheresis platforms is that once weight is entered into the system, the platform will revert to a slow flow rate for small patients (pediatric), something that cannot be overridden by the operator [34]. This latter point explains why procedures in children, though long, do not process a "large volume," because the length of the procedure corresponds to the final product volume, and longer procedures lead to larger product volumes, which can be more physiologically significant for a small patient. As a result, optimizing hematocrit prior to collection and priming the apheresis circuit with RBCs reduce changes to ECV and post-procedure hematocrit, translating into fewer adverse events [20, 33, 35].

Collections on new apheresis platforms can still be adjusted based on a colorimetric chart available with the equipment. Using this chart, collections can be modified to make them either lighter or darker (based on RBC content) to enrich for the desired cell layer (heavier-density leukocytes). On the other hand, lighter collections would be closer to the plasma layer, allowing for the collection of smaller cells. This ability to adjust has made it possible to penetrate deeply into the interface of plerixafor-mobilized adult sickle cell disease (SCD) patients to collect cells with much higher efficiency (82.2%), despite using a low collection preference. The only apparent drawback is that there is higher RBC contamination of the stem cell product [36]. This would also influence how a product may need to be processed, especially when transplants are performed across ABO blood group barriers [27]. Therefore, the operator retains the ability to optimize as needed and collect a darker product, which, though containing a higher presence of RBCs, can yield a much higher PBSC content in the collection bag [24, 37, 38].

As mentioned above, body weight considerations can raise concerns over procedures. PBSC collections in small children (<20 kg) can be challenging; however, results from studies looking at both autologous and allogeneic collections have indicated that these apheresis procedures can be performed safely while obtaining a sufficient number of cells for transplantation [39]. In older apheresis systems, pediatric patients weighing less than 20 kg frequently needed longer procedures to achieve cell targets [15]. These older systems depended more heavily on the operator for procedure adjustments, following a colorimetric scale to establish preference parameters for the desired collection—a method that is still in use in new platforms [23, 32]. Since collections are shorter in the newer, more efficient systems, platelet losses into the product have decreased, but they still occur, and losses depend on both the length and number of collections needed [40]. It is encouraging that even children weighing 8–15 kg have been collected with minimal adverse events when blood priming, and intravenous calcium and magnesium supplementation are given prior to and throughout collection [41, 42]. These collections are performed without increasing procedure time, negating the need for previously favored larger volume procedures, which, as stated earlier, result in a higher incidence of adverse events.

New systems, through their display and software management system, allow the operator real-time interface (buffy coat) monitoring, permitting adjustments [25, 43]. In cases when $CD34^+$ cells are collected from non-mobilized subjects, this can still be done with few contaminating granulocytes [44]. Platelet contamination/losses can also be reduced unless collecting lymphocytes, in which case the collection occurs closer to the platelet layer, leading to greater platelet removal [45, 46]. Due to high efficiency, these collections also do not need to be long [47]. Similarly, an added benefit of these collections is that when collecting lymphocytes, new systems do so without much RBC contamination [48]. Thus, fine adjustments to the collection still permit further reduction of contamination if so desired [49].

In the Spectra Optia (Terumo BCT), there are two ways in which PBSC collections can occur. The first is non-continuous, in which the machine empties the cells into an intermediate chamber before adjusting to continue the collection (mononuclear cells [MNCs]). In the second, this step does not occur, as the intermediate chamber is missing, and thus the collections continue without interruption (continuous MNCs [cMNCs]). Nevertheless, despite being non-continuous, the MNC setting returns platelets and the rest of the blood elements back to the patient [50]. In the MNC setting, filling of the intermediate chamber and overflow of cells triggers a sensor that empties the contents into the collection bag, with intermittent plasma flushes of the chamber. This cycle repeats itself throughout the collection, followed by auto-resetting of the collection, which can also be done manually by the operator [26]. This setting takes longer and may result in greater platelet removal but still meets the cell collection target.

23.3 CAR T-Cell Therapies

Lymphocytapheresis in recent years has become an increasingly important procedure. The ability of apheresis platforms to collect MNCs, specifically lymphocytes, for the manufacture of CAR T-cell therapies has resulted in the growth of these collections. In lymphoma patients, the Spectra Optia can readily collect $>2 \times 10^9$ nucleated cells and $CD3^+$ lymphocytes of $\geq 1 \times 10^9$ with improved cell viability, regardless of pretreatment or advanced patient age [51]. This platform collects a higher number of lymphocytes in shorter procedure run times with great efficiency. However, the limitation is that when the operator adjusts the cell composition of the final cell product, a greater number of platelets may be removed into the product [52]. These procedures have also been successful with an efficiency of >80% in young adult and pediatric patients requiring collections for leukemia and neuroblastoma [53]. Importantly, the frequency of adverse events is similar to what has been reported for PBSC collections.

In the field, there has been an attempt to find ways to determine, prior to lymphocytapheresis, when a patient is likely to meet a desired cell target or when this may not be the case. Efforts to develop prediction models for lymphocyte collections have been undertaken in patients with B-cell acute lymphoblastic leukemia and diffuse large B-cell lymphoma [54]. As seen in PBSC collections, it was established that to increase the procedure's efficiency and improve the success of a collection, a higher hematocrit, optimal circulating $CD3^+$ cell counts, and good platelet counts will influence the volume of blood needed to be processed to obtain sufficient cells for CAR T-cell therapy manufacturing [54]. These are important factors that, in many patients undergoing collection, may need to be improved through transfusion of platelets and/or RBCs to increase apheresis efficiency. Hopefully, future studies will shed light on the specific parameters (ranges) that need to be met for patients to undergo lymphocytapheresis.

23.4 Therapeutic Apheresis

Much of the care taken for PBSC and CAR T-cell therapy collections translates into the precautions needed for therapeutic procedures. Notably, the body of literature regarding therapeutic apheresis usage is expanding, which is evident from the need to regularly update the indications that can benefit from apheresis therapy based on evidence. Indeed, the number of diseases in which apheresis can be utilized has steadily grown, with over 90 diseases encompassing nearly 200 indications described [55]. On the other hand, pediatric apheresis literature has increased at a slower pace, perhaps due to the aforementioned difficulties of using the platforms in young patients. Nevertheless, hundreds of articles—mostly single-center studies—case reports, and case series are available, with only a minority of them (2%) involving actual clinical trials [56]. Despite this, it can be inferred that procedures in children are effective, as reports describe complete recovery in a majority of patients receiving TPE, with adverse events ranging from mostly allergic reactions to isolated cases of cardiac arrest and transfusion-related acute lung injury, which were reported in a minority of patients [57]. In this section, developments will be presented according to the type of procedure performed.

23.5 Leukocytapheresis (Leukodepletion)

This procedure has been reserved for patients presenting with hyperleukocytosis and symptoms associated with stasis and increased viscosity. Due to the limited number of patients treated via apheresis for significant hyperleukocytosis, no clinical trials comparing the effectiveness of leukocytapheresis with other therapies have been formally conducted. As a result, most apheresis use in this setting is empirical, with two main goals: first to reduce cell burden and avoid tumor lysis syndrome once chemotherapy is initiated and second to relieve symptoms related to stasis. It should be noted that, although a study reported a reduction in mortality when leukocytapheresis is used in leukemia [58], other reports have shown no effect on patient outcomes [59, 60] nor on long-term survival [60, 61]. On the contrary, data has indicated that outcomes were better when chemotherapy was initiated early, even without leukocytapheresis, despite cell count [62]. Thus, it remains to be determined whether performing these depletion procedures improves survival compared to the immediate initiation of chemotherapy, regardless of cell count.

23.6 TPE

Nowadays, TPE has become one of the most commonly used apheresis procedures to treat an expanding number of diseases [2, 63]. The growth in TPE use, along with the evidence supporting or not supporting its use, has resulted in better treatment of diseases that otherwise would have had much higher morbidity and, in some cases, mortality [64, 65]. The ASFA Guidelines have become one of the most up-to-date resources for evaluating the available evidence for the use of apheresis [2]. The guidelines classify diseases from Category I, in which apheresis is considered first-line therapy, to Category IV, in which apheresis has shown no benefit in the disease process or may be contraindicated.

TPE, unlike plasmapheresis, is performed by exchanging plasma from a patient and replacing it with donated plasma, a combination of plasma and albumin, or albumin alone. The vast majority of diseases effectively treated with TPE are caused by pathologic antibodies that, when removed over a series of procedures, improve both symptoms and reduce overall clinical complications [66–68]. Thus, it is well accepted by apheresis practitioners and in the literature that diseases that respond to TPE are those in which the offending antibody can be removed by apheresis [69]. The procedure is relatively well-tolerated, and adverse events are mostly mild, with the most common being secondary to the use of plasma (transfusion reactions), anticoagulation-associated hypocalcemia, or rapid fluid shifts (hypotension) [70, 71]. On the other hand, severe adverse events tend to be associated with the use of plasma as either part of or the sole replacement fluid [35]. Furthermore, once reactions occur during a procedure, extra care and higher doses of pre-medications may be needed, as the patient is at higher risk of additional reactions.

The efficiency of these procedures is good, exchanging plasma with minimal losses of cellular components, which mostly occur during longer procedures [72]. Specifically, longer-duration procedures can be associated with the potential worsening of anemia or thrombocytopenia [73, 74], as well as greater hypocalcemia-associated symptoms due to the increased need for ACD-A anticoagulation. This is why the vast majority of procedures will replace either 1–1.5 plasma volumes to avoid complications [75].

TPE is a nonselective process that removes and exchanges a patient's plasma. This can have unintended negative effects, as albumin use does not replace coagulation factors and non-pathogenic immunoglobulins are removed during the procedure. However, using plasma to account for this is also not helpful due to the inherent risks associated with blood components. This has led to efforts to find more specific methodologies that remove the offending antibody/mediator while leaving the rest of the patient's plasma elements intact. One possible approach is immunoadsorption apheresis; however, this technology has not been approved by the US Food and Drug Administration. In patients with myasthenia gravis (MG), the patient's plasma proteins are passed through a column that specifically removes offending antibodies while leaving the rest of the patient's plasma proteins untouched and returning them to the patient [76]. This approach has been reported to be more effective, leading to longer-lasting clinical improvement in MG patients compared to intravenous immunoglobulin [76]. Nevertheless, it remains to be determined how this procedure compares to traditional TPE in terms of clinical improvement or the duration of symptom-free recovery.

23.7 Apheresis and COVID-19

If there is one event that affected society more than any other in recent years, it is the COVID-19 pandemic. Among the many therapeutic approaches attempted to help patients with severe COVID-19 infection was the use of apheresis in patients with severe disease. This entirely investigational approach became a focus of research in the field. TPE had been reported to reduce the concentration of inflammatory mediators in COVID-19 patients admitted to the intensive care unit (ICU), sometimes resulting in the reversal of respiratory and multiorgan failure [77, 78]. Alternatively, selective removal of cells producing pro-inflammatory mediators was believed to be useful in the setting of severe COVID-19 [79]. Reviews on the subject have proposed that apheresis procedures in patients with severe COVID-19 infection and cytokine storm syndrome (CSS) can reduce interleukin-6 levels, C-reactive protein (CRP), ferritin, D-dimer, and fibrinogen while increasing lymphocyte counts through the immunomodulatory effect of TPE [80]. This potential role for TPE was perhaps supported by a report describing decreased mortality in moderate to critically ill COVID-19 patients treated with apheresis [81]. However, an open-label clinical trial evaluating the benefits of TPE in patients with severe COVID-19 showed that, although the procedures decreased the number of days on mechanical ventilation and ICU stay, they failed to reduce mortality [82]. As a result, it remains unclear whether there is a benefit to using TPE in the setting of COVID-19.

Immunoadsorption apheresis has been reported to help patients with severe COVID-19 symptoms, but this technology is not available in the US [83]. This approach is partly supported by the positive outcomes of using absorption apheresis procedures to remove CRP, which is produced in excess in patients with severe COVID-19 infection, to ameliorate symptoms even when significant organ damage had occurred [84, 85]. When used early, CRP-specific apheresis of patients requiring ventilation was reported to reverse symptoms [86]. Not surprisingly, this led to a form of this technology being tested during a multisite clinical trial in the US. It involved the use of the Depuro D2000 Adsorption Cartridge coupled with the TPE setup of the Spectra Optia [87]. This cartridge/column was designed to remove CSS-associated cytokines in COVID-19 patients with severe disease to prevent complications related to their accumulation. However, as of the writing of this text, results from this trial are not available, and it remains to be determined if this approach had any benefit for these patients. The potential use of apheresis in such settings has been reviewed by ASFA to determine the best ways in which, if called upon, apheresis services can treat such patients [88].

23.8 RCE and Erythrocytapheresis

The majority of patients needing RCEs are those with hemoglobinopathies in crisis due to critical levels of abnormal hemoglobin, requiring the exchange of affected RBCs and replacement with normal donated RBCs. SCD patients can present with a generalized crisis or with specific symptoms such as a cerebrovascular accident or hypoxia secondary to acute chest. This is due to the concentration of sickle cell hemoglobin (HbS), which causes sickling of RBCs, leading to reduced cell flow and poor gas exchange. Simple RBC transfusions can offer relief by improving oxygenation and reducing HbS concentration, but the chronic use of this approach leads over time to iron overload. For this reason, RBC exchanges—either modified partial (manual exchange) or automated RCE—are favored during a crisis, as they lead to greater reductions in HbS concentration, improving symptoms while maintaining iron neutrality [89, 90].

Mechanistically, apheresis platforms performing automated RCE are programmable not only to target a specific HbS level but also to adjust the final fraction of cells remaining (FCR) and the hematocrit of the patient [91]. In the procedure, RBC units are accessed one at a time and exchanged with an equal volume of the patient's RBCs. However, as the procedure continues, a proportion of RBCs given early during the RCE are removed and exchanged in the second half of the procedure. One consideration raised regarding the use of RCE in a chronic setting is that exposure to multiple RBC units per procedure could result in higher alloimmunization rates. However, this does not appear to be the case, as a proportion of cells from each unit are removed during the RCE, so the patient is exposed to a lower antigenic burden per unit [92]. Comparisons between manual and automated RCE have reported that the latter lowers HbS by 3% more per session, with the major caveat being that apheresis has a 74-fold higher cost [93].

A pressing challenge facing the performance of automated RCE is procuring a sufficient number of RBC units to carry out the procedures. Decreasing inventories are likely to represent an ongoing difficulty, which requires outreach efforts to the community, including the inclusion of donor groups that were until recently deferred. Adding to this challenge is the fact that in industrialized nations, there are ethnic differences between those donating and the patients needing units for RCE. One approach that has gathered attention in recent years is to use isovolemic hemodilution prior to performing RCE. This limited hemodilution involves replacing a predetermined volume of RBCs with normal saline, followed by automated RCE. This has been reported to result in a lower FCR, which can be as low as 30%, require fewer RBC units per procedure, greater time between exchanges, and fewer procedures annually per patient [94]. Importantly, isovolemic hemodilution is safe, with no higher incidence of adverse events [95, 96]. Since many patients benefit from receiving chronic RCE at regular intervals to prevent disease complications, this approach clearly helps preserve inventory while providing the benefits of apheresis to both adult and pediatric SCD patients [97, 98].

23.9 Thrombocytapheresis

This is one of the rarest apheresis therapeutic procedures, performed in patients with essential thrombocythemia. The rarity of this disease means that conducting a controlled clinical trial to evaluate the efficacy of platforms is unlikely.

When performed, modern apheresis systems reduce platelet counts, thereby improving thrombocytosis-associated symptoms [99]. However, this ability to collect platelets via apheresis technology has significantly increased the collection of platelet units from single donors, which now represent the majority of platelet units in the US [100]. Data on the safety and effectiveness of apheresis for platelet collection indicate that it is a safe procedure with few adverse events [101].

23.10 Extracorporeal Photopheresis

This procedure combines leukocytapheresis, treatment of cells with ultraviolet A (UVA) light after exposure to 8-methoxypsoralen, and reinfusion into the patient. This therapy is used in the treatment of autoimmune syndromes, cutaneous T-cell lymphoma, graft-versus-host disease, and cell-mediated rejection following solid-organ transplantation [102]. The use of psoralen and UVA light crosslinks nucleic acids, causing disruption of DNA transcription and replication [103]. Platforms can operate in an open circuit, requiring a second piece of equipment to perform the UVA irradiation, or in a closed system where the entire process is carried out by the same platform [104, 105]. Regardless of the setup, this procedure has been shown to effectively inactivate cells, leading to improvement in patients receiving this therapy.

23.11 Low-Density Lipoprotein (LDL) Apheresis

Familial hypercholesterolemia is a rare condition that leads to increased morbidity and early mortality in affected patients. LDL apheresis has been used to assist these patients by removing the high concentrations of LDL cholesterol from their plasma to prevent disease-associated complications. To achieve therapeutic benefit, patients need to undergo procedures at predetermined intervals to maintain low levels, especially when medication regimens have failed [106]. Two types of LDL apheresis have been described: one is heparin-induced extracorporeal LDL precipitation (HELP), and the second is dextran sulfate (DS) adsorption [107]. HELP systems isolate plasma, mixing it with acetic acid buffer followed by the addition of heparin, which causes LDL cholesterol to precipitate, and it is then removed using a polycarbonate membrane [107]. In contrast, DS adsorption systems use negatively charged DS columns to remove LDL cholesterol [107]. These technologies can be used interchangeably to treat patients, with HELP systems potentially removing LDL cholesterol to a greater extent [108]. Alternatively, TPE can also be used effectively to remove LDL cholesterol, but these procedures need to be repeated every few weeks to maintain low levels [109, 110].

23.12 Apheresis Research

The reach of modern apheresis systems and the greater utilization of procedures, from collections to therapeutic exchanges, continue to increase worldwide, as indicated by reports from sub-Saharan Africa, where more rare indications are among the diseases treated with increased frequency by TPE [111]. This broader use opens up possibilities for more research into the potential roles of apheresis in a wide range of etiologies. However, limitations significantly affecting apheresis research exist, as indicated by the fact that abstracts describing new apheresis developments often do not translate into published literature [112]. This is even more apparent when examining extended periods of submissions to the annual ASFA meeting, which show that most abstracts submitted (84%) failed to generate citable full-text manuscripts. What is more concerning is that even when abstracts are published in peer-reviewed journals, changes to their content often occur, leading to conclusions that differ markedly from those presented during the original submission to the meeting [113]. This lack of concordance not only affects how the results should be interpreted but also raises questions which conclusions should be considered when adjusting practices.

One of the newer disease settings in which a role for apheresis has been investigated is in sepsis patients. However, available data does not support the use of procedures unless they are employed as a last resort, once other therapies have failed [114]. In other cases, even when there is evidence favoring the use of TPE, such as in catastrophic antiphospholipid syndrome, the debate over what to use as the best replacement fluid during the procedure remains unresolved [115]. These challenges in apheresis research, coupled with efforts to use procedures without clear indications, as well as the use of blood components in situations where they may not be warranted, complicate further research into apheresis in a uniform and controlled manner.

As presented in a prior section of this chapter, the ability of apheresis systems to collect cells makes it possible to use them for research purposes in manufacturing cell therapy products. A possible source of cells is thrombocyte apheresis cassettes, which collect the undesired byproducts of SDP collections and have been shown to contain viable cells that respond to mitogens, as well as sufficient numbers of T cells that readily divide in response to cytokine stimulation [116]. Granulocyte collections can also serve as another potential source of cells for research, as these collections contain various white blood cells with minimal RBC and platelet contaminants [117]. Thus, depending on the need, apheresis systems can not only facilitate the study of new disease applications but, through its ability to segregate desired blood elements, provide plasma or cells for investigational purposes.

23.13 Summary

Apheresis has revolutionized the treatment of many diseases to date. Technological advances in both software and hardware have made current platforms highly efficient while increasing patient safety. Undoubtedly, there is a need to develop a structured scientific approach to performing procedures, and establishing which diseases are responsive to therapy will lead to a better understanding of the applications and limitations of the technology. Furthermore, there is a need to improve the literature presenting results from apheresis-based studies. The field continues to grow, and as the development of CAR T-cell therapies expands to treat a greater number of malignancies, increased apheresis use is expected. As the pace of developments accelerates, there is reason for optimism that higher remission rates and even cures are possible in the era of CAR T-cell therapies.

Disclosure of Conflicts of Interest No conflicts of interest to declare with this submission.

References

1. Freireich EJ, Judson G, Levin RH. Separation and collection of leukocytes. Cancer Res. 1965;25(9):1516–20.
2. Connelly-Smith L, Alquist CR, Aqui NA, Hofmann JC, Klingel R, Onwuemene OA, et al. Guidelines on the use of therapeutic apheresis in clinical practice—evidence-based approach from the writing Committee of the American Society for apheresis: the ninth special issue. J Clin Apher. 2023;38(2):77–278.
3. Maitta RW. Current state of apheresis technology and its applications. Transfus Apher Sci. 2018;57(5):606–13.
4. Ward DM. Conventional apheresis therapies: a review. J Clin Apher. 2011;26(5):230–8.
5. Liu HD, Su L, Winters JL, Thibodeaux SR, Park YA, Wu Y, et al. Considerations for immune effector cell therapy collections: a white paper from the American Society for Apheresis. Cytotherapy. 2022;24(9):916–22.
6. Rebersek K, Furlan T, Zver S, Podgornik H. Hematopoietic progenitor cell counting can optimize peripheral blood stem cell apheresis process. J Clin Apher. 2021;36(6):870–7.
7. Gratwohl A, Baldomero H, Horisberger B, Schmid C, Passweg J, Urbano-Ispizua A, et al. Current trends in hematopoietic stem cell transplantation in Europe. Blood. 2002;100(7):2374–86.
8. Brauninger S, Bialleck H, Seifried E, Bonig H. Asystole during stem cell apheresis in a young healthy female volunteer donor. Transfusion. 2011;51(7):1594–5.
9. Holig K, Kramer M, Kroschinsky F, Bornhauser M, Mengling T, Schmidt AH, et al. Safety and efficacy of hematopoietic stem cell collection from mobilized peripheral blood in unrelated volunteers: 12

years of single-center experience in 3928 donors. Blood. 2009;114(18):3757–63.
10. Halter J, Kodera Y, Ispizua AU, Greinix HT, Schmitz N, Favre G, et al. Severe events in donors after allogeneic hematopoietic stem cell donation. Haematologica. 2009;94(1):94–101.
11. Ohto H. Efficient and safe stem cell apheresis. Transfus Apher Sci. 2004;31(3):203–5.
12. Yuan S, Ziman A, Smeltzer B, Lu Q, Goldfinger D. Moderate and severe adverse events associated with apheresis donations: incidences and risk factors. Transfusion. 2010;50(2):478–86.
13. Cherqaoui B, Rouel N, Auvrignon A, Defachelles AS, Demeocq F, Kanold J, et al. Peripheral blood stem cell collection in low-weight children: retrospective comparison of two apheresis devices. Transfusion. 2014;54(5):1371–8.
14. Kara A, Turgut S, Cagli A, Sahin F, Oran E, Tunc B. Complications of therapeutic apheresis in children. Transfus Apher Sci. 2013;48(3):375–6.
15. Salazar-Riojas R, Garcia-Lozano JA, Valdes-Galvan M, Martinez-Gonzalez O, Cantu-Rodriguez OG, Gonzalez-Llano O, et al. Effective collection of peripheral blood stem cells in children weighing 20 kilogram or less in a single large-volume apheresis procedure. J Clin Apher. 2015;30(5):281–7.
16. Kanold J, Halle P, Berger M, Rapatel C, Palcoux JB, Rouzier C, et al. Large-volume leukapheresis procedure for peripheral blood progenitor cell collection in children weighing 15 kg or less: efficacy and safety evaluation. Med Pediatr Oncol. 1999;32(1):7–10.
17. Sauer H, Roland H, Ulla L, Ortrud D, Jurgen F. Leukapheresis in children weighing less than 20 kg. Pediatr Blood Cancer. 2012;58(4):627–9.
18. Orbach D, Hojjat-Assari S, Doz F, Pacquement H, Guillaume A, Mathiot C, et al. Peripheral blood stem cell collection in 24 low-weight infants: experience of a single centre. Bone Marrow Transplant. 2003;31(3):171–4.
19. Cooling L, Hoffmann S, Webb D, Meade M, Yamada C, Davenport R, et al. Procedure-related complications and adverse events associated with pediatric autologous peripheral blood stem cell collection. J Clin Apher. 2017;32(1):35–48.
20. Ohara Y, Ohto H, Tasaki T, Sano H, Mochizuki K, Akaihata M, et al. Comprehensive technical and patient-care optimization in the management of pediatric apheresis for peripheral blood stem cell harvesting. Transfus Apher Sci. 2016;55(3):338–43.
21. Michon B, Moghrabi A, Winikoff R, Barrette S, Bernstein ML, Champagne J, et al. Complications of apheresis in children. Transfusion. 2007;47(10):1837–42.
22. Moog R. Apheresis techniques for collection of peripheral blood progenitor cells. Transfus Apher Sci. 2004;31(3):207–20.
23. Flommersfeld S, Bakchoul T, Bein G, Wachtel A, Loechelt C, Sachs UJ. A single center comparison between three different apheresis systems for autologous and allogeneic stem cell collections. Transfus Apher Sci. 2013;49(3):428–33.
24. Ikeda K, Ohto H, Nemoto K, Yamamoto G, Kato K, Ogata T, et al. Collection of MNCs and progenitor cells by two separators for PBPC transplantation: a randomized crossover trial. Transfusion. 2003;43(6):814–9.
25. Reinhardt P, Brauninger S, Bialleck H, Thorausch K, Smith R, Schrezenmeier H, et al. Automatic interface-controlled apheresis collection of stem/progenitor cells: results from an autologous donor validation trial of a novel stem cell apheresis device. Transfusion. 2011;51(6):1321–30.
26. Ikeda K, Minakawa K, Muroi K, Fujiwara SI, Yamada-Fujiwara M, Fujimori Y, et al. Prospective randomized and crossover comparison of two apheresis machines for peripheral blood stem cell collection: a multicenter study. Transfusion. 2016;56(11):2839–47.
27. Brauninger S, Bialleck H, Thorausch K, Felt T, Seifried E, Bonig H. Allogeneic donor peripheral blood "stem cell" apheresis: prospective comparison of two apheresis systems. Transfusion. 2012;52(5):1137–45.
28. Golsorkhi M, Azarfar A, Abdipour A. Vascular access in therapeutic apheresis: one size does not fit all. Ther Apher Dial. 2022;26(4):694–716.
29. Empringham B, Chiang KY, Krueger J. Collection of hematopoietic stem cells and immune effector cells in small children. Transfus Apher Sci. 2018;57(5):614–8.
30. Male C, Chait P, Andrew M, Hanna K, Julian J, Mitchell L, et al. Central venous line-related thrombosis in children: association with central venous line location and insertion technique. Blood. 2003;101(11):4273–8.
31. McGee DC, Gould MK. Preventing complications of central venous catheterization. N Engl J Med. 2003;348(12):1123–33.
32. Even-Or E, Eden-Walker A, Di Mola M, McDougall E, Schechter T, Ali M, et al. Comparison of two apheresis systems for autologous stem cell collections in pediatric oncology patients. Transfusion. 2017;57(1):122–30.
33. Maitta RW, Vasovic LV, Mohandas K, Music-Aplenc L, Bonzon-Adelson A, Uehlinger J. A safe therapeutic apheresis protocol in paediatric patients weighing 11 to 25 kg. Vox Sang. 2014;107(4):375–80.
34. Gorlin JB, Humphreys D, Kent P, Galacki D, Kevy SV, Grupp S, et al. Pediatric large volume peripheral blood progenitor cell collections from patients under 25 kg: a primer. J Clin Apher. 1996;11(4):195–203.
35. Kundrapu S, Datla S, Griffin V, Maitta RW. Adverse events during apheresis: a 10-year experience at a tertiary academic medical center. J Clin Apher. 2019;34(5):528–36.
36. Sharma A, Leonard A, West K, Gossett JM, Uchida N, Panch S, et al. Optimizing haematopoietic stem and progenitor cell apheresis collection from

plerixafor-mobilized patients with sickle cell disease. Br J Haematol. 2022;198(4):740–4.
37. Knudsen LM, Nikolaisen K, Gaarsdal E, Johnsen HE. Kinetic studies during peripheral blood stem cell collection show CD34+ cell recruitment intra-apheresis. J Clin Apher. 2001;16(3):114–9.
38. Heuft HG, Dubiel M, Rick O, Kingreen D, Serke S, Schwella N. Inverse relationship between patient peripheral blood CD34+ cell counts and collection efficiency for CD34+ cells in two automated leukapheresis systems. Transfusion. 2001;41(8):1008–13.
39. Norooznezhad AH, Malek Mohammadi A, Fumani HK, Aminian P, Jalili M, Nikbakht M, et al. Peripheral blood stem cell apheresis in low-weight children: a single centre study. Transfus Apher Sci. 2019;58(3):300–3.
40. Ikeda K, Ohto H, Kanno T, Gonda K, Suzuki Y, Ono T, et al. Peripheral blood progenitor cell collection by two programs for autologous and allogeneic transplantation. Transfusion. 2014;54(5):1235–42.
41. Mohammadi AM, Norooznezhad AH, Aminian P, Nikbakht M, Chahardouli B, Rostami S, et al. An alternative method for custom prime: a case report of successful peripheral blood stem cell harvesting from two low-weight child donors. Transfus Apher Sci. 2017;56(6):886–8.
42. Greze V, Rouel N, Rochette E, Merlin E, Halle P, Plantaz D, et al. Peripheral blood stem cell collection in children with extremely low body weight (</=8 kg). What have we learned over the past 25 years and where are the limits? J Clin Apher. 2021;36(3):322–31.
43. Li Y, Li J, Reeves HM, Reyes R, Maitta RW. Comparison of two apheresis systems during hematopoietic progenitor stem cell collections at a tertiary medical center. Transfusion. 2016;56(11):2833–8.
44. Karafin MS, Graminske S, Erickson P, Walters MC, Scott EP, Carter S, et al. Evaluation of the Spectra Optia apheresis system for mononuclear cell (MNC) collection in G-CSF mobilized and nonmobilized healthy donors: results of a multicenter study. J Clin Apher. 2014;29(5):273–80.
45. Drezet A, Granata A, Lemarie C, Calmels B, Chabannon C. An intra-patient comparison of blood cell separators Spectra and Optia in patients and donors undergoing blood mononuclear cell collections at a single institution for subsequent autologous or allogeneic hematopoietic cell transplantation reveals comparable collection efficiencies. Bone Marrow Transplant. 2016;51(7):1007–9.
46. Lee SN, Sohn JY, Kong JH, Eom HS, Lee H, Kong SY. Comparison of two apheresis systems of COBE and Optia for autologous peripheral blood stem cell collection. Ann Lab Med. 2017;37(4):327–30.
47. Wuchter P, Hundemer M, Schmitt A, Witzens-Harig M, Pavel P, Hillengass J, et al. Performance assessment and benchmarking of autologous peripheral blood stem cell collection with two different apheresis devices. Transfus Med. 2017;27(1):36–42.
48. Schulz M, Bialleck H, Thorausch K, Bug G, Dunzinger U, Seifried E, et al. Unstimulated leukapheresis in patients and donors: comparison of two apheresis systems. Transfusion. 2014;54(6):1622–9.
49. Pham HP, Dormesy S, Wolfe K, Budhai A, Sachais BS, Shi PA. Potentially modifiable predictors of cell collection efficiencies and product characteristics of allogeneic hematopoietic progenitor cell collections. Transfusion. 2021;61(5):1518–24.
50. Brauninger S, Bialleck H, Thorausch K, Seifried E, Bonig H. Mobilized allogeneic peripheral stem/progenitor cell apheresis with Spectra Optia v.5.0, a novel, automatic interface-controlled apheresis system: results from the first feasibility trial. Vox Sang. 2011;101(3):237–46.
51. Harrer DC, Heidenreich M, Fante MA, Muller V, Haehnel V, Offner R, et al. Apheresis for chimeric antigen receptor T-cell production in adult lymphoma patients. Transfusion. 2022;62(8):1602–11.
52. Putensen D, Smith R, Pilcher L, Trandafir G. Comparison of the CMNC and MNC apheresis protocol for the collection of T-cells showed comparable outcome: an observational study in a single centre. J Clin Apher. 2018;33:349.
53. Ceppi F, Rivers J, Annesley C, Pinto N, Park JR, Lindgren C, et al. Lymphocyte apheresis for chimeric antigen receptor T-cell manufacturing in children and young adults with leukemia and neuroblastoma. Transfusion. 2018;58(6):1414–20.
54. Jo T, Yoshihara S, Hada A, Arai Y, Kitawaki T, Ikemoto J, et al. A clinically applicable prediction model to improve T cell collection in chimeric antigen receptor T cell therapy. Transplant Cell Ther. 2022;28(7):365.e1–7.
55. Pham HP, Schwartz J. New apheresis indications in hematological disorders. Curr Opin Hematol. 2016;23(6):581–7.
56. Meyer EK, Wong EC. Pediatric therapeutic apheresis: a critical appraisal of evidence. Transfus Med Rev. 2016;30(4):217–22.
57. Haque A, Sher G, Hoda M, Moiz B. Feasibility of pediatric plasma apheresis in intensive care settings. Ther Apher Dial. 2014;18(5):497–501.
58. Giles FJ, Shen Y, Kantarjian HM, Korbling MJ, O'Brien S, Anderlini P, et al. Leukapheresis reduces early mortality in patients with acute myeloid leukemia with high white cell counts but does not improve long-term survival. Leuk Lymphoma. 2001;42(1–2):67–73.
59. Chang MC, Chen TY, Tang JL, Lan YJ, Chao TY, Chiu CF, et al. Leukapheresis and cranial irradiation in patients with hyperleukocytic acute myeloid leukemia: no impact on early mortality and intracranial hemorrhage. Am J Hematol. 2007;82(11):976–80.
60. Choi MH, Choe YH, Park Y, Nah H, Kim S, Jeong SH, et al. The effect of therapeutic leukapheresis on early complications and outcomes in patients with acute leukemia and hyperleukocytosis: a propensity score-matched study. Transfusion. 2018;58(1):208–16.

61. Bug G, Anargyrou K, Tonn T, Bialleck H, Seifried E, Hoelzer D, et al. Impact of leukapheresis on early death rate in adult acute myeloid leukemia presenting with hyperleukocytosis. Transfusion. 2007;47(10):1843–50.
62. Korkmaz S. The management of hyperleukocytosis in 2017: do we still need leukapheresis? Transfus Apher Sci. 2018;57(1):4–7.
63. Stegmayr B, Ptak J, Wikstrom B, Berlin G, Axelsson CG, Griskevicius A, et al. World apheresis registry 2003-2007 data. Transfus Apher Sci. 2008;39(3):247–54.
64. Rock GA, Shumak KH, Buskard NA, Blanchette VS, Kelton JG, Nair RC, et al. Comparison of plasma exchange with plasma infusion in the treatment of thrombotic thrombocytopenic purpura. Canadian Apheresis Study Group. N Engl J Med. 1991;325(6):393–7.
65. Bukowski RM, King JW, Hewlett JS. Plasmapheresis in the treatment of thrombotic thrombocytopenic purpura. Blood. 1977;50(3):413–7.
66. Reeves HM, Winters JL. The mechanisms of action of plasma exchange. Br J Haematol. 2014;164(3):342–51.
67. Pons-Estel GJ, Salerni GE, Serrano RM, Gomez-Puerta JA, Plasin MA, Aldasoro E, et al. Therapeutic plasma exchange for the management of refractory systemic autoimmune diseases: report of 31 cases and review of the literature. Autoimmun Rev. 2011;10(11):679–84.
68. Rovira J, Cid J, Gutierrez-Garcia G, Pereira A, Fernandez-Aviles F, Rosinol L, et al. Fatal immune hemolytic anemia following allogeneic stem cell transplantation: report of 2 cases and review of literature. Transfus Med Rev. 2013;27(3):166–70.
69. Chegini A, Ahmadi Karvigh S, Rahbar M, Sharifi RA. Therapeutic apheresis in neurological, nephrological and gastrointestinal diseases. Transfus Apher Sci. 2019;58(3):266–72.
70. Shemin D, Briggs D, Greenan M. Complications of therapeutic plasma exchange: a prospective study of 1,727 procedures. J Clin Apher. 2007;22(5):270–6.
71. Norda R, Stegmayr BG, Swedish AG. Therapeutic apheresis in Sweden: update of epidemiology and adverse events. Transfus Apher Sci. 2003;29(2):159–66.
72. Weinstein R. Hypocalcemic toxicity and atypical reactions in therapeutic plasma exchange. J Clin Apher. 2001;16(4):210–1.
73. Perdue JJ, Chandler LK, Vesely SK, Duvall DS, Gilcher RO, Smith JW, et al. Unintentional platelet removal by plasmapheresis. J Clin Apher. 2001;16(2):55–60.
74. Wood L, Jacobs P. The effect of serial therapeutic plasmapheresis on platelet count, coagulation factors, plasma immunoglobulin, and complement levels. J Clin Apher. 1986;3(2):124–8.
75. Cid J, Molina JM, Mustieles MJ, Perianez M, Lozano M. Comparison of plasma exchange procedures using three apheresis systems. Transfusion. 2015;55(5):1001–7.
76. Yasuda M, Uzawa A, Ozawa Y, Kojima Y, Onishi Y, Akamine H, et al. Immunoadsorption apheresis versus intravenous immunoglobulin therapy for exacerbation of myasthenia gravis. Scand J Immunol. 2022;95(2):e13122.
77. Xanthi Z, Vasiliki P, Stavros A. Apheresis and COVID-19 in intensive care unit (ICU). Transfus Apher Sci. 2022;61(6):103593.
78. Iannaccone G, Scacciavillani R, Del Buono MG, Camilli M, Ronco C, Lavie CJ, et al. Weathering the cytokine storm in COVID-19: therapeutic implications. Cardiorenal Med. 2020;10(5):277–87.
79. Kanekura T, Kawahara K. Adsorptive granulocyte and monocyte apheresis: a potentially relevant therapeutic option for COVID-19. Int J Infect Dis. 2020;99:1–2.
80. Beraud M, Hashami SA, Lozano M, Bah A, Keith P. Role of therapeutic plasma exchange in the management of COVID-19-induced cytokine storm syndrome. Transfus Apher Sci. 2022;61(4):103433.
81. Qin J, Wang G, Han D. Benefits of plasma exchange on mortality in patients with COVID-19: a systematic review and meta-analysis. Int J Infect Dis. 2022;122:332–6.
82. Faqihi F, Alharthy A, Abdulaziz S, Balhamar A, Alomari A, AlAseri Z, et al. Therapeutic plasma exchange in patients with life-threatening COVID-19: a randomised controlled clinical trial. Int J Antimicrob Agents. 2021;57(5):106334.
83. Tseke P, Griveas I. Immunoadsorption and covid 19 pandemic. Transfus Apher Sci. 2022;61(6):103599.
84. Esposito F, Matthes H, Schad F. Seven COVID-19 patients treated with C-reactive protein (CRP) apheresis. J Clin Med. 2022;11(7).
85. Kayser S, Kunze R, Sheriff A. Selective C-reactive protein apheresis for Covid-19 patients suffering from organ damage. Ther Apher Dial. 2021;25(2):251–2.
86. Ringel J, Ramlow A, Bock C, Sheriff A. Case report: C-reactive protein apheresis in a patient with COVID-19 and fulminant CRP increase. Front Immunol. 2021;12:708101.
87. Faqihi F, Alharthy A, Alodat M, Asad D, Aletreby W, Kutsogiannis DJ, et al. A pilot study of therapeutic plasma exchange for serious SARS CoV-2 disease (COVID-19): a structured summary of a randomized controlled trial study protocol. Trials. 2020;21(1):506.
88. Yamada C, Hofmann JC, Witt V, Gupta GK, Winters JL, Taskforce AC-. The report from ASFA COVID-19 taskforce: considerations and prioritization on apheresis procedures during the SARS-CoV-2 coronavirus disease (COVID-19) pandemic. J Clin Apher. 2021;36(6):878–81.
89. Uchida K, Rackoff WR, Ohene-Frempong K, Kim HC, Reilly MP, Asakura T. Effect of erythrocytapheresis on arterial oxygen saturation and hemo-

globin oxygen affinity in patients with sickle cell disease. Am J Hematol. 1998;59(1):5–8.
90. Adams RJ, McKie VC, Hsu L, Files B, Vichinsky E, Pegelow C, et al. Prevention of a first stroke by transfusions in children with sickle cell anemia and abnormal results on transcranial Doppler ultrasonography. N Engl J Med. 1998;339(1):5–11.
91. Quirolo K, Bertolone S, Hassell K, Howard T, King KE, Rhodes DK, et al. The evaluation of a new apheresis device for automated red blood cell exchange procedures in patients with sickle cell disease. Transfusion. 2015;55(4):775–81.
92. Wahl SK, Garcia A, Hagar W, Gildengorin G, Quirolo K, Vichinsky E. Lower alloimmunization rates in pediatric sickle cell patients on chronic erythrocytapheresis compared to chronic simple transfusions. Transfusion. 2012;52(12):2671–6.
93. Koehl B, Sommet J, Holvoet L, Abdoul H, Boizeau P, Ithier G, et al. Comparison of automated erythrocytapheresis versus manual exchange transfusion to treat cerebral macrovasculopathy in sickle cell anemia. Transfusion. 2016;56(5):1121–8.
94. Sarode R, Matevosyan K, Rogers ZR, Burner JD, Rutherford C. Advantages of isovolemic hemodilution-red cell exchange therapy to prevent recurrent stroke in sickle cell anemia patients. J Clin Apher. 2011;26(4):200–7.
95. Kim J, Joseph R, Matevosyan K, Sarode R. Comparison of spectra Optia and COBE spectra apheresis systems' performances for red blood cell exchange procedures. Transfus Apher Sci. 2016;55(3):368–70.
96. Matevosyan K, Anderson C, Sarode R. Isovolemic hemodilution-red cell exchange for prevention of cerebrovascular accident in sickle cell anemia: the standard operating procedure. J Clin Apher. 2012;27(2):88–92.
97. Driss F, Moh-Klaren J, Pela AM, Tertian G. Regular automated erythrocytapheresis in sickle cell patients. Br J Haematol. 2011;154(5):656–9.
98. Duclos C, Merlin E, Paillard C, Thuret I, Demeocq F, Michel G, et al. Long-term red blood cell exchange in children with sickle cell disease: manual or automatic? Transfus Apher Sci. 2013;48(2):219–22.
99. Malachowski R, Grzybowska-Izydorczyk O, Besson N, Szmigielska-Kaplon A, Nowicki M, Wierzbowska A. Safety and feasibility of therapeutic platelet depletion with Spectra Optia in a pregnant woman. Transfus Apher Sci. 2017;56(4):563–5.
100. Perseghin P, Mascaretti L, Speranza T, Belotti D, Baldini V, Dassi M, et al. Platelet activation during plasma-reduced multicomponent PLT collection: a comparison between COBE Trima and Spectra LRS turbo cell separators. Transfusion. 2004;44(1):125–30.
101. Keklik M, Eser B, Kaynar L, Sivgin S, Keklik E, Solmaz M, et al. Comparison of plateletpheresis on the Fenwal Amicus, Fresenius COM.TEC, and Trima Accel cell separators. J Clin Apher. 2015;30(3):171–5.
102. Marques MB, Adamski J. Extracorporeal photopheresis: technique, established and novel indications. J Clin Apher. 2014;29(4):228–34.
103. Raval JS, Ratcliffe NR. Extracorporeal photopheresis and personalized medicine in the 21st century: the future's so bright! J Clin Apher. 2018;33:461.
104. Brosig A, Hahnel V, Orso E, Wolff D, Holler E, Ahrens N. Technical comparison of four different extracorporeal photopheresis systems. Transfusion. 2016;56(10):2510–9.
105. Piccirillo N, Putzulu R, Massini G, Fiore AG, Chiusolo P, Sica S, et al. Mononuclear cell collection for extracorporeal photopheresis: concentrate characteristics for off-line UV-A irradiation procedure. J Clin Apher. 2017;33:217.
106. Thompson GR, Group H-ULAW. Recommendations for the use of LDL apheresis. Atherosclerosis. 2008;198(2):247–55.
107. Drouin-Chartier JP, Tremblay AJ, Bergeron J, Pelletier M, Laflamme N, Lamarche B, et al. Comparison of two low-density lipoprotein apheresis systems in patients with homozygous familial hypercholesterolemia. J Clin Apher. 2016;31(4):359–67.
108. Empen K, Otto C, Brodl UC, Parhofer KG. The effects of three different LDL-apheresis methods on the plasma concentrations of E-selectin, VCAM-1, and ICAM-1. J Clin Apher. 2002;17(1):38–43.
109. Dann EJ, Shamir R, Mashiach T, Shaoul R, Badian A, Stravets T, et al. Early-onset plasmapheresis and LDL-apheresis provide better disease control for pediatric homozygous familial hypercholesterolemia than HMG-CoA reductase inhibitors and ameliorate atherosclerosis. Transfus Apher Sci. 2013;49(2):268–77.
110. Stefanutti C, Di Giacomo S, Labbadia G. Timing clinical events in the treatment of pancreatitis and hypertriglyceridemia with therapeutic plasmapheresis. Transfus Apher Sci. 2011;45(1):3–7.
111. Poole C, Strydom C, van der Berg K, Vrielink H. Taking therapeutic apheresis services to patients in South Africa: an eight year review of SANBS mobile therapeutic apheresis service, 2013-2020. Transfus Apher Sci. 2021;60(3):103167.
112. Pham HP, Jiang N, Pan Z, Williams LA 3rd, Marques MB. Apheresis research-more abstracts should be published as full manuscripts to provide more evidence for clinical practice guidelines. J Clin Apher. 2016;31(4):353–8.
113. Simmons SC, Bui CM, Kim CH, Feldman AZ, Staley EM, Pham HP. Frequency of alterations in apheresis-related abstracts prior to publications as peer-reviewed articles. Ther Apher Dial. 2020;24(2):215–20.

114. Aydin K, Korkmaz S, Erkurt MA, Sarici A, Ekinci O, Baysal NA, et al. Apheresis in patients with sepsis: a multicenter retrospective study. Transfus Apher Sci. 2021;60(5):103239.
115. Ozgur G, Beyan C. Therapeutic apheresis in the treatment of catastrophic antiphospholipid syndrome. Transfus Apher Sci. 2018;57(1):13–5.
116. Cunningham S, Buchele V, Brox R, Strasser E, Hackstein H. Thrombocyte apheresis cassettes as a novel source of viable peripheral blood mononuclear cells. Transfusion. 2020;60(7):1500–7.
117. Thorausch K, Schulz M, Bialleck H, Luxembourg B, Seifried E, Bonig H. Granulocyte collections: comparison of two apheresis systems. Transfusion. 2013;53(12):3262–8.

24 The Role of Therapeutic Plasma Exchange (Plasmapheresis) in Aging

D. Kiprov, R. Rohe, M. Conboy, and I. Conboy

24.1 Introduction

People worldwide are living longer. According to the World Health Organization (WHO), by 2050, the global population aged 60 or older is projected to reach two billion, up from 900 million in 2015 [1]. Although longer life expectancy brings personal, familial, and societal opportunities, older age is associated with various physical and mental disorders. Age-related diseases are the leading causes of death and healthcare costs. Slowing the aging process could yield significant medical and financial benefits.

Population aging and public health expenditures dedicated to older, dependent individuals pose major challenges for all countries, with substantial implications for their economies and labor markets. Sustainable economic development depends on maintaining a well-balanced workforce comprising both younger and older individuals. As this balance increasingly shifts toward older populations, productivity tends to decline while demand for healthcare services rises [2].

Geroscience, a new interdisciplinary field focused on understanding the relationship between aging and chronic age-related diseases as well as geriatric syndromes, is opening avenues for mechanisms to slow aging. The anti-aging market is projected to reach $90 billion by 2030 [3].

24.2 Aging and Disease

The longstanding question of whether old age itself is a disease has been debated since ancient times. The Roman playwright Terentius claimed, "senectus ipsa est morbus" (old age itself is a disease), while Cicero, writing decades later in *De Senectute*, argued, "pugnandum, tamquam contra morbum sic contra senectutem" (we must fight against aging as we do against a disease). These quotations encapsulate a long-held view of aging and old age that has been explored by numerous scholars. With the advent of modern medicine in the nineteenth century, this notion was somewhat set aside as the focus shifted toward defining specific medical entities (diseases and syndromes) and their causes (e.g., infections, genetics, degenerative processes, and inflammation). While some still view aging and disease as separate phenomena, most scientists today recognize that aging, age-related diseases, and geriatric syndromes exist on a continuum and share the same fundamental molecular and cellular mechanisms. Aging is a major risk factor for most diseases and conditions that limit healthspan [4].

D. Kiprov (✉) · R. Rohe
Global Apheresis, Inc., Mill Valley, CA, USA

M. Conboy · I. Conboy
Department of Bioengineering and GB Institute, University of California, Berkeley, CA, USA

I. Kozanoglu (ed.), *Problem Solving in Apheresis Medicine*,
https://doi.org/10.1007/978-3-031-74081-7_24

Pharmaceutical research, driven by advances in molecular genetics (e.g., pharmacogenomics, DNA microarrays), has focused on individual diseases of old age. However, these efforts have yet to yield unequivocal clinical breakthroughs. Similarly, attempts to treat most age-related diseases with antioxidant supplements have largely been disappointing, despite the well-documented benefits of a healthy diet [4].

24.3 Current Understanding of the Aging Process

Aging can be described as a detrimental loop that begins with damage to macromolecules and cells. This, in turn, leads to impaired activation of tissue-resident stem cells, resulting in a lack of tissue maintenance and repair. Ultimately, this loop causes tissue pathologies, with typical age-associated features including adiposity, fibrosis, and chronic inflammation. Aging tissues also release a secretome composed of adipose, fibrotic, and inflammatory cells, along with senescent cells. These secreted proteins are collectively referred to as the senescence-associated secretory phenotype (SASP) and enter the circulation [5].

With aging, the circulation contains numerous signals of tissue damage, many of which are reduced by therapeutic plasma exchange (TPE). These include self-molecules, cellular debris, micro-RNAs, lipofuscins, advanced glycation end-products, tau protein aggregates, α-synuclein fibrils, and amyloid-β (Aβ) peptides. These factors are present in bodily fluids, partly within extracellular vesicles, and can spread from inflamed or unrepaired organ sites to distant cells and tissues [5].

24.4 Heterochronic Parabiosis

Heterochronic parabiosis models in mice (two animals sharing circulatory systems) have demonstrated that blood sharing between young and old individuals leads to multi-tissue rejuvenation (Figs. 24.1 and 24.2) [6]. The intuitive conclusion that factors in young blood are solely responsible for the rejuvenation has been challenged by further experiments involving plasma exchange in both mice and humans [7]. Plasma exchange

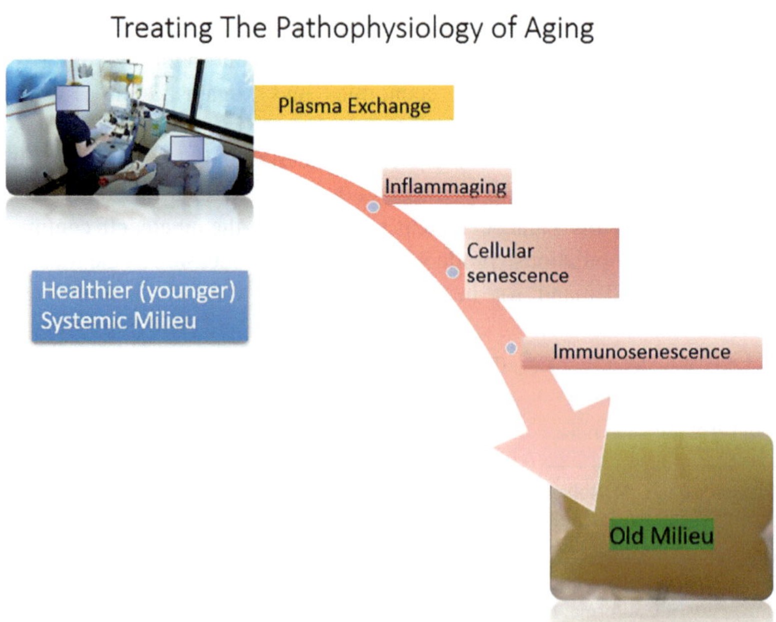

Fig. 24.1 Plasmapheresis affects all aspects of the pathophysiology of aging by replacing the old systemic milieu with a new one and reestablishing homeostasis

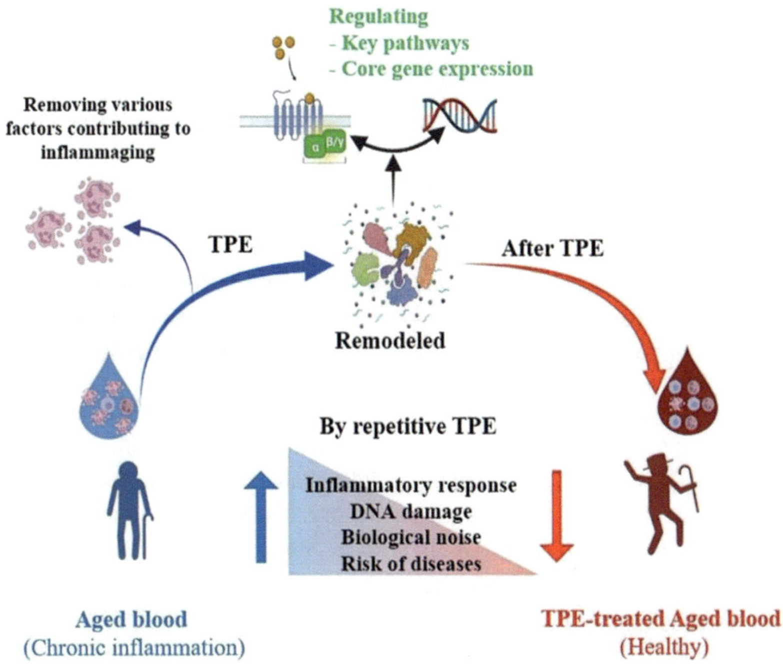

Fig. 24.2 The effect of repetitive TPE on aged blood. Aged blood exhibits characteristics of chronic inflammation (inflammaging), increased PBMC DNA damage and senescence, and immune deregulation, all of which contribute to a heightened risk of diseases. TPE resets the systemic milieu to a younger state by significantly diluting the age-elevated inhibitors of canonical signaling pathways that regulate tissue maintenance and repair. The immediate effect is a reduction in inflammation, followed by improvements in cellular and molecular homeostasis through calibrated cell-cell signing crosstalks and a reduction in biological noise, as defined in this study. (*First published in GeroScience (2022) 44:2701–2720.* D Kim, D Kiprov, C Luellen, M Lieb, C Liu, E Watanabe, X Mei, K Cassaleto, L Kramer, M Conoy, I Conboy. *Old plasma dilution reduces human biological age: a clinical study.* http://creativecommons.org/licenses/by/4.0/)

has been proposed as a heterochronic parabiosis model in humans [8]. Using neutral saline and/or albumin as plasma replacement fluids achieved or even exceeded the rejuvenation effects observed in the parabiosis model [9].

24.5 TPE and the Aging Process

TPE is a medical procedure that uses blood cell separators to exchange a patient's plasma with physiological fluids such as 5% albumin or fresh frozen plasma (FFP). TPE effectively removes pathogenic circulatory factors, including autoantibodies, cytokines, triglycerides, and others. It is widely used in the treatment of many autoimmune diseases. Adverse reactions to TPE are observed in 4–7% of treatments when 5% albumin is used as the replacement fluid. These reactions are usually mild and primarily related to hypocalcemia induced by citrate, the anticoagulant used during the procedure. However, when FFP is used as the replacement fluid, the rate of adverse reactions increases to 27%, according to our experience with 17,000 procedures [6].

Three primary physiological mechanisms contribute to the aging process: cellular senescence, immunosenescence, and chronic inflammation—collectively referred to as "inflammaging." Studies in both mice and humans show that TPE affects all three mechanisms.

24.6 Cellular Senescence and TPE

Cellular senescence is characterized by cell cycle arrest and the activation of a hypersecretory phenotype known as SASP [10].

SASP involves the production of growth factors, chemokines, cytokines, proteases, bioactive lipids, and extracellular vesicles, many of which are pro-inflammatory. These factors negatively impact distant tissue health and repair, accelerating the aging process at the organismal level by perpetuating a chronic inflammatory response [11–13]. These factors include, but are not limited to, interleukin (IL)-1α, IL-2, IL-6, IL-8, growth-related oncogene (GRO)-α, and GRO-β, various members of the chemokine (C-C motif) ligand (CCL) and chemokine (C-X-C motif) ligand (CXCL) families, granulocyte-macrophage colony-stimulating factor, macrophage-stimulating factor, insulin-like growth factor-binding proteins, and extracellular remodeling proteins such as matrix metalloproteinases and serine proteases [4]. TPE effectively removes all SASP-associated proteins and chemokines [6].

24.7 Immunosenescence and TPE

Immunosenescence refers to the gradual, age-associated functional decline of the immune system, which contributes to an increased risk of morbidity and mortality. This decline is associated with an altered inflammatory response and impaired stem cell function. Older individuals are more susceptible to infections and exhibit poor responses to vaccines due to an inefficient immune system [5].

Common effects of immune system aging include a decline in the production of fresh naïve T cells, a less expansive T-cell receptor (TCR) repertoire, and weaker T-cell activation. Clonal populations of CD8+ T cells expand with age, limiting their diversity. In addition to removing pathogenic pro-inflammatory factors, TPE has been shown to affect cellular immunity. TPE normalizes the CD4/CD8 ratio in patients with autoimmune diseases and influences the Th1/Th2 ratio as well as cytokine production by these cells.

Repeated TPE has also been shown to increase CD4+/CD25+ T cells, correlating with clinical improvement in patients with systemic lupus erythematosus (SLE) [6].

24.8 Systemic Chronic Inflammation (SCI) (Inflammaging) and TPE

Chronic inflammatory diseases are recognized as the leading cause of death worldwide. More than 50% of all deaths are attributed to chronic inflammatory diseases, including ischemic heart disease, stroke, cancer, type-2 diabetes, chronic kidney disease, nonalcoholic fatty liver disease (NAFLD), and autoimmune and neurodegenerative disorders. Acute inflammation is usually triggered by infections. Once an infection resolves, regulatory molecules signal the cessation of the acute inflammatory response.

In contrast, SCI is triggered in the absence of an acute infection by "sterile" agents, such as physical, chemical, or metabolic noxious stimuli. The most common causes of SCI include physical inactivity, obesity, diet, intestinal dysbiosis, stress, social isolation, and disturbed circadian rhythm (sleep). These are referred to as the exposome. Chronic infections may also contribute to SCI. For example, chronic infection with cytomegalovirus (CMV) has been associated with the so-called immune risk phenotype, which has been predictive of early mortality in longitudinal studies. SCI increases with age, as indicated by higher levels of circulating cytokines, chemokines, and acute-phase proteins, as well as greater expression of genes involved in inflammation. Cellular senescence is also a major contributor to SCI, with the continuous release of pro-inflammatory SASP [5].

Age-related defects that lead to persistent inflammation include unrepaired damaged macromolecules, mis-adaptation to stress, and altered metabolism. This is accompanied by changes in the immune system that favor the innate inflammatory response when adaptive immunity becomes deficient. The biomarkers of inflammation are strong predictors of morbidity and mortality in older individuals. Among the inflammatory mediators, IL-6, CRP, and interferon (IFN)-γ are of particular interest. TPE has the capacity to diminish circulatory inflammaging directly by diluting systemic pro-inflammatory proteins, through the antioxidant and sequestering activities of albumin, and by resetting or modifying the immune system [14].

Our recent study demonstrated that plasmapheresis in mice and humans caused a molecular resetting of the systemic signaling milieu, where the levels of many positive determinants of tissue homeostasis and regeneration, such as "young" angiogenic growth factors and immune modulators, were upregulated after treatment [14].

24.9 DNA Damage and Epigenetics

DNA damage associated with aging affects not only cell health but also cell fate, leading to a loss of tissue homeostasis, chronic inflammation, and other dysfunctions. In particular, immune cells with damaged DNA interfere with productive immune responses and the homeostatic immunity-inflammation axis, contributing to inflammaging [15]. Changes in cell fate during hematopoiesis trigger lymphoid/myeloid skewing, resulting in inefficient immunity. When the immunity-inflammation axis is imbalanced, the risks of autoimmune diseases, neurodegenerative diseases, or cancer increase [16]. Thus, the younger lymphoid/myeloid balance promoted by TPE in aged peripheral blood mononuclear cells (PBMCs), along with the lower DNA damage and senescence observed in these cells, may be either limited or synergistic, with implications for improving immune responses and reducing age-related flares of infections and cancers [17].

In line with the age-related increase in cancers, our data show that the levels of many cancer-related proteins were elevated in the aged blood before TPE. For example, SDF-1 is expressed in various cancers, such as ovarian, breast, thyroid, and lung cancers, and contributes to metastasis [18]. TGF-α plays a key role in promoting carcinogenesis and malignancy progression. The expression of kinase insert domain-containing receptor (KDR) contributes to cancer development through vascularity and is associated with metastasis in colon and breast cancers [19]. Notably, the age-increased cancer-related factors, including the proteins mentioned above, were downregulated after the multiple rounds of TPE. The protein-protein interaction (PPI) network analysis with cancer-related terms identified six proteins—TGFBR2, TGF-α, FGF21, SMAD4, TGFBR1, and FZD3—all of which are involved in tumor development. Moreover, profiling the PBMCs revealed that the tumor suppressors p21 and p53 were increased by TPE, while no change was observed in the expression of the oncogene c-Myc. Overall, these data suggest that TPE may decrease the propensity for cancer.

The mechanism underlying the rejuvenating effects of repetitive TPE is suggested by the results of longitudinal comparative proteomics, which identify key interactive signaling pathways with TLR4 as their central node. Moreover, gene expression analysis of larger datasets confirms that the levels of TLR4 increase with age, emphasizing the significance of its TPE-related attenuation [5]. TLR4 participates in the production of inflammatory cytokines through NF-KB signaling, but it also has many other pleiotropic activities. The expression of TLR4 is elevated in the aged brain, which may contribute to the development of neurodegenerative disorders. The effects of age-specific pathways on tissue maintenance and repair, senescence, apoptosis, DNA repair, and cell fate determination in blood lineages are well known. We show that this pivotal network is reset by TPE to a younger state. Notably, each of the age-specific pathways influenced by TPE is morphogenic and multifunctional, exerting different effects based on their intensity and the overall signaling landscape. Thus, it is important that our study identified the specific proteins within these pathways that were deregulated in the aged blood and gradually, yet stably, normalized after rounds of TPE, in correlation with the rejuvenated PBMCs [14].

TPE has been tested for treating Alzheimer's disease, as the pathogenic Aβ peptides circulate in the blood and bind to serum albumin. Removing these peripheral Aβ peptides may allow more brain Aβ peptides to be cleared into the blood [20].

In recent work [14], we show that TDP43 is elevated in the serum of relatively healthy older adults and is stably attenuated by rounds of TPE. These data add to previously published reports that TDP43 is a key trigger of various neurological diseases and becomes elevated in the cerebrospinal fluid and plasma of patients with age-associated neurodegenerative disorders. Attenuation of TDP43 by rounds of TPE in undiagnosed adults further suggests a preventive capacity against age-associated neurological diseases.

24.10 Discussion

Aging contributes to the development of systemic chronic inflammation, leading to tissue degeneration, metabolic pathologies, perturbed molecular and cellular homeostasis, and the development of age-related diseases, including cardiovascular disease, type-2 diabetes, neurodegenerative diseases, and cancer [5]. Until now, efforts by the medical establishment and the pharmaceutical industry have focused on treating individual age-related diseases. These efforts have been successful, allowing people to live longer, but they are heavily dependent on lifelong medical care and suffer from multiple disabilities. As the aging population exponentially increases, the socioeconomic effects will become unsustainable [2]. Therefore, it is urgent to recognize aging as a disease entity and develop medical interventions to ameliorate the aging process. Pharmaceutical efforts have been unsuccessful so far. The most likely reason is that aging is an extraordinarily complex process involving multiple mechanisms, and targeting a single molecular pathway is unlikely to be effective. Recently, TPE has emerged as a potential medical intervention capable of affecting multiple pathophysiologies of aging—such as inflammaging, immunosenescence, and cellular senescence. Although initial studies have been promising, sham-controlled clinical trials are needed to establish TPE as treatment and/or prevention for aging. One such trial was recently completed (https://doi.org/10.1101/2024.08.02.24310303). A large, controlled clinical trial of TPE in Alzheimer's disease was recently published [21]. It demonstrated that TPE was able to arrest the progression of the disease in patients with moderate to severe disease in over 60% of treated patients. More importantly, patients with mild Alzheimer's disease showed no progression (100%) and experienced neurophysiological and quality of life improvements, suggesting that TPE may delay the development of the disease and possibly prevent it.

References

1. Garza A. The aging population: the increasing effects on health care. Pharm Times. 2016;82(1).
2. Cristea M, Noja GG, Stefea P, Sala AL. The impact of population aging and public health support on EU labor markets. Int J Environ Res Public Health. 2020;17:1439. https://doi.org/10.3390/ijerph17041430.
3. Anti-ageing drugs market size worth $90.2 billion by 2030 at 7.10% CAGR—report by market research future (MRFR), market research future. 2022. https://www.marketresearchfuture.com/sample_request/30504.
4. Franceschi C, Garagnani P, Morsiani C, et al. The continuum of aging and age-related diseases: common mechanisms but different rates. Front Med. 2018;5:61.
5. Furman D, Campisi J, Verdin E, et al. Chronic inflammation in the etiology of disease across the life span. Nat Med. 2019;25:1822–32.
6. Mehdipour M, Etienne J, Liu C, et al. Attenuation of age-elevated blood factors by repositioning plasmapheresis: a novel perspective and approach. Transfus Apher Sci. 2021;60:103162.
7. Conboy IM, Conboy MJ, Wagers AJ, Girma ER, Weissman IL, Rando TA. Rejuvenation of aged progenitor cells by exposure to a young systemic environment. Nature. 2005;433:760.
8. Kiprov DD. Intermittent heterochronic plasma exchange as a modality for delaying cellular senescence—a hypothesis. J Clin Apher. 2013;28:387–9. https://doi.org/10.1002/jca.21.286.

9. Mehdipour M, Mehdipour T, Skinner CM, et al. Plasma dilution improves cognition and attenuates neuroinflammation in old mice. GeroScience. 2021;43:1.
10. Borghesan M, Hoogaars WMH, Varela-Eirin M, et al. A senescence-centric view of aging: implications for longevity and disease. Trends Cell Biol. 2020;s30:777–91. https://doi.org/10.1016/j.tcb.2020.07.002.
11. Coppe J-P, Desprez P-Y, Krtolica A, Campisi J. The senescence-associated secretory phenotype: the dark side of tumor suppression. Annu Rev Pathol. 2021;5:99–118. https://doi.org/10.1146/annurev-pathol-121808-102144.
12. Coppe J-P, Patil CK, Rodier F, et al. Senescence-associated secretory phenotypes reveal cell-nonautonomous functions of oncogenic RAS and the p53 tumor suppressor. PLoS Biol. 2008;6:2853–69. https://doi.org/10.1371/journal.pbio.0060301.
13. Van Deursen JM. The role of senescent cells in ageing. Nature. 2014;509:439–46. https://doi.org/10.1038/nature13193.
14. Kim D, Kiprov D, Luellen C, et al. Old plasma dilution reduces human biological age: a clinical study. GeroScience. 2022;44:2701–20. https://doi.org/10.1007/s11357-022-00645-w.
15. Schumacher B, Pothof J, Vijg J, et al. The central role of DNA damage in the ageing process. Nature. 2021;592(7856):695.
16. Lopez-Otin C, Clasco MA, Partridge L, et al. Hallmarks of aging: an expanding universe. Cell. 2023;153:1194.
17. Howlander N, Noone AM, Krapcho M, et al. SEER cancer statistics review, 1975–2017. National Cancer Institute. https://seer.cancer.gov.cse/1975_2017/. Accessed Apr 2020.
18. Muller A, Homey B, Soto H, et al. Involvement of chemokine receptors in breast cancer metastasis. Nature. 2001;410(6824):50.
19. Takagi H, Sharp R, Takayama H, et al. Collaboration between growth factors and diverse chemical carcinogens in hepatocarcinogenesis of transforming growth factor alpha transgenic mice. Cancer Res. 1993;53:4329–36.
20. Boada M, Lopez OL, Olazaran J, et al. A randomized, controlled clinical trial of plasma exchange with albumin replacement for Alzheimer's disease: preliminary results of the AMBAR study. Alzheimers Dement. 2020;16:1412. https://doi.org/10.1002/alz.12137.
21. Boada M, Lopez OL, Olazaran J, et al. Neuropsychological, neuropsychiatric, and quality-of-life assessments in Alzheimer's disease patients treated with plasma exchange with albumin replacement from the randomized AMBAR study. Alzheimers Dement. 2022;18(7):1314–2324. https://doi.org/10.1002/alz.12477.

Apheresis and COVID-19

25

Funda Tanrikulu

25.1 Introduction

The novel coronavirus disease (COVID-19) is an infectious disease that first appeared in China in late 2019 and quickly spread world, leading the World Health Organization to declare it a global pandemic. The causative agent of the disease, which presents with respiratory symptoms such as fever, cough, and shortness of breath, has been identified as the severe acute respiratory syndrome coronavirus 2 (SARS-CoV-2) [1]. Since the outbreak of the pandemic, many promising treatment options have been tested, but few have proven effective. Vaccination against SARS-CoV-2 has dramatically reduced the spread of the virus, but emerging variants continue to infect people, some of whom become severely ill [2]. Mortality rates in critically ill patients, however, remain high, and improved treatment strategies beyond antiviral drugs are needed [3]. Apheresis services offer some options to achieve optimal outcomes, especially for critically ill COVID-19 patients. The proposed apheresis methods are summarized in Table 25.1 and will be discussed in this chapter.

Table 25.1 Proposed apheresis methods for patients with COVID-19

Apheresis method	Patient group	Targeted mechanism	Reference
Therapeutic plasma exchange	Patients with cytokine release syndrome	Elimination of inflammatory cytokines, reversing coagulopathy	[20]
Convalescent plasma therapy	Patients in need of passive immunization against COVID-19	Viral neutralization by given antibodies	[9]
Immunoadsorption	Patients with cytokine release syndrome	Elimination of inflammatory cytokines	[24]
Selective CRP[a] apheresis	Patients with high CRP[a] levels	Elimination of CRP[a]	[27]

[a] *CRP* C-reactive protein

F. Tanrikulu (✉)
University of Turkish Ministry of Health, Adana City Education and Research Hospital, Adult Hematology Clinic, Adana, Turkey

I. Kozanoglu (ed.), *Problem Solving in Apheresis Medicine*,
https://doi.org/10.1007/978-3-031-74081-7_25

25.2 Convalescent Plasma Therapy

Convalescent plasma therapy is a passive antibody therapy. Passive antibody therapy involves the use of pooled immunoglobulin preparations containing high concentrations of specific antibodies. In convalescent plasma therapy, the source of these specific antibodies is plasma from patients who have recovered from the infection. It is an emerging treatment option when a vaccine or specific therapy is not yet available for new viruses [4].

Convalescent plasma therapy was used during the SARS-CoV-1 outbreak in 2003 and has also been reported to be effective against Middle East respiratory syndrome coronavirus (MERS-CoV) [5, 6]. Although the exact mechanism of action is not fully defined, the main effect of convalescent plasma is thought to be viral neutralization. The neutralizing antibodies present in the plasma help decrease viral load, while non-neutralizing antibodies also play a role in recovery [7]. Based on these experiences, convalescent plasma therapy was used during the COVID-19 pandemic. There was an urgent need and no time to produce immunoglobulin preparations. Plasma containing anti-SARS-CoV-2 antibodies was collected from recovered patients using apheresis machines and stored in blood banks for use in other patients with active disease [8].

Following the discovery of the vaccine and its rapid introduction into large communities, the number of COVID-19 cases has progressively declined. Currently, the use of convalescent plasma therapy has fallen out of focus, not only because of the decline in the pandemic but also because available evidence does not support a clear role for convalescent plasma in patients with severe disease [9]. However, it should still be considered in individuals with immunocompromising conditions or antibody production deficits, such as those on anti-CD20 therapy for hematological malignancies [10, 11].

All centers equipped with apheresis technology can collect convalescent plasma, and its administration carries risks similar to those of plasma transfusion. There is also a theoretical risk of transmission of SARS-CoV-2 via plasma, but there is no evidence to date to support the transmission of SARS-CoV-2 via blood transfusion [12].

25.3 Therapeutic Plasma Exchange

During the COVID-19 pandemic, clinicians used many complementary therapeutic approaches to save lives, and therapeutic plasma exchange (TPE) is one of the more promising treatments used in critically ill patients [13]. It is a well-known therapeutic procedure used in many diseases and is considered an alternative supportive treatment in severe sepsis. Although the results for the use of TPE in sepsis are conflicting, some studies support its role in improving hemodynamic parameters and coagulation imbalance in septic patients [14, 15].

COVID-19 shares similarities with sepsis in that the severity of the infection depends on the host response, and there is an excessive release of cytokines. This uncontrolled cytokine release, also known as a cytokine storm, promotes acute respiratory distress syndrome and multiple organ dysfunction, ultimately leading to death after physiological deterioration. Timely control of the cytokine storm in the early stages has been shown to reduce mortality in COVID-19 patients with severe disease [16]. Currently, immunomodulators and cytokine antagonists are used for this purpose, but TPE is faster and nonselective in eliminating inflammatory cytokines [17].

In addition, COVID-19 patients experience coagulopathy, not only directly induced by the SARS-CoV-2 virus but also as a result of inflammation. Systemic inflammation leads to acquired ADAMTS13 deficiency, and the increase in abnormal von Willebrand factor multimers eventually results in microthrombotic disease [18, 19]. Therefore, TPE with fresh frozen plasma provides additional benefits by replacing some of the missing factors, such as ADAMTS13, and helps to reverse the coagulopathy.

TPE is a procedure that can be associated with potential complications, but studies have shown that it is well tolerated in COVID-19 patients.

The main limitation is the limited availability of equipment and professional staff [20]. If available, it is recommended to start TPE in the early stages of inflammation when there is a very high concentration of inflammatory cytokines but relatively less organ damage. Serum markers of inflammation and coagulation may be used to guide the decision to initiate the process, as they are also considered indicators of cytokine release syndrome. The clinical application is thought to be similar to that in sepsis: daily TPE sessions for 1–14 days or until symptom resolution, with the exchange of 1–1.5 plasma volumes [14].

Some studies have suggested that plasma exchange may also reduce viral load in COVID-19 patients, but there is no published literature confirming the reduction of SARS-CoV-2 viral load by TPE. At present, the main use of TPE in COVID-19 patients is to reduce cytokine load and help treat coagulopathy.

25.4 Immunoadsorption

Immunoadsorption is a blood purification method in which plasma, after separation from the blood, is passed through a medical device capable of removing selected immunoglobins, immune complexes, or antibodies by binding to selective ligands. It has been used in patients with severe sepsis to remove certain cytokines and/or exotoxins and has been reported to result in objective improvements in both clinical and biochemical parameters [21]. In addition, leukocytes, mainly activated monocytes and neutrophils, have also been reported to be adsorbed by this procedure [22].

The major advantage over TPE is that immunoadsorption is a selective apheresis, which allows for the massive removal of specific molecules in the first session without affecting other important plasma constituents. There is also no need for fluid substitution with plasma, albumin, or other colloid solutions [23].

As mentioned above, severe COVID-19 infection shares similarities with sepsis in terms of cytokine storm, and based on experience with septic patients, immunoadsorption has also been used in critically ill COVID-19 patients with uncontrolled cytokine release [24]. Although the available literature on this topic is limited to small case series, the results are promising, and immunoadsorption should be considered as an option when appropriate.

25.5 C-Reactive Protein Apheresis

C-reactive protein (CRP) is an acute-phase protein and a well-known marker of inflammation. During COVID-19 infection, CRP levels rise significantly and remain elevated, especially in critically ill patients with a high risk of death [25]. CRP itself also mediates tissue damage and contributes to irreversible tissue destruction, such as pulmonary fibrosis [26]. Unfortunately, there is no way to reduce its synthesis, but selective CRP apheresis has been proposed as a method to reduce its levels in COVID-19 patients during the pandemic. It has been used in a small group of reported patients, and the results suggest that CRP could be a therapeutic target in severe COVID-19 patients [27]. Although the number of patients in the literature is small, CRP apheresis is a treatment option that should be considered in the early stages of the disease, when there is little or no irreversible organ damage.

25.6 Post-COVID-19 Apheresis

Post-COVID is defined as signs or symptoms that develop during or after a COVID-19 infection and persist for more than 12 weeks [28]. The most common post-COVID symptoms are fatigue, depression, and restless sleep [29]. The underlying mechanism has not been clearly defined but is thought to be heterogeneous, involving a combination of factors such as COVID-19-induced autoimmunity, infection-induced rheological abnormalities (deformation of red blood cells and increased blood viscosity), and latent viral reactivation [30].

To date, various forms of apheresis have been used to treat post-COVID patients, but no published data on outcomes are available [31]. It has been postulated that apheresis may reduce autoantibodies and thereby alleviate symptoms. However, in the absence of efficacy data confirmed by well-designed trials, more evidence is needed before recommending its use in routine clinical practice.

25.7 Summary

In summary, extracorporeal apheresis was frequently discussed as an adjunctive therapeutic modality to improve patient outcomes during the COVID-19 pandemic. Although convalescent plasma therapy was the most widely advertised, other modalities—mainly aimed at eliminating inflammatory mediators—have been reported, such as TPE, immunoadsorption, and selective CRP apheresis. These methods should be considered early during a cytokine storm to help prevent organ damage and improve survival. There are no absolute contraindications for apheresis in COVID-19 patients, and its use in selected cases should always be considered when applicable.

References

1. Gorbalenya AE, Baker SC, Baric RS, de Groot RJ, Drosten C, Gulyaeva AA, et al. Severe, acute respiratory syndrome-related coronavirus; the species and its viruses—a statement of the coronavirus study group. Nat Microbiol. 2020:536–44.
2. Fernandes Q, Inchakalody VP, Merhi M, Mestiri S, Taib N, Moustafa Abo El-Ella D, et al. Emerging COVID-19 variants and their impact on SARS-CoV-2 diagnosis, therapeutics and vaccines. Ann Med. 2022;54(1):524–40.
3. Cummings MJ, Baldwin MR, Abrams D, Jacobson SD, Meyer BJ, Balough EM, et al. Epidemiology, clinical course, and outcomes of critically ill adults with COVID-19 in New York City: a prospective cohort study. Lancet. 2020;395(10239):1763–70.
4. Marano G, Vaglio S, Pupella S, Facco G, Catalano L, Liumbruno GM, et al. Convalescent plasma: new evidence for an old therapeutic tool? Blood Transfus. 2016;14(2):152–7.
5. Soo YO, Cheng Y, Wong R, Hui DS, Lee CK, Tsang KK, et al. Retrospective comparison of convalescent plasma with continuing high-dose methylprednisolone treatment in SARS patients. Clin Microbiol Infect. 2004;10(7):676–8.
6. Ko JH, Seok H, Cho SY, Ha YE, Baek JY, Kim SH, et al. Challenges of convalescent plasma infusion therapy in Middle East respiratory coronavirus infection: a single centre experience. Antivir Ther. 2018;23(7):617–22.
7. Van Erp EA, Luytjes W, Ferwerda G, van Kasteren PB. Fc-mediated antibody effector functions during respiratory syncytial virus infection and disease. Front Immunol. 2019;10:548.
8. Brown BL, McCullough J. Treatment for emerging viruses: convalescent plasma and COVID-19. Transfus Apher Sci. 2020;59(3):102790.
9. Piechotta V, Chai KL, Valk SJ, Doree C, Monsef I, Wood EM, et al. Convalescent plasma or hyperimmune immunoglobulin for people with COVID-19: a living systematic review. Cochrane Database Syst Rev. 2020;7(7):CD013600.
10. Senefeld JW, Franchini M, Mengoli C, Cruciani M, Zani M, Gorman EK, et al. COVID-19 convalescent plasma for the treatment of immunocompromised patients: a systematic review and meta-analysis. JAMA Netw Open. 2023;6(1):e2250647.
11. Thompson MA, Henderson JP, Shah PK, Rubinstein SM, Joyner MJ, Choueiri TK, et al. COVID-19 and cancer consortium. Association of convalescent plasma therapy with survival in patients with hematologic cancers and COVID-19. JAMA Oncol. 2021;7(8):1167–75.
12. Katz LM. Is SARS-CoV-2 transfusion transmitted? Transfusion. 2020;60(6):1111–4.
13. Keith PD, Scott LK, Weaver KE, Day M, Choe C, Perkins L, et al. Treatment of critically ill coronavirus disease 2019 patients with adjunct therapeutic plasma exchange: a single-center retrospective case series. Crit Care Explor. 2020;2(9):e0223.
14. Padmanabhan A, Connelly-Smith L, Aqui N, Balogun RA, Klingel R, Meyer E, et al. Guidelines on the use of therapeutic apheresis in clinical practice—evidence-based approach from the writing Committee of the American Society for apheresis: the eighth special issue. J Clin Apher. 2019;34(3):171–354.
15. Rimmer E, Houston BL, Kumar A, Abou-Setta AM, Friesen C, Marshall JC, et al. The efficacy and safety of plasma exchange in patients with sepsis and septic shock: a systematic review and meta-analysis. Crit Care. 2014;18(6):699.
16. Ye Q, Wang B, Mao J. The pathogenesis and treatment of the 'cytokine storm' in COVID-19. J Infect. 2020;80(6):607–13.
17. Mehta P, McAuley DF, Brown M, Sanchez E, Tattersall RS, Manson JJ, HLH Across Specialty Collaboration, UK. COVID-19: consider cytokine storm syndromes and immunosuppression. Lancet. 2020;395(10229):1033–4.
18. Chang JC. Acute respiratory distress syndrome as an organ phenotype of vascular microthrombotic disease: based on hemostatic theory and endothelial molecular pathogenesis. Clin Appl Thromb. 2019;25:1076029619887437.

19. Bockmeyer CL, Claus RA, Budde U, Kentouche K, Schneppenheim R, Lsche W, et al. Inflammation-associated ADAMTS13 deficiency promotes formation of ultra-large von Willebrand factor. Haematologica. 2008;93(1):137–40.
20. Beraud M, Hashami SA, Lozano M, Bah A, Keith P. Role of therapeutic plasma exchange in the management of COVID-19-induced cytokine storm syndrome. Transfus Apher Sci. 2022;61(4):103433.
21. Schefold JC, von Haehling S, Corsepius M, Pohle C, Kruschke P, Zuckermann H, et al. A novel selective extracorporeal intervention in sepsis: immunoadsorption of endotoxin, interleukin 6, and complement-activating product 5a. Shock. 2007;28:418–25.
22. Rimmelé T, Kaynar AM, McLaughlin JN, Bishop JV, Fedorchak MV, Chuasuwan A, et al. Leukocyte capture and modulation of cell-mediated immunity during human sepsis: an ex vivo study. Crit Care. 2013;17:R59.
23. Sanchez AP, Cunard R, Ward DM. The selective therapeutic apheresis procedures. J Clin Apher. 2013;28(1):20–9.
24. Chen H, Zhang L, Zhang W, Liu L, Dai Z, Chen M, Zhang D. Blood purification in severe and critical COVID-19 patients: a case series of 5 patients. Front Public Health. 2021;9:741125. https://doi.org/10.3389/fpubh.2021.741125.
25. Chen G, Wu D, Guo W, Cao Y, Huang D, Wang H, et al. Clinical and immunological features of severe and moderate coronavirus disease 2019. J Clin Invest. 2020;130(5):2620–9.
26. Ries W, Heigl F, Garlichs C, Sheriff A, Torzewski J. Selective C-reactive protein-apheresis in patients. Ther Apher Dial. 2019;23:570–4.
27. Esposito F, Matthes H, Schad F. Seven COVID-19 patients treated with C-reactive protein (CRP) apheresis. J Clin Med. 2022;11(7):1956.
28. National Institute for Health and Care Excellence: clinical guidelines. In: COVID-19 rapid guideline: managing the long-term effects of COVID-19. NICE Guideline, No.188. London: National Institute for Health and Care Excellence (NICE) Copyright NICE; 2020. https://www.ncbi.nlm.nih.gov/books/NBK567261/.
29. Huang L, Li X, Gu X, Zhang H, Ren L, Guo L, et al. Health outcomes in people 2 years after surviving hospitalisation with COVID-19: a longitudinal cohort study. Lancet Respir Med. 2022;10(9):863–76.
30. Choutka J, Jansari V, Hornig M, Iwasaki A. Unexplained post-acute infection syndromes. Nat Med. 2022;28(5):911–23.
31. Steenblock C, Walther R, Tselmin S, Jarzebska N, Voit-Bak K, Toepfner N, et al. Post COVID and apheresis—where are we standing? Horm Metab Res. 2022;54(11):715–20.

GPSR Compliance

The European Union's (EU) General Product Safety Regulation (GPSR) is a set of rules that requires consumer products to be safe and our obligations to ensure this.

If you have any concerns about our products, you can contact us on ProductSafety@springernature.com

In case Publisher is established outside the EU, the EU authorized representative is:

Springer Nature Customer Service Center GmbH
Europaplatz 3
69115 Heidelberg, Germany

Batch number: 09640328

Printed by Printforce, the Netherlands